KU-439-761

Neurology: Neonatology Questions and Controversies

Neurology

Neonatology Questions and Controversies

Series Editor

Richard A. Polin, MD
Professor of Pediatrics
College of Physicians and Surgeons
Columbia University
Director, Division of Neonatology
Morgan Stanley Children's Hospital of New York - Presbyterian
Columbia University Medical Center
New York, New York

Other Volumes in the Neonatology Questions and Controversies Series

Neurology
Neonatology Questions and Controversies

Jeffrey M. Perlman, MB, ChB
Professor of Pediatrics
Division of Newborn Medicine
Department of Pediatrics
Weill Cornell Medical College
Division Chief, Newborn Medicine
New York Presbyterian Hospital
New York, New York

Consulting Editor
Richard A. Polin, MD
Professor of Pediatrics
College of Physicians and Surgeons
Columbia University
Director, Division of Neonatology
Morgan Stanley Children's Hospital of New York - Presbyterian
Columbia University Medical Center
New York, New York

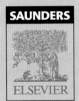

SAUNDERS

ELSEVIER

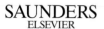
SAUNDERS
ELSEVIER

1600 John F. Kennedy Blvd.
Suite 1800
Philadelphia, PA 19103-2899

NEUROLOGY: Neonatology Questions and Controversies ISBN: 978-1-4160-3157-4
Copyright © 2008 by Saunders, an imprint of Elsevier Inc.

All rights reserved. No part of this publication may be reproduced or transmitted in any form or by any means, electronic or mechanical, including photocopying, recording, or any information storage and retrieval system, without permission in writing from the publisher. Permissions may be sought directly from Elsevier's Rights Department: phone: (+1) 215 239 3804 (US) or (+44) 1865 843830 (UK); fax: (+44) 1865 853333; e-mail: healthpermissions@elsevier.com. You may also complete your request on-line via the Elsevier website at http://www.elsevier.com/permissions.

Notice

Knowledge and best practice in this field are constantly changing. As new research and experience broaden our knowledge, changes in practice, treatment and drug therapy may become necessary or appropriate. Readers are advised to check the most current information provided (i) on procedures featured or (ii) by the manufacturer of each product to be administered, to verify the recommended dose or formula, the method and duration of administration, and contraindications. It is the responsibility of the practitioner, relying on their own experience and knowledge of the patient, to make diagnoses, to determine dosages and the best treatment for each individual patient, and to take all appropriate safety precautions. To the fullest extent of the law, neither the Publisher nor the Authors assumes any liability for any injury and/ or damage to persons or property arising out of or related to any use of the material contained in this book.

The Publisher

Library of Congress Cataloging-in-Publication Data

Neurology: neonatology questions and controversies/[edited by] Jeffrey Perlman;
consulting editor, Richard A. Polin.—1st ed.
    p.; cm
  Includes bibliographical references.
  ISBN: 978-1-4160-3157-4
  1. Pediatric neophrology. 2. Newborn infants—Diseases I. Perlman, Jeffrey. II. Polin, Richard A. (Richard Alan), 1945-
  [DNLM: 1. Infant, Newborn, Diseases. 2. Nervous System Diseases. 3. Infant, Newborn. WS 320 N4941 2008]
  RJ290.N466 2008
  618.92′8—dc22

2007044204

Publishing Director: Judith Fletcher
Developmental Editor: Lisa Barnes
Associate Development Editor: Bernard Buckholtz
Senior Project Manager: David Saltzberg
Design Direction: Karen O'Keefe-Owens

Working together to grow libraries in developing countries

www.elsevier.com | www.bookaid.org | www.sabre.org

ELSEVIER   **BOOK AID** International   Sabre Foundation

Printed in China

Last digit is the print number: 9 8 7 6 5 4 3 2 1

Contents

Contributors

Rowena G. Cayabyab, MD
Assistant Professor of Pediatrics
USC Division of Neonatal Medicine
Department of Pediatrics
Women's and Children's Hospital
LAC+USC Medical Center and
Children's Hospital Los Angeles
Keck School of Medicine
University of Southern California
Los Angeles, California
Cerebral Circulation and Hypotension in the Premature Infant: Diagnosis and Treatment

Keung-kit Chan, MBBS, MRCPCH
Resident Specialist
Department of Pediatrics
Kwong Wah Hospital
Kowloon, Hong Kong
Neonatal Hypotonia

Basil T. Darras, MD
Associate Neurologist-in-Chief
Professor of Neurology – Pediatrics
Harvard Medical School
Director, Residency Training Program
Director, Neuromuscular Program
Department of Neurology
Children's Hospital Boston
Boston, Massachusetts
Neonatal Hypotonia

Gabrielle de Veber, MD
Director, Children's Stroke Program
Division of Neurology
Hospital for Sick Children
Toronto, Ontario
Stroke in the Fetus and Neonate

Petra S. Hüppi, MD

Professor of Pediatrics
Department of Pediatrics
University Children's Hospital
Geneva, Switzerland

Magnetic Resonance Imaging's Role in the Care of the Infant at Risk for Brain Injury

David Kaufman, MD

Associate Professor of Pediatrics
Department of Pediatrics
University of Virginia Medical School
University of Virginia Children's Hospital
Charlottesville, Virginia

Neonatal Meningitis: Current Treatment Options

Abbot R. Laptook, MD

Medical Director
Neonatal Intensive Care Unit
Women and Infants' Hospital of Rhode Island
Professor of Pediatrics
Department of Pediatrics
Warren Alpert Medical School at Brown University
Providence, Rhode Island

Brain Cooling for Neonatal Encephalopathy: Potential Indications for Use

Claire W. McLean, MD

Assistant Professor of Pediatrics
Keck School of Medicine
University of Southern California
USC Division of Neonatal Medicine
Attending Neonatologist
Children's Hospital Los Angeles
Los Angeles, California

Cerebral Circulation and Hypotension in the Premature Infant: Diagnosis and Treatment

Caroline C. Menache, MD

Pediatric Neurologist
Department of Pediatrics
University Children's Hospital
Geneva, Switzerland

Magnetic Resonance Imaging's Role in the Care of the Infant at Risk for Brain Injury

Laura R. Ment, MD

Professor
Departments of Pediatrics and Neurology
Associate Dean for Admissions
Yale University School of Medicine
New Haven, Connecticut

Stroke in the Fetus and Neonate

Shahab Noori, MD

Assistant Professor of Pediatrics
Neonatal Perinatal Medicine
Department of Pediatrics
University of Oklahoma, College of Medicine
The Children's Hospital
Oklahoma City, Oklahoma

Cerebral Circulation and Hypotension in the Premature Infant: Diagnosis and Treatment

Koray Özduman, MD

Research Fellow
Yale School of Medicine
Department of Neurosurgery
New Haven, Connecticuit

Stroke in the Fetus and Neonate

Jeffrey M. Perlman, MB, ChB

Professor of Pediatrics
Division of Newborn Medicine
Department of Pediatrics
Weill Cornell Medical College
Division Chief, Newborn Medicine
New York Presbyterian Hospital
New York, New York

Intraventricular Hemorrhage and White Matter Injury in the Preterm Infant

General Supportive Management of the Term Infant with Neonatal Encephalopathy Following Intrapartum Hypoxia-Ischemia

Kenneth J. Poskitt, MD

Assistant Professor
Department of Radiology
Faculty of Medicine
BC Children's Hospital
Vancouver, Canada

Glucose and Perinatal Brain Injury: Questions and Controversies

Pablo J. Sánchez, MD

Professor of Pediatrics
University of Texas Southwestern Medical Center
Department of Pediatrics
Parkland Health and Hospital System
Children's Medical Center Dallas
Dallas, Texas

Neonatal Meningitis: Current Treatment Options

Mark S. Scher, MD

Chief, Division of Pediatric Neurology
Director, Programs of Fetal/Neonatal Neurology
Rainbow Babies and Children's Hospital
University Hospitals Case Medical Center
Professor, Pediatrics and Neurology
Case Western Reserve University
Cleveland, Ohio

Diagnosis and Treatment of Neonatal Seizures

Istvan Seri, MD, PhD

Professor of Pediatrics
Keck School of Medicine
University of Southern California
Head, USC Division of Neonatal Medicine
Director, Center for Fetal and Neonatal Medicine and
The Institute for Maternal-Fetal Health
Children's Hospital Los Angeles and
Women's and Children's Hospital
LAC+USC Medical Center
Los Angeles, California

Cerebral Circulation and Hypotension in the Premature Infant: Diagnosis and Treatment

Steven M. Shapiro, MD

Professor of Neurology, Pediatrics, Physical Medicine and Rehabilitation,
Otolaryngology, and Physiology
Vice Chairman
Division of Child Neurology
Department of Neurology
Medical College of Virginia Campus
Virginia Commonwealth University Medical Center
Richmond, Virginia

Hyperbilirubinemia and the Risk for Brain Injury

Betty R. Vohr, MD

Director, Neonatal Follow Up
Women and Infants' Hospital of Rhode Island
Professor of Pediatrics
Warren Alpert Medical School at Brown University
Providence, Rhode Island

Long-term Follow-up of Very Low Birth Weight Infants

Andrew Whitelaw, MD, FRCPCH

Professor of Neonatal Medicine and Consultant Neonatologist
University of Bristol Medical School
Southmead Hospital
Bristol, United Kingdom

Posthemorrhagic Hydrocephalus Management Strategies

Jerome Y. Yager, MD

Professor and Director
Division of Pediatric Neurology
Head - Section of Pediatric Neurosciences
Department of Pediatrics
Stollery Children's Hospital
University of Alberta
Edmonton, Alberta

Glucose and Perinatal Brain Injury: Questions and Controversies

Santina Zanelli, MD

Assistant Professor of Pediatrics
University of Virginia School of Medicine
and University of Virginia Medical Center
Charlottesville, Virginia

Neonatal Meningitis: Current Treatment Options

Series foreword

Learn from yesterday, live for today, hope for tomorrow. The important thing is not to stop questioning.

ALBERT EINSTEIN

The art and science of asking questions is the source of all knowledge.

THOMAS BERGER

In the mid 1960s W.B. Saunders began publishing a series of books focused on the care of newborn infants. The series was entitled *Major Problems in Clinical Pediatrics*. The original series (1964–1979) consisted of ten titles dealing with problems of the newborn infant (*The Lung and its Disorders in the Newborn Infant* edited by Mary Ellen Avery, *Disorders of Carbohydrate Metabolism in Infancy* edited by Marvin Cornblath and Robert Schwartz, *Hematologic Problems in the Newborn* edited by Frank A. Oski and J. Lawrence Naiman, *The Neonate with Congenital Heart Disease* edited by Richard D. Rowe and Ali Mehrizi, *Recognizable Patterns of Human Malformation* edited by David W. Smith, *Neonatal Dermatology* edited by Lawrence M. Solomon and Nancy B. Esterly, *Amino Acid Metabolism and its Disorders* edited by Charles L. Scriver and Leon E. Rosenberg, *The High Risk Infant* edited by Lula O Lubchenco, *Gastrointestinal Problems in the Infant* edited by Joyce Gryboski and *Viral Diseases of the Fetus and Newborn* edited by James B Hanshaw and John A. Dudgeon). Dr. Alexander J. Schaffer was asked to be the consulting editor for the entire series. Dr. Schaffer coined the term "neonatology" and edited the first clinical textbook of neonatology entitled *Diseases of the Newborn*. For those of us training in the 1970s, this series and Dr. Schaffer's textbook of neonatology provided exciting, up-to-date information that attracted many of us into the subspecialty. Dr. Schaffer's role as "consulting editor" allowed him to select leading scientists and practitioners to serve as editors for each individual volume. As the "consulting editor" for *Neonatology: Questions and Controversies*, I had the challenge of identifying the topics and editors for each volume in this series. The six volumes encompass the major issues encountered in the neonatal intensive care unit (newborn lung, fluid and electrolytes, neonatal cardiology and hemodynamics, hematology, immunology and infectious disease, gastroenterology and neurology). The editors for each volume were challenged to combine discussions of fetal and neonatal physiology with disease pathophysiology and selected controversial topics in clinical care. It is my hope that this series (like *Major Problems in Clinical Pediatrics*) will excite a new generation of trainees to question existing dogma (from my own generation) and seek new information through scientific investigation. I wish to congratulate and thank each of the volume editors (Drs. Bancalari, Oh, Guignard, Baumgart, Kleinman, Seri, Ohls, Yoder, Neu and Perlman) for their extraordinary effort and finished products. I also wish to acknowledge Judy Fletcher at Elsevier who conceived the idea for the series and who has been my "editor and friend" throughout my academic career.

Richard A. Polin, MD

Preface

The discipline of newborn neurology has expanded substantially over the past two decades. This has involved both basic and clinical research. As a consequence, great strides have been made in our understanding of the mechanisms contributing to brain injury. This has facilitated the introduction of targeted strategies in several instances. This volume addresses many neurological conditions and has focused on several important mechanisms that may contribute to neonatal brain injury as well as enhancements in diagnostic capabilities. The contributing authors are all outstanding clinicians who, through training, investigative research, and practice, have developed expertise that relates either directly or indirectly to neonatal neurologic problems.

Although this volume is not all-inclusive, the goal is that the information contained within will facilitate patient care and serve as a stimulus for future research.

Jeffrey M. Perlman, MB, ChB

Chapter 1

Introduction

Jeffrey M. Perlman, MB, ChB

The perinatal period represents a time of great vulnerability for the developing brain, with the potential for devastating injury as a consequence of a diverse group of causes with the possibility of long lasting profound neurocognitive deficits. Over the past two decades great strides have been made in the understanding of the basic mechanisms contributing to brain injury. This has facilitated the introduction of targeted strategies in several instances. This book tries to address some of the prominent factors/events contributing to brain injury as well as describing some of the novel treatment options that have been introduced.

Given the prominent important role of cerebral perfusion in the genesis of both hemorrhagic and ischemic cerebral injury, Chapter 2 in this book is devoted to neonatal hypotension and the relevance to brain injury. Discussion is focused on different treatment options in maintaining blood pressure and thus cerebral perfusion. Specifically in the preterm infant disturbances in cerebral perfusion have been associated with intraventricular hemorrhage as well as white matter injury and is discussed in Chapter 3. However it has become clear that the developing brain is also vulnerable to free radicals, excitatory amino acids, as well as cytokines. Interestingly while the incidence of severe intraventricular hemorrhage has declined over time, particularly in those infants whose mothers received a course of steroid prior to delivery, injury to white matter is being identified with increasing frequency on a magnetic resonance imaging study usually performed prior to discharge. Moreover in such cases there is often an associated reduction in gray matter volume as well as a reduction in cerebellar volumes. Thus it is not surprising that cognitive deficits are being identified in substantial numbers even in infants with normal sonograms. The management of posthemorrhagic hydrocephalus, a major complication of intraventricular hemorrhage, is discussed in Chapter 4. Recognition that hypoxic-ischemic cerebral injury is an evolving process initiated at the time of the insult and extending through post recovery is a secondary phase of injury, termed reperfusion injury, has led to a major therapeutic advance, i.e., the introduction of modest hypothermia either selective or systemic in infants at high risk for developing neonatal encephalopathy. Hypothermia has been shown to dampen many of the processes contributing to reperfusion injury. Brain cooling has been associated with a significant reduction in the incidence of cerebral palsy and/or death at 18-month follow-up in a subset of those infants treated. While exciting, there are large gaps in knowledge that limits its introduction into routine practice and these concerns are discussed in Chapter 5. In Chapter 6 supportive management strategies for infants with neonatal encephalopathy are discussed, including the importance of optimizing ventilation, monitoring glucose, and promptly treating seizures. Focal cerebral infarction remains an enigma for the clinician. Its onset is unpredictable, and the primary cause is often not clear thus limiting the potential for prevention as well as treatment following diagnosis. These issues as well as gaps in knowledge are discussed in Chapter 7. Neonatal seizures remain an important clinical problem. The more frequent use of video monitoring has repeatedly demonstrated the common finding of electrographic seizures without a clinical correlate. Treatment has remained relatively unchanged over time, although the most frequently used anticonvulsants, e.g., Phenobarbital, are only effective about 50% of the time in the effective elimination of seizures. This is discussed in Chapter 8. Hypoglycemia remains a concern for the developing brain and the diagnosis and management of this condition is discussed in Chapter 9. The clinical approach to the hypotonic neonate is clearly delineated in Chapter 10. Of particular note is the increasing number of conditions that can be localized to a particular chromosome segment. This has facilitated the diagnosis and has helped with parent counseling. The management of the infant with hyper-bilirubinemia is discussed in Chapter 11. Particular emphasis is focused on the treatment of those infants who are at great risk for developing kernicterus. In Chapter 12 the issue of neonatal meningitis is extensively covered. In Chapter 13 the role of advanced neuroimaging in the diagnosis and assessment of brain injury in both preterm as well as term infants is clearly delineated. The importance of neonatal follow-up is highlighted in Chapter 14.

It is the goal of this book that after reading each chapter the reader will have a clearer management strategy that is based on an understanding of the underlying pathophysiology. In addition a desired goal is that the highlighted gaps in knowledge will serve as a strong stimulus for future research.

Chapter 2

Cerebral Circulation and Hypotension in the Premature Infant: Diagnosis and Treatment

Claire W. McLean, MD • Rowena G. Cayabyab, MD
• Shahab Noori, MD • Istvan Seri, MD, PhD

Introduction

Definition of Hypotension

Pathogenesis and Diagnosis of Pathologic Cerebral Blood Flow

Treatment Strategies

Summary and Recommendations

CASE HISTORY

A 956 g male infant is born via emergent cesarean section for a non-reassuring fetal heart tracing at 27- and 2/7 weeks gestation to a 29-year-old, G2; P 1 mother with an unremarkable medical history, previous and current pregnancy, and prenatal laboratory studies. She had presented to her obstetrician that morning complaining of abdominal pain. The mother received one dose of betamethasone less than an hour prior to the delivery. Membranes were ruptured at delivery with clear fluid. The baby was born somewhat depressed with Apgars of 4 and 7 at 1 and 5 minutes, respectively. He was intubated immediately and responded to careful bag ventilation with improvement of the heart rate, color, and tone. He was transported to the NICU where he received surfactant within 20 minutes after delivery. Subsequently he was weaned rapidly to low mean airway pressures and room air on synchronized intermittent mandatory ventilation. He had umbilical venous and arterial lines placed and he was started on intravenous fluids. Initial laboratory studies were significant for white blood cell and platelet counts of 3000/μL and 80 000/μL, respectively, and he had a hematocrit of 51%. A blood culture was sent and antibiotics were started. Spinal tap was not performed due to the low platelet count. The mother had a fever after delivery to 39.8°C, and the placental pathology later confirmed chorioamnionitis. The infant developed hypotension at 4 hours after delivery with a mean arterial blood pressure (MABP) between 21 and 24 mmHg. The hypotension initially responded to dopamine administration titrated up to 20 mcg/kg/min in a stepwise manner. Although dopamine could be weaned off by 28 hours, the baby developed increasing FiO$_2$ requirements and recurrence of hypotension with a MABP of 21–24 mmHg and diastolic blood pressures between 12 and 16 mmHg within 12 hours. An echocardiogram was performed at this time, which confirmed the presence of the suspected widely open patent ductus arteriosus (PDA) with almost all left-to-right shunting. He received a course of indomethacin, and follow-up echocardiogram on postnatal day 4 revealed no PDA. He continued to require somewhat higher ventilatory support and FiO_2, and by that time placental cultures were positive for *E. coli*, sensitive to the antibiotics the baby had been receiving. A spinal tap was performed upon the positive placental culture on postnatal day 4 despite the mild ongoing coagulopathy treated with repeated platelet transfusions and fresh frozen plasma. The spinal tap showed no evidence of meningitis. Throughout this acute period, urine output and other indirect indicators of end-organ perfusion were adequate including normal lactate levels on two occasions. Cranial ultrasound on postnatal day 4 revealed a left Grade II and a right Grade I peri/intraventricular hemorrhage (P/IVH). Follow-up head ultrasounds at 1 week and 1 month of age showed no evidence for periventricular echogenicity or cystic lesions in the periventricular white matter. However, an MRI study showed diffuse as well as minimal focal periventricular white matter injury (PWMI) at 34 weeks postmenstrual age without evidence of notable ventriculomegaly or gray matter injury. Patient was discharged home on nasal cannula oxygen and full feedings and with appropriate growth parameters at 36 weeks postmenstrual age. In follow-up clinic at 2 years of age he had evidence of mild bilateral lower extremity spastic diplegia. He walked at 22 months of age. By school age, language and other cognitive milestones had been met adequately but he had ongoing mild gross and fine motor delays.

INTRODUCTION

The preceding case study illustrates a fairly typical course for a 27-week preterm infant who had not benefited from antenatal steroid exposure. It also highlights the complexity of determining causation for both radiographic brain abnormalities and long-term neurodevelopmental deficits seen in this patient population. Several questions should be asked regarding the pathogenesis of the central nervous system injury in this patient. Did the injury occur as a result of the inflammatory process associated with the chorioamnionitis, or was it caused by the severe and repeated episodes of hypotension and the associated periventricular white matter hypoperfusion followed by reperfusion upon normalization of the blood pressure? Or did both pathogenetic factors contribute to the outcome? If it was primarily or also due to the hypoperfusion–reperfusion injury, at what point did the injury occur? Finally, how should the practicing neonatologist monitor for all these factors known to cause brain injury, and how should appropriate interventions be chosen when these risk factors are present?

As the field of neonatology has progressed over the last few decades, better monitoring and more effective interventions have been developed for supporting the respiratory, fluid and electrolyte, and nutritional abnormalities frequently encountered in very low birth weight (VLBW) infants. However, our ability to effectively and continuously monitor the hemodynamic changes at the level of organ blood flow and tissue perfusion remains very limited despite the recent advances achieved with the use of functional echocardiography and other bedside organ and tissue perfusion monitoring modalities. With the improvements in hemodynamic monitoring and a better understanding of the principles of developmental cardiovascular physiology has come the realization of how little we actually know about circulatory compromise and its effect on organs (especially the brain), blood flow, and long-term outcomes. Although we can continuously and reliably monitor systemic blood pressure and we have myriad interventions for "normalizing" it, blood pressure is only one component of the hemodynamic parameters determining tissue perfusion. Indeed, in addition to monitoring and maintaining perfusion pressure (blood pressure), our goal is to preserve normal blood flow and tissue oxygenation, especially to the vital organs, i.e., to the brain, heart, and adrenals. In this regard, when it comes to the brain, we are at an even greater disadvantage. For instance, measuring cerebral blood flow (CBF) is much more difficult than measuring systemic blood flow (left ventricular output). It is of note, however, that even assessment of systemic blood flow becomes very complicated when shunting through the fetal channels (ductus arteriosus and foramen ovale) occurs during the first few postnatal days in the VLBW neonate. In addition, we cannot detect clinical evidence of ischemia in the brain as easily as we can for other organs, for example the heart, liver, or kidneys. Seizure activity is a clear sign of a pathologic process, but these can also be difficult to recognize in the VLBW population. In addition, by the time seizures are present, irreversible injury may have already occurred. Thus, we are facing the formidable task to effectively support and protect the enormously complex developmental processes that are occurring in the brain of a VLBW infant. Yet we even have difficulties in detecting changes in CBF and cerebral function in a timely manner and have very little understanding of how to manage the hemodynamic disturbances potentially affecting brain function and structure and ultimately neurodevelopmental outcome.

The intent of this chapter is to review the available information on the definition of systemic hypotension and the pathogenesis, diagnosis, and treatment of early cerebral perfusion abnormalities in the VLBW infant that have been shown to precede intracranial hemorrhage and PWMI. Because CBF and cerebral oxygenation in this population is such a complex topic, we will focus our discussion on the first postnatal days, during which the cardiorespiratory transition from fetal to extrauterine life occurs. We will discuss some of the modalities that are being explored for identifying decreased CBF and cerebral oxygenation at the bedside. Once a pathologic process is identified, provision of a coherent, safe, and effective means of treating it is crucial. We will present a rationale treatment for the pathologic processes underlying clinically evident brain injury in the VLBW infant based on the most up-to-date monitoring and clinical evidence available. In an area as controversial and complex as this one, it is important to always highlight what we do not know. Our goal is to provide the practitioner with recommendations for diagnosis and treatment that should be considered guidelines only. Finally, although our understanding of both normal and pathologic processes in the preterm brain is improving, evidence for a definitive clinical approach remains scant.

DEFINITION OF HYPOTENSION

Hypotension occurs in up to 50% of VLBW infants admitted to the neonatal intensive care unit. As in the case in this chapter, hypotension in the immediate postnatal period is thought to be one of the major factors contributing to central nervous system injury and eventual cerebral palsy and poor long-term neurological outcome in VLBW neonates. Indeed, the *association* between hypotension and brain injury and poor neurodevelopmental outcome is well documented (1–8) and forms the basis of our therapeutic efforts to normalize blood pressure. However, *causation* has never been demonstrated between hypotension and poor neurodevelopment.

In clinical practice, hypotension is usually defined as the blood pressure value below the 5th or 10th percentile for the gestational- and postnatal age-dependent normative blood pressure values (9–11) (Fig. 2-1). In general, however, there is no consensus among neonatologists about the acceptable lower limit of systemic mean or systolic arterial blood pressure and most units have different guidelines for the initiation of treatment of hypotension.

From a pathophysiologic standpoint, there are three levels of functional alterations of increasing severity that can be used to guide the definition of hypotension

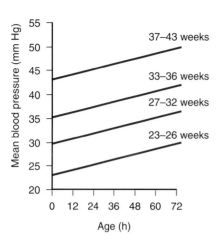

Figure 2-1 Gestational- and postnatal age-dependent normogram for mean blood pressure values in preterm and term neonates during the first three postnatal days. The normogram is derived from continuous arterial blood pressure measurements obtained from 103 neonates with gestational ages between 23 and 43 weeks. As each line represents the lower limit of 80% confidence interval of mean blood pressure for each gestational age group, 90% of infants for each gestational age group will have a mean blood pressure equal or greater than the value indicated by the corresponding line (the lower limit of confidence interval). (From Nuntnarumit P, Yang W, Bada-Ellzey HS. Blood pressure measurements in the newborn. Clin Perinatol 26:981–96, 1999 with permission.)

based on recent findings in the literature (Fig. 2-2). However, it is important to keep in perspective that there is no prospectively collected information available on mortality and morbidity associated with these different thresholds of hypotensive blood pressure values.

First, the mean blood pressure value associated with the loss of CBF autoregulation is the generally accepted definition of hypotension (*autoregulatory blood pressure threshold*) (12, 13). Indeed, there is considerable information in the literature indicating that CBF autoregulation is functional in normotensive but not in hypotensive VLBW neonates in the immediate postnatal period (Fig. 2-3) (5, 13, 14). Autoregulation is the property of arteries to constrict or dilate in response to an increase or decrease, respectively, in the transmural pressure to maintain blood flow relatively constant within a range of arterial blood pressure changes (Fig. 2-2). However, in the neonate, this response has a limited capacity. In addition, the autoregulatory blood pressure range is narrow in the neonatal patient population and the 50th percentile of the mean blood pressure is relatively close to the lower autoregulatory blood pressure threshold. In other words, small decreases in blood pressure may result in loss of CBF autoregulation especially in the preterm infant (13). Recent findings suggest that the autoregulatory blood pressure threshold is around 28–30 mmHg even in the extremely low birth weight (ELBW) neonate during the first postnatal day (13, 15) (Fig. 2-4). At this blood pressure, however, cellular function and structural integrity are unlikely to be affected as increased cerebral fraction oxygen extraction (CFOE), microvascular vasodilation, and a shift in the hemoglobin–oxygen dissociation curve to the left can maintain tissue oxygen delivery at levels appropriate to sustain cellular function and integrity (16, 17).

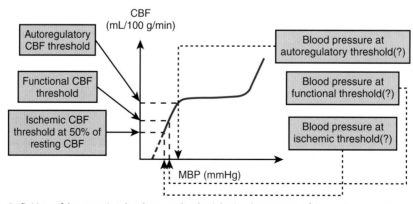

Figure 2-2 Definition of hypotension by three pathophysiologic phenomena of increasing severity: autoregulatory, functional and ischemic thresholds of hypotension.

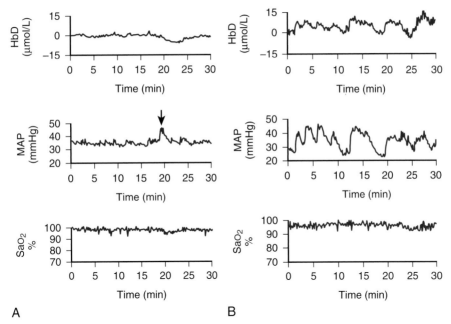

Figure 2-3 Intact and compromised CBF autoregulation in VLBW neonates in the immediate postnatal period. Changes in cerebral intravascular oxygenation (HbD = HbO$_2$−Hb) correlate with changes in CBF (5). (A) Changes in HbD (i.e., CBF), mean arterial pressure (MAP), and oxygen saturation (SaO$_2$) in a 1-day-old 28-week gestation preterm infant whose subsequent head ultrasound remained normal. No change occurs in CBF in relation to the sudden increase in MAP associated with endotracheal tube suctioning (arrow). (B) Changes in HbD (CBF), MAP, and SaO$_2$ in a 1-day-old 27-week GA preterm infant whose subsequent head ultrasound revealed the presence of PWMI. Changes in blood pressure are clearly associated with changes in CBF. (From Tsuji M, Saul PJ, duPlessis A et al. Cerebral intravascular oxygenation correlates with mean arterial pressure in critically ill premature infants. Pediatrics 106:625, 2000 with permission.)

However, if blood pressure continues to fall, it reaches a value at which cerebral function becomes compromised (*functional blood pressure threshold*). Recent data suggest that the functional blood pressure threshold may be around 22–24 mmHg in the VLBW neonate during the first postnatal days (16, 17) (Fig. 2-5). However, caution is needed when interpreting these findings obtained in a small number of preterm infants as their clinical relevance is unclear. Furthermore, the relationship among cerebral electrical activity, neurodevelopmental outcome, and the threshold of CBF associated with impaired brain activity is not known.

Finally, if blood pressure decreases even further, it reaches a value at which structural integrity becomes compromised (*ischemic blood pressure threshold*). Based on findings in developing animals, it is assumed that the ischemic CBF threshold is around 50% of the resting CBF (13). Although it is unclear at what blood pressure value represents the ischemic CBF threshold in the VLBW neonate during the first postnatal day, this number may be below 20 mmHg (18, 19) (Fig. 2-2). It is important to emphasize that the situation is further complicated by the fact that these numbers represent moving targets for the individual patient. Indeed, several factors such as PaCO$_2$ levels, the presence of acidosis, preexisting insults (asphyxia), and the underlying pathophysiology (sepsis, anemia) have an impact on the critical blood pressure value at which perfusion pressure and cerebral oxygen delivery cannot satisfy cellular oxygen demand to sustain autoregulation, then cellular function and finally structural integrity.

At present, continuous monitoring of blood pressure and assessment of indirect signs of tissue perfusion (urine output, capillary refill time (CRT), lactic acidosis) remain the basis of identifying the presence of a cardiovascular compromise. However, adequate blood pressure may not always guarantee adequate organ

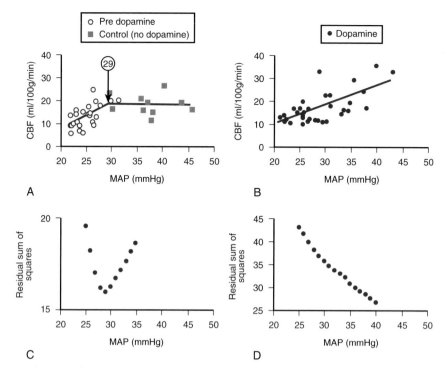

Figure 2-4 Relationship between CBF and mean arterial pressure (MAP) in hypotensive and normotensive ELBW neonates during the first postnatal day and the effect of dopamine on this relationship. (A, B) MAP (mmHg) and CBF (mL/100 g/min) measured by NIRS in normotensive ELBW neonates not requiring dopamine ("Control," filled squares; $n = 5$) and hypotensive ELBW neonates before dopamine administration ("Pre-dopamine," open circles; $n = 12$). The lower threshold of the CBF autoregulatory blood pressure limit (29 mmHg; A) is identified as the minimum of residual sum of squares of the bilinear regression analysis (B). (C, D) MAP (mmHg) and CBF (mL/100 g/min) in the formerly hypotensive ELBW neonates after dopamine treatment (filled circles). No breakpoint is evident in the CBF–MAP curve in ELBW neonates on dopamine (C), because there is no minimum identified by the bilinear regression analysis (D). (From Munro MJ, Walker AM, Barfield CP. Hypotensive extremely low birth weight infants have reduced cerebral blood flow. Pediatrics 114:1591, 2004 with permission.)

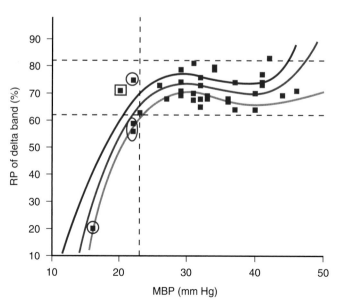

Figure 2-5 Relationship between mean blood pressure (MBP) and cerebral electrical activity in VLBW neonates during the first 4 postnatal days. Relationship between MBP and the relative power (RP) of the delta band of the EEG, showing line of best fit with 95% confidence interval ($N = 35$; $R^2 = 0.627$; $p < 0.001$). Horizontal dotted lines represent the normal range of the relative power of the delta band (10th–90th percentile) while the vertical dotted line identifies the point of intercept. The open square identifies the infant with abnormal CFOE and the abnormal EEG records are circled. (From Victor S, Marson AG, Appleton RE et al. Relationship between blood pressure, cerebral electrical activity, cerebral fractional oxygen extraction and peripheral blood flow in very low birth weight newborn infants. Pediatr Res 59:314–19, 2006 with permission.)

perfusion in VLBW neonates during the first postnatal day (20). Indeed, blood pressure, the product of systemic blood flow and systemic vascular resistance, only weakly correlates with superior vena cava (SVC) flow in VLBW neonates during the immediate postnatal adaptation (21). SVC flow has been used as a surrogate of systemic blood flow in the VLBW neonate during the immediate postnatal period when shunting through the fetal channels prohibits the use of left ventricular (LV) output to assess systemic blood flow (22). The finding that adequate blood pressure may not always guarantee adequate systemic blood flow in these patients may be explained at least in part by the notion that the vascular bed of the forebrain, especially of the 1-day-old ELBW neonate, may not be of high priority and thus it will constrict rather than dilate in response to a decrease in the perfusion pressure (23, 24) (discussed in detail below).

PATHOGENESIS AND DIAGNOSIS OF PATHOLOGIC CEREBRAL BLOOD FLOW

Fluctuations in CBF are implicated in the pathogenesis of P/IVH and PWMI in the VLBW infant (1). Both systemic and local (intracerebral) factors play a role in the pathogenesis of these central nervous system injuries, and therefore are important in diagnosis. In addition, the level of maturity, postnatal age, and intercurrent clinical factors (infection/inflammation, vasopressor-resistant hypotension, etc.) need to be considered. In this section, we will briefly discuss monitoring parameters that are currently in widespread clinical use (systemic arterial pressure and arterial blood gas sampling) and then delve into the emerging field of bedside monitoring of CBF and brain activity. We will review most of the existing technologies, including Doppler ultrasound and functional echocardiography, near-infrared spectroscopy (NIRS) and amplitude-integrated EEG, and discuss the applicability and limitations of these modalities. We will not discuss the use of MRI for assessing CBF in the neonatal patient population as this topic is addressed elsewhere in this book in detail.

A logical place to begin the discussion on monitoring CBF in the VLBW infant is to ask, "What is the normal CBF in the VLBW infant?" Several investigators have addressed this issue. It is clear from these studies that CBF is lower in preterm infants than adults matching the lower metabolic rate of the preterm brain. Greisen using ^{133}Xe clearance found that in 42 preterm infants with a mean gestational age of 31 weeks, CBF was 15.5 ± 7.2 mL/100 g/min during the first postnatal week; a value three to four times lower than that in adults (25). Interestingly, patients enrolled in this study receiving mechanical ventilation had lower CBF than their nonventilated counterparts or those receiving continuous positive airway pressure (11.8 ± 3.2 vs. 19.8 ± 5.3 and 21.3 ± 12 mL/100 g/min, respectively). Cerebral blood flow in this study was not consistently affected by postnatal age, gestational age, birth weight, mode of delivery, $PaCO_2$, hemoglobin concentration, mean blood pressure, or Phenobarbital therapy. In contrast, subsequent publications investigating CBF reactivity in preterm infants during the first three postnatal days showed that, as expected, $PaCO_2$ and hemoglobin concentration affect CBF in this patient population (26–28).

Using positron emission tomography (PET) to measure CBF, Altman et al. found lower values for CBF in preterm and term neonates compared to those obtained by the use of ^{133}Xe clearance (29). More importantly, they reported that out of one term and five preterm infants with a CBF between 4.9 and 10 mL/100 g/min, the term neonate and three preterm infants had normal neurodevelopmental outcome at 24 months (29). Therefore, the lower limit of CBF not necessarily associated with ischemic brain damage in the neonate may be between 5 and 10 mL/100 g/min. Finally, as CBF is affected by many factors other than blood pressure, it is not yet possible to define the blood pressure value consistently associated with a decrease of CBF below this range resulting in ischemic brain injury.

Kluckow and Evans (22) used SVC blood flow as a surrogate for systemic blood flow and CBF in well preterm neonates <30 weeks gestation receiving minimal ventilatory support, and established normal values of SVC flow during the first 48 postnatal hours. Of note is that the extent to which SVC flow is representative of systemic or cerebral blood flow in preterm neonates during the first postnatal days is not known. In a subsequent study that included sick preterm infants less than 30 weeks gestation, the same group found that 38% of infants had a period of low SVC in the first 24 (mostly 12) postnatal hours (20). The incidence of low SVC flow was significantly related to the level of immaturity and was over 70% in very preterm neonates with a gestational age of <27 weeks. The sudden increase in the peripheral vascular resistance caused by the loss of the low-resistance placental circulation, the complex process of cardiorespiratory transition to the postnatal circulatory pattern, and myocardial and autonomic central nervous system immaturity have been proposed to contribute to these findings. Indeed, these factors may explain why many of these very preterm neonates struggle to maintain normal systemic blood flow during the first 12–24 postnatal hours. Importantly, a proportion of the very preterm babies with catastrophic SVC flow were found to have systemic blood pressures in the "normal range" (i.e., equal or greater than their gestational age in weeks), a finding supported by subsequent studies of this group of researchers (20, 30, 31). As normal blood pressure and decreased organ blood flow to nonvital organs are the hallmarks of the compensated phase of shock and since a portion of SVC flow represents blood returning from the brain, a vital organ, it is conceivable that the vascular beds of the cerebral cortex and white matter are low-priority vessels and function as those of nonvital organs in the very preterm neonate during the immediate postnatal period. This hypothesis is supported by recent observations (23, 24) and may explain why SVC blood flow may be decreased in some very preterm neonates who have normal systemic blood pressure. Most babies with documented low SVC flow in the first 24–48 hours that do not go on to develop P/IVH or PWMI are more mature (28 weeks vs. 25–26 weeks). Thus, for preterm babies <30 weeks gestation, low systemic blood flow (and CBF) may be necessary but not sufficient to cause intracranial pathology. Importantly, all patients studied had an increase in SVC flow by 24 to 36 hours, and all P/IVH occurred after the SVC flow had increased. This finding implicates ischemia–reperfusion cycle in the pathogenesis of P/IVH.

The methods used to assess systemic and cerebral blood flow in VLBW neonates in the immediate transitional period have significant limitations. For the use of SVC flow to assess systemic and cerebral blood flow, the limitations include operator-dependence due to the uncertainties associated with the accurate measurement of vessel diameter and flow velocity. The fluctuations in vessel size during the cardiac cycle and the pattern of low flow velocity in the SVC are the major factors contributing to these technical difficulties. In addition, the shape of the SVC, the lack of data on the magnitude of the contribution of CBF to SVC flow, and the lack of a documented association between $PaCO_2$ and SVC flow in this patient population call for some caution when interpreting these interesting findings.

Kehrer et al. (32) measured blood flow in both internal carotid and vertebral arteries and used the sum of the blood flows in the four arteries supplying the brain to assess the changes in CBF volume in preterm infants of 28–35 weeks gestation over the first 2 postnatal weeks. Although the technique has its significant limitations, the findings suggest that a steep rise in CBF occurs from the first to the second postnatal day and this pattern is independent of gestational age. Thereafter, CBF continues to gradually rise (Fig. 2-6). Because there is not a significant increase in brain weight during the first 48 postnatal hours, the authors inferred that the

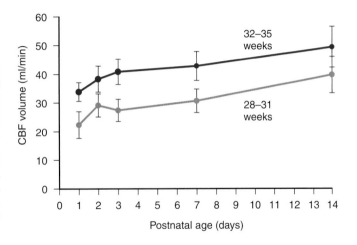

Figure 2-6 Changes in CBF volume in preterm neonates during the first 14 days after delivery. Development of CBF volume with increasing postnatal age in two different gestational age groups (28–31 and 32–35 weeks). Mean and 95% confidence interval are shown (ANOVA; $n = 29$, $p < 0.0001$).(From Kehrer M, Blumenstock G, Ehehalt S et al. Development of cerebral blood flow volume in preterm neonates during the first two weeks of life. Pediatr Res 58:927–30, 2005 with permission.)

observed increase in CBF during that period was secondary to increased cerebral perfusion per unit weight of tissue. On the other hand, the more gradual increase over the ensuing two weeks is likely due to a combination of both increased brain weight and increased perfusion (32). The investigators only studied "healthy" preterm infants with normal brains, whereas the series of investigations by Kluckow and Evans (20, 21, 30, 31) included preterm infants who, as a group, were sicker, and a percentage of who had significant intracranial pathology. Nevertheless, the results of the two groups are complementary as they provide evidence for a decreased CBF in the first postnatal day, followed by a significant increase by the second postnatal day. It is tempting to speculate that the low CBF in the study by Kehrer et al. (32) during the first postnatal day represents a decrease from that in the fetus and that the increase in the second postnatal day corresponds to the return of CBF to the normal levels following the establishment of a more stable postnatal circulatory pattern, as described by Kluckow and Evans (20, 21). Taken together, these studies suggest that low CBF in the first postnatal day and perhaps the ensuing "reperfusion" is a physiologic phenomenon occurring in most if not all very preterm neonates and that this phenomenon is a necessary but not sufficient cause of intracranial pathology (P/IVH or PWMI) in this patient population.

Our ultimate goal is to improve neurodevelopmental outcome in preterm infants, and since low SVC flow in the early postnatal period has been implicated not only in the development of P/IVH and PWMI but also in impaired neurologic outcome at 3 years (6), we need to identify those infants most at risk in the immediate postnatal period. It is clear from the large number of epidemiological and the above-cited hemodynamic studies that the level of immaturity is one of the most important predisposing factors for more abrupt changes in CBF during postnatal adaptation and for poor neurologic outcome. Therefore, assessment of CBF during the first 24 to 48 postnatal hours in the most immature and thus vulnerable patients is important. However, due to the technical difficulties associated with reliable and continuous assessment of CBF, clinical practice currently relies upon indirect measures for diagnosis of changes in cerebral perfusion. For instance, the notion that a "pressure-passive" cerebral circulation exists in most sick preterm neonates has led to the use of systemic blood pressure as the only surrogate measure for cerebral perfusion. However, as discussed earlier, in the compensated phase of shock, maintenance of normal systemic blood pressure is not the equivalent of adequate nonvital organ blood flow and the forebrain may not be a vital organ especially in the 23- to 26-week gestation neonate immediately after delivery. Therefore, the sole reliance upon blood pressure in the assessment of CBF in this patient population during the first postnatal day may not be adequate.

Nevertheless, recent data also suggest that a mean arterial pressure less than the gestational age during the immediate postnatal transitional period is likely to be close to the "functional and ischemic blood pressure thresholds" leading to functional abnormalities and permanent tissue injury, respectively (18, 19). Clearly, maintenance of systemic blood pressure at levels higher than the ischemic threshold is fundamental. Unfortunately and as discussed earlier, while there is some evidence that the CBF autoregulatory and functional blood pressure thresholds are around 28–30 and 22–24 mmHg in the very preterm neonate, respectively, the cerebral ischemic blood pressure threshold is not known.

In addition to blood pressure, monitoring of the indirect clinical indicators of tissue perfusion such as urine output, CRT, and acid–base status may be of importance. While these indirect clinical indicators by themselves are fairly nonspecific for detecting low systemic flow, the combined use of blood pressure and CRT increases their sensitivity. Indeed, when blood pressure and CRT are <30 mmHg and ≥3 seconds, respectively, the sensitivity to detecting low systemic blood flow is close to 80% (33). In addition, because of its direct effect on CBF, careful monitoring of $PaCO_2$ and avoidance of both hypo- and hypercapnia are of utmost importance.

If the monitoring we commonly use now in the clinical practice at the bedside is not sufficient to tell the whole story on CBF, what can be added? Fortunately, most of the interest in organ blood flow monitoring has focused on the cerebral circulation, in part because we cannot use indirect indices of perfusion such as urine output, liver function, or feeding tolerance for the assessment of CBF as we do for other organs. This interest has led to the development of a multitude of techniques for monitoring CBF, including Doppler ultrasound (the most popular, easily implemented, and widely researched), NIRS, amplitude-integrated EEG (aEEG), and newer MRI techniques (arterial spin-labeling, gadolinium). We will briefly discuss each of these modalities in the following sections with a primary focus on those that can be done noninvasively at the bedside.

Doppler Ultrasound

Velocity of blood flow can be measured using the Doppler principle, which states that the change in frequency of reflected sound is proportional to the velocity of the passing object (in this case, blood). The calculated velocity needs to be corrected for the angle between the vessel and the emitted sound beam ("angle of insonation"), and the straightforward idea is complicated by the fact that arterial blood is pulsatile and its speed varies within the vessel (i.e., it is faster in the center of the vessel). It is important to recognize that speed of blood (distance traveled per unit time) in a vessel means little by itself; we are really interested in the absolute blood flow (volume per unit time). Thus, volumetric measurements are crucial. Investigators have used several different volumetric indices, including SVC, internal carotid artery, and vertebral artery flow as previously discussed (22, 32). The limitations of SVC flow measurements were discussed earlier. In general, major technical problems with volumetric measurements include but are not restricted to the small size of the vessels, the motion of vessel wall and whether or not an angle of insonation of <20° can be achieved. In addition to volumetric measurements of vessel blood flow, right ventricular (RV) and LV outflow have been studied. Both are fraught with pitfalls in the very preterm neonate in the immediate postnatal period, as the patent foramen ovale (PFO) and PDA create shunts that confound the measurements for the RV and LV output, respectively. It is felt that RV output may be a more reliable indicator of systemic blood flow during the immediate postnatal period with the fetal channels open, because PFO shunting is less significant than ductal shunting during the first 24 hours after delivery (34). Indeed, RV output and systemic blood pressure have recently been correlated with EEG parameters (brain function) in VLBW infants in the immediate postnatal period (35).

Ultrasound techniques are noninvasive and widely accessible in the intensive care setting and can be done at the bedside. However, all ultrasound measurements are dependent on operator skill and have their significant limitations. As for the issues related to operator skills, centers utilizing these methods to diagnose pathologic CBF in neonates must have a rigorous quality control system in place with neonatologists well trained in functional echocardiography and available at the bedside at all times (36).

With regard to the limitations to the use of vascular Doppler in assessing organ blood flow, the most important limitation is the small size of the artery of interest (e.g., middle or anterior cerebral artery), which precludes accurate measurement of its diameter. Since the estimation of blood flow (Q) depends on assessment of mean velocity of the blood (V) and the vessel diameter (D) ($Q = V\pi D^2 \times 60$), any small error in measuring the diameter will translate into a significant error in estimating the actual blood flow. Therefore, instead of directly measuring blood flow, investigators often use changes in various Doppler-derived indices such as mean blood flow velocity or the pulsatility or resistance index as a surrogate for changes in blood flow. This approach is based on the premise that the vessel diameter remains constant despite the changes in blood flow. However, this concept in not universally accepted (37). Nevertheless, both animal and human studies have shown an acceptable correlation between these indices and other measures of blood flow (38–42).

As for the technical aspect of vascular Doppler, one must pay special attention to consistently Doppler the same segment of the vessel with the same angle of insonation. As the vessel diameter may vary at different sites, the measured velocity may also be different. With regard to the Doppler angle of insonation, one should try not to exceed 20°, as with a higher angle the velocity is significantly underestimated. Although most new ultrasound systems have the capability to correct for the angle of insonation, using the same angle of insonation for repeated measurements will ensure a better reproducibility of the data. Finally, although normative data for the Doppler-derived indices for various vessels are available, because of the above limitations one must be very cautious in interpreting a single measurement. Rather, repeated measurements and the use of trends over time are thought to be more informative of the hemodynamic status and the changes in organ blood flow.

Near-infrared Spectroscopy

This modality has received much attention since its first use in newborns in 1985 (43), and numerous papers have been published since then describing its use. Basically, it involves light of a specific wavelength (NIR range, 600–900 nm) being emitted from one optode, traveling through tissue, and being detected on the other side by another optode. Because of the presence of compounds whose absorption of NIR light is oxygen status dependent ("chromophores" such as hemoglobin and cytochrome aa3), absorption during passage through brain can be measured and oxygenation indices calculated. The newborn skull and tissues overlying the brain are thin, so most of the signal received will be representative of brain tissue. In the VLBW neonate, the biparietal diameter is such that essentially the whole brain can be "seen" by the traveling light and results can be interpreted as "global." Different wavelengths of light can be used to assess different parameters such as oxyhemoglobin, deoxyhemoglobin, and cytochrome aa3 oxidase. By inducing a small but rapid change in arterial oxygen saturation in the subject, CBF can be calculated using Fick's principle. This assumes that during the measurement period cerebral blood volume (CBV) and cerebral oxygen extraction remain constant.

Because the measurement depends on inducing a small but sudden change in arterial oxygen concentration, the technique may not be feasible in babies with severe lung disease (no change in oxygen saturation with an increased FiO_2) and in infants with normal lungs who saturate at 100% on room air. To get around this problem, an injected tracer dye such as indocyanine green has been used instead of oxygen with similar results (44). Newer instruments use an index called the tissue oxygenation index (TOI), which is the weighted average of arterial, capillary, and venous oxygenation and theoretically allows the measurement of cerebral hemoglobin-oxygen saturation without manipulating FiO_2 or using dye. However, this index also has significant potential for inaccuracy with an intrameasurement agreement in a single subject as large as -17 to $+17\%$ (45). Indeed, reproducibility of NIRS measurements in general has been an ongoing issue for investigators, especially in the detection of focal changes in cerebral hemodynamics (46). This is a significant problem, as focal hemodynamic changes are at least as likely to contribute to neuropathology as are global changes.

Despite these limitations, NIRS has been validated using comparison to ^{133}Xe clearance in human newborns (47). [133]Xe clearance is the experimental model "gold standard," utilizing ateriovenous difference in an inert radioisotope and giving a global measurement of CBF. Although NIRS potentially represents a practical solution, it is not ready yet for use in general clinical practice. Accumulation of more descriptive data in many patients, repeated measurements in the same patient, and prospective studies looking at both short- and long-term outcomes are likely to be the key in transitioning NIRS from the experimental arena to standard clinical monitoring.

Amplitude-integrated EEG (Cerebral Function Monitoring)

There is evidence to support the use of aEEG in asphyxiated infants in the first several hours after birth, as it is one of the most accurate bedside methods to establish a neurologic prognosis (48, 49). For this reason, it has been used to select candidates for enrollment in head-cooling neuroprotection trials. This technology uses a single-channel EEG recording with biparietal electrodes. Frequencies less than 2 Hz and greater than 15 Hz are filtered selectively, and the amplitude of the signal is integrated. The signal is then recorded semilogarithmically with slow speed, effectively compressing hours of EEG recording into shorter segments that reflect global background activity and major deviations from baseline (e.g., seizures). Studies have shown that aEEG correlates well with conventional EEG (50) and has the distinct advantage of being easily applied and interpreted by nonneurologists. More recently, normal aEEG in the first 72 postnatal hours in asphyxiated term neonates has been shown to be prognostic of normal neurologic outcome at 2 years of age (51). Coupled with early neurologic examination, simultaneous aEEG improved specificity and positive predictive value of an abnormal exam for abnormal neurologic outcome at 18 months of age (52).

Significantly less information has been gathered using aEEG in the preterm population. However, some typical patterns of background activity for preterm infants have been established, and a number of studies exist that point to its applicability in this group. For instance, low CBF (measured by ^{133}Xe clearance) correlates with discontinuous aEEG activity in ventilated preterm neonates of 27–33 weeks of gestation (53) and in preterm infants with a large P/IVH, aEEG during the first postnatal week is predictive of survival and intermediate-term neurologic outcome (54).

Before aEEG can be incorporated into routine clinical use, data on tracings in normal premature infants in the immediate postnatal period as well as longitudinal development of mature brain activity must be collected and evaluated. Two recent studies by a group of investigators have attempted to do just that (55, 56). A group of clinically and ultrasonographically normal infants with gestational ages between 23 and 29 weeks were studied with aEEG in the first 2 postnatal weeks. With increasing gestational and postnatal age, the occurrence of continuous activity increased and discontinuous low-voltage activity was less likely to be seen. The number of bursts per hour also decreased with increasing gestational age. Although the authors offered these findings as a foundation for neurodevelopmental prognosis in VLBW infants, it also represents an important starting point for cerebral function monitoring in the immediate postnatal period.

A recent study examined the relationships between echocardiographic blood flow findings, mean arterial blood pressure and aEEG in the first 48 hours after birth in <30 weeks gestation preterm infants (35). The authors found that low RV output used as a surrogate for systemic blood flow in neonates with shunting across the fetal channels at 12 hours of postnatal life correlated with low aEEG amplitude while low mean blood pressure (<31 mmHg) correlated with low EEG continuity. However, there was no relationship between aEEG and SVC flow. Although preliminary in nature, this study at least succeeds in drawing an association between a parameter in wide clinical use (blood pressure monitoring) and two more experimental modes of CBF monitoring (Doppler ultrasound and aEEG). Taken together with evidence that early aEEG in preterm infants can be helpful in predicting long-term neurodevelopmental outcome, it is reasonable to suggest that aEEG merits further study in the VLBW population as a means of identifying infants at risk for low CBF and/or for pathologic fluctuations in CBF.

In summary, methods capable of diagnosing altered CBF in the VLBW population in the first hours to days after delivery are still largely in the experimental arena. However, experimental technologies are giving us an insight into more commonly used monitoring parameters, and as experience with and understanding of these new methods expand, it is likely that some will be incorporated into routine clinical use in the not too distant future.

TREATMENT STRATEGIES

In the previous section we focused on newer experimental modalities for monitoring CBF in the VLBW neonate, with a primary emphasis on those that could be performed at the bedside noninvasively. As mentioned earlier, Doppler, functional echocardiography, NIRS, and aEEG are not yet currently appropriate for widespread routine clinical use for CBF monitoring, as their application and interpretation require specialized technology and further study to determine the significance and reproducibility of results and that their use affects outcome. However, results of studies using these experimental strategies can be useful for tailoring routine care as they allow us a glimpse of how mean arterial pressure and systemic blood flow affect CBF. This section will focus on how routinely monitored indices such as arterial blood pressure, acid–base status, and oxygenation as well as commonly used medications, presence of a PDA, and intercurrent infection may impact CBF as suggested by studies using the aforementioned CBF monitoring techniques. We will discuss management options, including evidence for when and how to treat systemic hypotension and clinical signs of systemic organ hypoperfusion. Ultimately we will propose a rational treatment strategy for maintaining brain perfusion and oxygenation in the VLBW infant in the first few postnatal days.

Systemic Hypotension

As mentioned previously, questions have recently arisen about the nature of the relationship between systemic blood pressure and systemic blood flow and CBF in

VLBW neonates during the immediate postnatal period (20). However, given what we understand about the development of cerebrovascular autoregulation, the autoregulatory, functional, and ischemic thresholds of systemic blood pressure, the presentation of "pressure-passive" cerebral circulation in many critically ill VLBW infants, and the available evidence on the impact of blood pressure on CBF, cerebral function, and structural integrity and outcomes (1–8, 15, 18, 19, 30, 57–60), it is prudent to carefully consider the possible effects of systemic blood pressure fluctuations in these babies. Ultimately, both blood pressure and systemic blood flow are important, as blood pressure ensures the appropriate organ perfusion pressure necessary to drive systemic blood flow to the tissues.

As mentioned briefly earlier, autoregulation is a process by which arterial blood flow to the given organ is kept constant over a range of perfusion pressures (Fig. 2-2). If perfusion pressure decreases within the autoregulatory range, the vessel dilates; if pressure increases, the vessel constricts. Outside the "autoregulatory window" where this process functions, a drop in pressure will lead to decrease in blood flow. "Static" autoregulation applies to the steady state, and "dynamic" autoregulation describes the time course of the return of the blood flow to baseline after an abrupt change in perfusion pressure. A number of studies have suggested that *static autoregulation* is intact even in very premature infants without significant cardiovascular compromise or evidence of severe lung disease (61–63), and that the lower threshold of the autoregulatory window for these babies is somewhere around 28–30 mmHg (15). In contrast to these findings, it appears that premature babies who go on to develop P/IVH have impaired static autoregulation before the bleeding occurs (14). It is generally accepted that impaired autoregulation is contributory to or even causative of P/IVH or PWMI in a subset of premature infants. Indeed, a correlation has been found between mean arterial pressure and cerebral intravascular oxygenation by NIRS in preterm neonates who went on to develop intracranial pathologies (5) (Fig. 2-2). However, dynamic autoregulation seems to be absent even in well preterm infants (64). Furthermore, several studies have shown that in hypotensive preterm infants treated with dopamine, there is an increase in CBF as blood pressure increases (15, 59) (see below), while in normotensive preterm neonates, dopamine does not affect CBF even if its administration results in an increase in the blood pressure (62). So, how should the clinician apply the findings of these studies when deciding how to treat systemic hypotension?

There are several clinical approaches to diagnose and treat neonatal hypotension. First, as mentioned earlier, in a small group of ELBW infants, Munro et al. (15) (Fig. 2-4) identified a mean arterial pressure of 28–30 mmHg as a "breakpoint" below which autoregulation appeared to be absent. Use of dopamine to raise the mean blood pressure resulted in a normalization of the CBF in these hypotensive infants. Thus, treatment of hypotension with dopamine quickly restores normal blood pressure and CBF. However, CBF autoregulation was not immediately restored. Indeed, findings of an earlier study suggest that it may take up to an hour until CBF autoregulation is restored following treatment of systemic hypotension (65). However, if a mean blood pressure of $\geq$28–30 mmHg is considered normal in all infants, many will be treated that may not require treatment based on their overall hemodynamic status or may receive a treatment modality (volume, vasopressor/inotropes or inotropes) that does not specifically address the underlying pathophysiology of their cardiovascular compromise. In weighing the risks and benefits of the different treatment modalities of neonatal circulatory compromise, it is important to keep in mind that there is no evidence that treatment affects outcome.

The most widespread approach to the definition and treatment of hypotension in the VLBW neonate during the immediate transitional period is using a mean blood pressure that equals to the gestational age in numbers. There are two major concerns with this approach. First, if the autoregulatory blood pressure breakpoint is truly at 28–30 mmHg for this patient population, blood pressure at the level of the gestational age in the more immature and thus vulnerable preterm neonates will be out of the autoregulatory range. Second, as discussed earlier, some of these immature neonates even with "normal" blood pressure will have low systemic and presumably cerebral blood flow (20) as their cerebral vasculature may constrict rather than dilate in the compensated phase of shock (23, 24). Since low CBF in the first postnatal day is a known risk factor for P/IVH and poor neurodevelopmental outcome (6), it is important to identify these babies at risk, and this cannot be done by using blood pressure monitoring alone. As discussed earlier, the combined use of blood pressure and indirect clinical signs of tissue hypoperfusion (blood pressure ≤ 30 mmHg and CRT ≥ 3 seconds (33)) may help to identify patients with low systemic and thus cerebral blood flow. If functional echocardiography is available, VLBW neonates that are "normotensive" (their blood pressure is equal or higher than their gestational age) but have low systemic blood flow may be identified. As this presentation mostly occurs during the first 6–12 hours postnatally, targeted use of functional echocardiography to measure SVC blood flow may be the best direct approach presently available to detect low systemic perfusion. However, even if one can diagnose low systemic blood flow during the first hours after delivery, at present we do not have a truly effective treatment modality to improve systemic blood flow in this patient population (31). In addition, as mentioned earlier, hypotension defined by the gestational age-based criterion in VLBW neonates appears to be a risk factor for poor neurodevelopmental outcome and treatment with vasopressors or inotropes may indeed not ameliorate the risk (60). Thus one could speculate that these hypotensive babies may have been treated too late to make a difference or that the most widely applied treatment approach is ineffective in ameliorating the hypotension- and/or low CBF-associated brain injury.

Finally, due to the uncertainties surrounding the definition of hypotension and the relationship between blood pressure and CBF in the VLBW neonate in the immediate postnatal period, as well as to the potential side effects of vasopressor use and the lack of evidence that treatment of hypotension improves neurodevelopmental outcome, some advocate that hypotension in the VLBW neonate during the first postnatal day(s) should only be treated if there is clear evidence of organ hypoperfusion (i.e., lactic acidosis). We would argue, however, that by the time lactic acidosis can be detected, cerebral ischemia is likely to have occurred provided that the brain has also contributed to the production of lactate. Therefore, this approach carries the theoretical risk of significant cerebral hypoperfusion occurring. However, most neonatologists agree that once the fetal channels are closed and the blood pressure–CBF relationship is restored after the first few days following delivery, blood pressure becomes a more reliable indicator of vital organ perfusion even in the most immature neonate, and hypotension should be treated promptly with careful titration of the most appropriate vasopressor/inotrope or inotrope to avoid sudden changes in systemic blood pressure and blood flow.

Treatment of Hypotension Associated with a PDA

A PDA with significant left-to-right shunting often manifests as hypotension (34, 66) and this is a common presentation in VLBW infants in the immediate postnatal transition period. It has been recently demonstrated that shunting through a non-constricting PDA in the first 6 hours after delivery is primarily left to right and highly associated with a low SVC flow state (20, 67). Treatment of the PDA before 6 hours of postnatal life with indomethacin induces ductal constriction by 2 hours of the drug administration but this effect is not associated with simultaneous improvements in systemic blood flow (68). Indomethacin decreases CBF via a direct cerebrovascular vasoconstrictive effect that is independent of the drug's inhibitory action on prostaglandin synthesis (69). It is possible that the documented decrease in severe P/IVH with early indomethacin use is due to this localized cerebral vasoconstrictive effect during a time when reperfusion may occur (68) and has less to do with improving the preceding low systemic blood flow state by closure of the ductus. However, this notion is not supported by the findings of a recent meta-analysis comparing the effectiveness, side effects, and hemodynamic effects of indomethacin to ibuprofen (70). According to the findings of the meta-analysis, although ibuprofen does not induce cerebral vasoconstriction to a degree comparable to that seen with indomethacin, there is no difference in the incidence of P/IVH between VLBW neonates treated with indomethacin or ibuprofen.

Cardiovascular management of the hemodynamically unstable, hypotensive VLBW neonate with a large PDA should focus on measures that induce stepwise and reversible increases in pulmonary vascular resistance until pharmacological or, if this fails, surgical closure of the PDA takes place. Such measures may include the avoidance of hyperventilation and respiratory (or metabolic) alkalosis and maintenance of oxygen saturations at the lower end of the acceptable range. It should also be remembered that high doses of vasopressors might preferentially increase systemic vascular resistance and thus left-to-right shunting through the ductus and, although blood pressure may be maintained in an acceptable range, systemic perfusion could become even more compromised. Therefore, administration of high doses of dopamine or epinephrine should be avoided unless systemic blood flow can be repeatedly assessed by the use of functional echocardiography.

Treatment of Hypotension Associated with Other Causes Such as Sepsis, Adrenal Insufficiency, or Hypovolemia

For hypotension due to causes such as septic shock, adrenal insufficiency, or hypovolemia, every effort should be made to treat the underlying cause and support the cardiovascular status. Although there is very little experimental data regarding the response of CBF to vasopressor medications in the hypotensive VLBW infant, some evidence is accumulating.

Dopamine is the first-line medication of choice for many neonatologists because of its beneficial cardiovascular and renal effects (71). It effectively increases blood pressure in the preterm infant, but its effect on organ blood flow is less well described. As mentioned earlier, recent evidence indicates that despite its effect on increasing blood pressure and renal perfusion, in normotensive VLBW neonates, dopamine does not have a selective vasoactive action on the cerebral circulation (62, 72). However, in hypotensive VLBW infants, the dopamine-induced increase in blood pressure is associated with an increase in CBF (15, 59, 65). This finding suggests once again that in hypotensive preterm infants cerebrovascular autoregulation is impaired and that effective treatment of hypotension is associated with an increase in CBF and a delay in the restoration of CBF autoregulation (see above).

Are other vasopressors more effective in restoring "normal" CBF in this population than dopamine? A recent randomized controlled trial compared the cerebrovascular, hemodynamic, and metabolic effects of dopamine and epinephrine using a stepwise titration of the two medications to achieve optimum blood pressure in VLBW neonates in the first 24 postnatal hours (59). Both medications increased cerebral perfusion in the medium dose range, with epinephrine being slightly more effective in infants <28 weeks gestation and dopamine being more effective in those >28 weeks gestation. As both medications were effective at increasing blood pressure and CBF and since this is the only peer-reviewed publication available on the cerebrovascular effects of epinephrine in VLBW neonates, there is no reason for choosing one over the other vasopressor for this particular application.

As for inotropes and lusitropes, there has been an increasing interest in the potential use of milrinone, a selective phosphodiesterase-III inhibitor, in neonates and infants following cardiac surgery and in VLBW neonates with low systemic blood flow during the first postnatal day. Milrinone effectively decreases the incidence of low cardiac output in infants following cardiac surgery (73, 74). Since the low-flow state in preterm infants immediately after birth is in many ways similar to the low cardiac output syndrome in postoperative cardiac patients, this drug has potential both as treatment for and as prophylaxis of low systemic blood flow (and presumably low CBF) in the VLBW patient population. A recent pilot study examined the safety, efficacy, and optimal dosing of milrinone in infants <29 weeks gestation during the first hours of postnatal life (75). At the applied dose, milrinone appears to be relatively safe in the 1-day-old VLBW neonate (75). However, as the findings of the recently completed randomized controlled trial revealed that milrinone is ineffective to prevent the occurrence of low systemic blood flow in the 1-day-old VLBW neonate (N. Evans and M. Kluckow, personal communication, 2007), the routine use of milrinone in this population cannot be recommended. Dobutamine, another sympathomimetic amine with direct positive inotropic and mild vasodilatory effects, effectively increases cardiac output and blood pressure in the VLBW neonate especially when the cardiovascular compromise is caused by myocardial dysfunction (76, 77). There are virtually no data available on the cerebrovascular effects of dobutamine in the VLBW neonate patient.

Beyond the presentation of different forms of neonatal shock treated by vasopressor/inotropes, inotropes, and lusitropes, there has been increasing recognition that "vasopressor-resistant" hypotension frequently develops in the VLBW population. This presentation is thought to be due to cardiovascular adrenergic receptor downregulation and the increased incidence of relative adrenal insufficiency in the VLBW neonate (78–81). A recent prospective observational study examined the hemodynamic effects of low-dose hydrocortisone administration in preterm neonates with vasopressor resistance and borderline hypotension and found no independent effect of this treatment modality on CBF in this patient population (81).

Impact of Provision of Intensive Care on Systemic and Cerebral Hemodynamics

In addition to the impact of the hemodynamic changes on CBF during the postnatal transition, we must consider the effects of our interventions at all times. This includes ventilatory maneuvers, the use of medications other than vasopressor/inotropes or inotropes, and invasive procedures. Premature infants with a median gestational age of 31 weeks have been reported to have a decrease in CBF velocity (and thus presumably in CBF) in response to transient hyperoxia (82). This occurs without a decrease in $PaCO_2$, implicating hyperoxia directly in the decrease in CBF. *Hypocarbia* is a well-described cause of cerebral vasoconstriction, and a negative association between $PaCO_2$ and CBF and cerebral oxygen extraction has been demonstrated in VLBW infants during the first postnatal days (23, 83, 84). In addition, lower levels of $PaCO_2$ are associated with slowing of the EEG, likely induced by decreased cerebral oxygen delivery (84). These effects are most significant in the first 24 postnatal hours, less evident on the second day, and gone by the third postnatal day. These findings support the notion that the first hours of postnatal life represent a period of heightened vulnerability to CBF fluctuations. Not surprisingly, severe hypocapnia in VLBW neonates during the immediate transitional period is associated with PWMI and cerebral palsy (85).

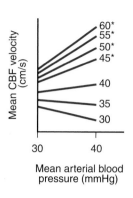

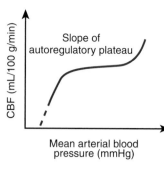

Figure 2-7 Effect of hypercapnia on CBF autoregulation in 43 ventilated VLBW neonates during the first two postnatal days. Left panel: lines represent the estimated mean slopes of the autoregulatory plateau from 30 to 60 mmHg $PaCO_2$ with mean blood pressure values between 30 and 40 mmHg. Horizontal line at slope zero indicates intact autoregulation with lines at 30, 35, and 40 mmHg being not significantly different from zero. The estimated means of the slope of the autoregulatory plateau (cm/s/mmHg) increased as $PaCO_2$ increased from 40 mmHg ($p = 0.004$). $*= p < 0.05$ vs. zero.

Importantly, it appears that *hypercapnia* may also have an impact on cerebral hemodynamics as $PaCO_2$ levels beyond 45 mmHg during the first two postnatal days are associated with compromised CBF autoregulation (86) (Fig. 2-7). If this finding is confirmed, the use of permissive hypercapnia during the immediate postnatal period might also place the VLBW neonate at higher risk for cerebral injury.

Finally, high mean airway pressures in the immediate postnatal period have also been implicated in low systemic and thus cerebral blood flow and a predilection for P/IVH (21). Beyond ventilatory maneuvers and interventions, commonly used medications such as midazolam and morphine have also been associated with potentially harmful changes in CBF (87) and even umbilical arterial blood sampling could have an effect on cerebral hemodynamics in these tiny infants (88).

The preceding paragraphs emphasize how changes in ventilatory management, administration of commonly used medications, or simple interventions in the VLBW infant, especially during the first postnatal days, can have negative and potentially devastating effects on CBF and cerebral oxygenation acutely, and on neurodevelopmental outcome ultimately. The mainstays of treatment have been, and should remain at this point, maintenance of homeostasis and avoidance of potentially harmful interventions and abrupt hemodynamic changes in this most vulnerable patient population.

SUMMARY AND RECOMMENDATIONS

As discussed in this chapter, the management of hypotension and low systemic and cerebral blood flow in the VLBW infant during the first postnatal days presents a significant challenge as both immaturity and postnatal transition affect the hemodynamic response to pathological processes and interventions. Because of these factors and the lack of evidence on how treatment affects mortality and short- and long-term morbidity, straightforward recommendations on the treatment of cardiovascular compromise cannot be given in the VLBW neonate during the period of transition to postnatal life.

Therefore, the following approach to diagnosis and treatment represents the view of the authors and should only be considered as such especially since, as discussed in this chapter, evidence on the effectiveness of the treatment of shock in the VLBW neonate during the first postnatal days is not available.

Diagnosis of Hypotension

1. We use the gestational age equivalent mean blood pressure as the definition of hypotension and initiate treatment at this point as long as signs of tissue

hypoperfusion cannot be detected at higher mean blood pressure values. This approach is supported by recent findings, and we maintain mean blood pressure at ≥24 mmHg even in the most immature ELBW neonate during the first postnatal day since cerebral electrical activity appears to be depressed at blood pressure values below this level.

2. Whenever there is indirect or direct evidence of poor tissue perfusion, we monitor both systemic blood flow and blood pressure closely and attempt to maintain appropriate systemic blood flow without much fluctuation in the blood pressure. Since a blood pressure breakpoint of the CBF autoregulatory curve may exist at 28–30 mmHg and since >90% of even ELBW neonates not receiving vasopressor support maintain their mean blood pressure ≥30 mmHg by the third postnatal day, we slowly increase mean blood pressure during the first three postnatal days and maintain it in the 28–30 mmHg range. However, it must be kept in mind that an increase in blood pressure during this period does not necessarily ensure rapid normalization of systemic and cerebral blood flow and that there are no data that this approach improves long-term neurodevelopmental outcome.

3. Although most neonatologists would agree with the approach described above, there is another less frequently practiced approach, which needs to be mentioned. Neonatologists using this approach initiate cardiovascular support only if there is evidence of poor systemic perfusion as long as mean blood pressure is at or higher than 20 mmHg or so in the ELBW neonate during the first postnatal day. Since within the first 24 hours it is hard to define poor perfusion especially without the use of functional echocardiography and since lactic acidosis heralds the presence of (ongoing or previously present) tissue ischemia, we do not practice this diagnostic and treatment philosophy. However, there is no direct evidence at present that the use of "permissive hypotension" as an approach to diagnose and manage cardiovascular compromise in VLBW neonates during the immediate postnatal period leads to increased mortality or morbidity.

Treatment of Hypotension

With regard to the kind of treatment utilized, the most appropriate strategy requires identification of the underlying pathogenesis of hypotension. As described earlier, the most frequent etiological factors are inappropriate peripheral vasoregulation and dysfunction of the myocardium complicated by the presence of a large PDA in VLBW neonates during the first postnatal days. Although the following may be recommended and is being practiced by the authors, it must be emphasized again that there is no evidence that treatment of hypotension in this patient population improves mortality, morbidity, or long-term neurodevelopmental outcome.

1. In the case of hypotension, since low to moderate doses of dopamine (or epinephrine) improve both blood pressure and CBF, we carefully titrate dopamine in a stepwise manner using 3- to 5-minute cycles and make every effort to avoid inducing significant rapid changes in blood pressure. If low systemic blood flow is detected with low-normal to normal blood pressure during the first postnatal day, we add dobutamine to low-dose dopamine and monitor for indirect (CRT, urine output, base deficit) and direct (functional echocardiography) signs of improvement in systemic perfusion.

2. In the presence of a hemodynamically significant PDA, immediate closure of the ductus arteriosus with a cyclooxygenase inhibitor (we use indomethacin) is

the ultimate solution along with appropriate supportive care. If pharmacologic closure fails in patients with a hemodynamically significant PDA, while waiting for surgical closure to take place, our goal is to decrease the left-to-right shunting across the ductus. As briefly described earlier, we attempt to achieve this goal by carefully increasing pulmonary resistance in a stepwise manner. Using this approach we frequently are successful at increasing pulmonary vascular resistance and the associated decrease in left-to-right shunting results in improvement of systemic blood flow and blood pressure. We avoid using high doses of dopamine or epinephrine in babies with a hemodynamically significant PDA because the drug-induced peripheral vasoconstriction may increase systemic vascular resistance more than pulmonary vascular resistance, potentially resulting in worsening of the left-to-right shunt. We only add dobutamine in the presence of impaired myocardial function since most VLBW neonates with a PDA after the first postnatal day have normal or hyperdynamic cardiac function. Indeed, the use of dobutamine in these patients may compromise myocardial filling and diastolic function. Finally, volume administration must be restricted because excessive (or even liberal) use of volume is associated with increased mortality and morbidity in this patient population.

3. Finally, as $PaCO_2$ is a much more potent mediator of cerebral vascular tone than blood pressure, we make every effort to keep $PaCO_2$ within the 45–50 mmHg range. We hope that by maintaining $PaCO_2$ relatively constant we minimize the

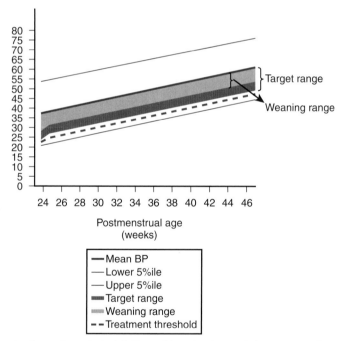

Figure 2-8 Postmenstrual age-dependent definition of hypotension and the target and weaning blood pressure ranges. Hypotension is defined as the treatment threshold, which is 1–3 points above the 5th percentile for postmenstrual age (10,11,79). Below the treatment threshold, the authors usually initiate treatment of hypotension. The target range is defined where mean blood pressure is intended to be kept. The target range is between 2 and 3 mmHg above the treatment threshold and the 50% percentile of the mean blood pressure (10,11,79). Finally, the weaning range is defined as the mean blood pressure range where careful weaning of vasopressor/inotropes and/or inotropes is commenced. This range is between 5 mmHg above the lower limits of target range and the 50 percentile of the mean blood pressure. Note that the upper limit of the target range does not exceed the 50 percentile of the mean blood pressure in order to decrease the risk of achieving an increase in blood pressure by causing significant increases in systemic vascular resistance and thus potentially decreases in cardiac output when vasopressor/inotropes are being administered. This graph was developed in collaboration with the "Under Pressure" hemodynamic group created as part of a Vermont-Oxford Network (VON) initiative for 2004–06. (One of the authors (IS) served as the "VON expert on hemodynamics" for this initiative.)

incidence of the hypocapnia-associated increased incidence of PWMI and cerebral palsy as well as the potential negative impact of hypercapnia on the integrity of CBF autoregulation.

Finally, Figure 2-8 illustrates our postmenstrual age-dependent approach to the diagnosis and treatment of hypotension in preterm and term neonates. It is important to note that our definition of hypotension (dotted line) and the target and weaning ranges have all been arbitrarily defined using epidemiologic data and extrapolation of hemodynamic findings and the data on the association between blood pressure and systemic and cerebral blood flow. As this approach, just like any other approach to manage the cardiovascular compromise in the neonatal patient population is not evidenced based, it cannot be recommended in general and only illustrates one of the many options in the diagnosis and treatment of neonatal hypotension. At present, the diagnosis and treatment of neonatal circulatory compromise requires careful monitoring of the appropriate hemodynamic parameters and a thorough understanding of developmental cardiovascular physiology and the pathophysiology of neonatal shock.

REFERENCES

1. Perlman JM, McMenamin JB, Volpe JJ. Fluctuating cerebral blood flow velocity in respiratory distress syndrome. Relation to the development of intraventricular hemorrhage. N Engl J Med 309(4):204–9, 1983.
2. Van Bel F, Van de Bor M, Stijnen T, et al., Aetiological role of cerebral blood flow alterations in development and extension of peri-intraventricular hemorrhage. Dev Med Child Neurol 29(5):601–14, 1987.
3. Miall-Allen VM, de Vries LS, Whitelaw AG. Mean arterial pressure and neonatal cerebral lesions. Arch Dis Child 62:1068–9, 1987.
4. Bada HS, Korones SB, Perry EH, et al., Mean arterial blood pressure changes in premature infants and those at risk for intraventricular hemorrhage. J Pediatr 117:607–14, 1990.
5. Tsuji M, Saul PJ, duPlessis A, et al., Cerebral intravascular oxygenation correlates with mean arterial pressure in critically ill premature infants. Pediatrics 106:625, 2000.
6. Hunt R, Evans N, Rieger I, et al., Low superior vena cava flow and neurodevelopment at 3 years in very preterm infants. J Pediatr 145:588–92, 2004.
7. Goldstein RF, Thompson RJ Jr, Oehler JM, et al., Influence of acidosis, hypoxemia, and hypotension on neurodevelopmental outcome in very low birth weight infants. Pediatrics 95:238–43, 1995.
8. Damman O, Allred EN, Kuban KCK, et al., Systemic hypotension and white matter damage in preterm infants. Dev Med Child Neurol 44:82–90, 2002.
9. Nuntnarumit P, Yang W, Bada-Ellzey HS. Blood pressure measurements in the newborn. Clin Perinat 26(4):981–96, 1999.
10. Report of a Joint Working Group of the British Association of Perinatal Medicine and the Research Unit of the Royal College of Physicians. Development of audit measures and guidelines for good practice in the management of neonatal respiratory distress syndrome. Arch Dis Child 67:1221–7, 1992.
11. Engle WD. Blood pressure in the very low birth weight neonate. Early Human Dev 62:97–130, 2001.
12. Seri I. Circulatory support of the sick newborn infant. Semin Neonatol 6:85–95, 2001.
13. Greisen G. Autoregulation of cerebral blood flow in newborn babies. Early Human Dev 81:423–8, 2005.
14. Milligan DWA. Failure of autoregulation and intraventricular haemorrhage in preterm infants. Lancet i:896–9, 1980.
15. Munro MJ, Walker AM, Barfield CP. Hypotensive extremely low birth weight infants have reduced cerebral blood flow. Pediatrics 114:1591, 2004.
16. Kissack CM, Garr R, Wardle SP, Weindling AM. Cerebral fractional oxygen extraction is inversely correlated with oxygen delivery in the sick, newborn preterm infant. J Cerebr Blood Flow Metab 25:545–53, 2005.
17. Weindling AM and Victor NM. Definition of hypotension in very low birth weight infants during the immediate neonatal period. NeoReviews 8(1):c32–c43, 2007.
18. Victor S, Marson AG, Appleton RE, et al., Relationship between blood pressure, cerebral electrical activity, cerebral fractional oxygen extraction and peripheral blood flow in very low birth weight newborn infants. Pediatr Res 59:314–19, 2006.
19. Victor S, Appleton RE, Beirne M, et al., The relationship between cardiac output, cerebral electrical activity, cerebral fractional oxygen extraction and peripheral blood flow in premature newborn infants. Pediatr Res 60:1–5, 2006.
20. Kluckow M, Evans N. Low superior vena cava flow and intraventricular haemorrhage in preterm infants. Arch Dis Child 82:188–94, 2000.

21. Kluckow M, Evans N. Relationship between blood pressure and cardiac output in preterm infants requiring mechanical ventilation. J Pediatr 129:506, 1996.
22. Kluckow M, Evans N. Superior vena cava flow in newborn infant: a novel marker of systemic blood flow. Arch Dis Child Fetal Neonatal Ed 82:182–7, 2000.
23. Kissack CM, Garr R, Wardle SP, et al., Cerebral fractional oxygen extraction in very low birth weight infants is high when there is low left ventricular output and hypocarbia but is unaffected by hypotension. Pediatr Res 55:400–5, 2004.
24. Seri I. Hemodynamics during the first two postnatal days and neurodevelopment in preterm neonates. J Pediatr 145:573–5, 2004.
25. Greisen G. Cerebral blood flow in preterm infants during the first week of life. Acta Paediatr Scand 75:43–51, 1986.
26. Pryds O, Andersen E, Hansen BF. Cerebral blood flow reactivity in spontaneously breathing infants shortly after birth. Acta Paediatr Scand 79:391–6, 1990.
27. Pryds O, Greisen P. Effect of $PaCO_2$ and haemoglobin concentration on day to day variation of CBF in preterm neonates. Acta Paediatr Scand 360:33–6, 1989.
28. Greisen G, Trojaborg W. Cerebral blood flow, $PaCO_2$ changes and visual evoked potentials in mechanically ventilated preterm infants. Acta Paediatr Scand 76:394–400, 1987.
29. Altman DI, Powers WJ, Perlman JM, et al., Cerebral blood flow requirement for brain viability in newborn infants is lower than in adults. Ann Neurol 24:218–26, 1988.
30. Kluckow M, Evans N. Low systemic blood flow and hyperkalemia in preterm infants. J Pediatr 139:227–32, 2001.
31. Osborn D, Evans N, Kluckow M. Randomised trial of dopamine and dobutamine in preterm infants with low systemic blood flow. J Pediatr 140:183–91, 2002.
32. Kehrer M, Blumenstock G, Ehehalt S, et al., Development of cerebral blood flow volume in preterm neonates during the first two weeks of life. Pediatr Res 58:927–30, 2005.
33. Osborn D, Evans N, Kluckow M. Clinical detection of low upper body blood flow in very premature infants using blood pressure, capillary refill time and central peripheral temperature difference. Arch Dis Child Fetal Neonatal Ed 89:168–73, 2004.
34. Evans N, Iyer P. Longitudinal changes in the diameter of the ductus arteriosus in ventilated preterm infants: correlation with respiratory outcomes. Arch Dis Child Fetal Neonatal Ed 72:F156–61, 1995.
35. West CR, Groves AM, Williams CE, et al., Early low cardiac output is associated with compromised electroencephalographic activity in very preterm infants. Pediatr Res 59:610–15, 2006.
36. Kluckow M, Seri I, Evans N. Functional echocardiography: an emerging clinical tool for the neonatologist. J Pediatr 150(2):125–30, 2007.
37. Gilbert RD, Pearce WJ, Ashwal S, Longo LD. Effects of hypoxia on contractility of isolated fetal lamb cerebral arteries. J Dev Physiol 13:199–203, 1990.
38. Hansen NB, Stonestreet BS, Rosenkrantz TS, Oh W. Validity of Doppler measurements of anterior cerebral artery blood flow velocity: correlation with brain blood flow in piglets. Pediatrics 72:526–31, 1983.
39. Greisen G, Johansen K, Ellison PH, et al., Cerebral blood flow in the newborn: comparison of Doppler ultrasound and [133]xenon clearance. J Pediatr 104:411–18, 1984.
40. Raju TN. Cerebral Doppler studies in the fetus and the newborn infant. J Pediatr 119:165–74, 1991.
41. van der Linden J, Wesslen O, Ekroth R, et al., Transcranial Doppler-estimated versus thermodilution-estimated cerebral blood flow during cardiac operations. Influence of temperature and arterial carbon dioxide tension. J Thorac Cardiovasc Surg 102:95–102, 1991.
42. Bassan H, Gauvreau K, Newburger JW, et al., Identification of pressure passive cerebral perfusion and its mediators after infant cardiac surgery. Pediatr Res 57:35–41, 2005.
43. Brazy JE, Lewis DV, Mitnisk MH, et al., Noninvasive monitoring of cerebral oxygenation in preterm infants: preliminary observation. Pediatrics 75:217–25, 1985.
44. Patel J, Marks K, Roberts I, et al., Measurement of cerebral blood flow in newborn infants using near infrared spectroscopy with indocyanine green. Pediatr Res 43:34–9, 1998.
45. Dullenkopf A, Kolarova A, Schulz G, et al., Reproducibility of cerebral oxygenation measurement in neonates and infants in the clinical setting using the NIRO 300 oximeter. Pediatr Crit Care Med 6:344–7, 2005.
46. Boas DA, Gaudette T, Strangman G, et al., The accuracy of near infrared spectroscopy and imaging during focal changes in cerebral hemodynamics. NeuroImage 13:76–90, 2001.
47. Bucher HU, Edwards AD, Lipp AE, et al., Comparison between near infrared spectroscopy and [133]xenon clearance for estimation of cerebral blood flow in critically ill preterm infants. Pediatr Res 33:56–60, 1993.
48. Toet MC, Hellstrom-Westas L, Groenendaal F, et al., Amplitude integrated EEG 3 and 6 hours after birth in full term neonates with hypoxic-ischaemic encephalopathy. Arch Dis Child Fetal Neonatal Ed 81:F19–F23, 1999.
49. Hellstrom-Westas L. Comparison between taper-recorded and amplitude-integrated EEG monitoring in sick newborn infants. Acta Paediatr 81:812–19, 1992.
50. Toet MC, van der Mei W, de Vries LS, et al., Comparison between simultaneously recorded amplitude-integrated electroencephalogram (cerebral function monitor) and standard electroencephalogram in neonates. Pediatrics 109:772–9, 2002.
51. Ter Horst HJ, Sommer C, Bergman KA, et al., Prognostic significance of amplitude-integrated EEG during the first 72 hours after birth in severely asphyxiated neonates. Pediatr Res 55:1026–33, 2004.

52. Shalak LF, Laptook AR, Velaphi SC, et al., Amplitude-integrated electroencephalography coupled with an early neurologic examination enhances prediction of term infants at risk for persistent encephalopathy. Pediatrics 111:351–7, 2003.

53. Greisen G, Pryds O. Low CBF, discontinuous EEG activity, and periventricular brain injury in ill, preterm neonates. Brain Dev 11:164–8, 1989.

54. Hellstrom-Westas L, Klette H, Thorngren-Jerneck K, et al., Early prediction of outcome with aEEG in preterm infants with large intraventricular hemorrhages. Neuropediatrics 32:319–24, 2001.

55. Olischar M, Klebermass K, Kuhle S, et al., Reference values for amplitude-integrated electroencephalographic activity in preterm infants younger than 30 weeks' gestational age. Pediatrics 113:e61–6, 2004.

56. Klebermass K, Kuhle S, Olischar M, et al., Intra-and extrauterine maturation of amplitude-integrated electroencephalographic activity in preterm infants younger than 30 weeks of gestation. Biol Neonate 89:120–125, 2006.

57. Woodward LJ, Anderson PJ, Austin NC, et al., Neonatal MRI to predict neurodevelopmental outcomes in preterm infants. N Engl J Med 255:685–94, 2006.

58. Miller SP, Ferriero DM, Leonard C, et al., Early brain injury in premature newborns detected with magnetic resonance imaging is associated with adverse early neurodevelopmental outcome. J Pediatr 147:609–16, 2005.

59. Pellicer A, Valverde E, Elorza MD, et al., Cardiovascular support for low birth weight infants and cerebral hemodynamics: a randomized blinded clinical trial. Pediatrics 115:1501, 2005.

60. Fanaroff JM, Wilson-Costello DE, Newman NS, et al., Treated hypotension is associated with neonatal morbidity and hearing loss in extremely low birth weight infants. Pediatrics 117:1131–5, 2006.

61. Pryds O, Greisen G, Lou H, et al., Heterogeneity of cerebral vasoreactivity in preterm infants supported by mechanical ventilation. J Pediatr 115:638–4, 1982.

62. Seri I, Abbasi S, Wood DC, et al., Regional hemodynamic effects of dopamine in the sick preterm neonate. J Pediatr 133:728–34, 1998.

63. Pryds O, Andersen GE, Friis-Hansen B. Cerebral blood flow reactivity in spontaneously breathing, preterm infants shortly after birth. Acta Paediatr Scand 79:391–6, 1990.

64. Boylan GB, Young K, Panerai RB, et al., Dynamic cerebral autoregulation in sick newborn infants. Pediatr Res 48:12–17, 2000.

65. Seri I, Rudas G, Bors Z, et al., Effects of low dose dopamine infusion on cardiovascular and renal functions, cerebral blood flow and plasma catecholamine levels in sick preterm neonates. Pediatr Res 34:742–9, 1993.

66. Evans N, Moorcraft J. Effect of patency of the ductus arteriosus on blood pressure in very preterm infants. Arch Dis Child 67:1169, 1992.

67. Kluckow M, Evans N. Early echocardiographic prediction of symptomatic patent ductus arteriosus in preterm infants undergoing mechanical ventilation. J Pediatr 127:774–9, 1995.

68. Osborn DA, Evans N, Kluckow M. Effect of early, targeted indomethacin on the ductus arteriosus and blood flow to the upper body and brain in the preterm infant. Arch Dis Child Fetal Neonatal Ed 88:477–82, 2003.

69. Yanowitz TD, Yao AC, Werner JC, et al., Effects of prophylactic low-dose indomethacin on hemodynamics in very low birth weight infants. J Pediatr 132:28–34, 1998.

70. Thomas RL, Parker GC, Van Overmeire B, et al., A meta-analysis of ibuprofen versus indomethacin for closure of patent ductus arteriosus. Eur J Pediatr 164:135–40, 2005.

71. Seri I. Cardiovascular, renal and endocrine actions of dopamine in neonates and children. J Pediatr 126:333–44, 1995.

72. Lundstrom K, Pryds O, Greisen G. The haemodynamic effects of dopamine and volume expansion in sick preterm infants. Early Hum Dev 57:157–63, 2000.

73. Chang AC, Atz A, Wernovsky G, et al., Milrinone: systemic and pulmonary hemodynamic effects in neonates after cardiac surgery. Crit Care Med 23:1907–11, 1995.

74. Hoffman TM, Wernovsky G, Atz AM, et al., Efficacy and safety of milrinone in preventing low cardiac output syndrome in infants and children after corrective surgery for congenital heart disease. Circulation 107:996–1002, 2003.

75. Paradisis M, Evans N, Kluckow M, et al., Pilot study of milrinone for low systemic blood flow in very preterm infants. J Pediatr 148:306–13, 2006.

76. Roze JC, Tohier C, Maingureneau C, et al., Response to dobutamine and dopamine in the hypotensive very preterm infant. Arch Dis Child 69:59–63, 1993.

77. Noori S, Friedlich P, Seri I. Cardiovascular and renal effects of dobutamine in the neonate. NeoReviews 5:E22–6, 2004.

78. Ng PC, Lee CH, Lam CWK, et al., Transient adrenocortical insufficiency of prematurity and systemic hypotension in very low birth weight infants. Arch Dis Child Fetal Neonatal Ed 89:F119–26, 2004.

79. Fernandez E, Schrader R, Watterberg. Prevalence of low cortisol values in term and near-term infants with vasopressor-resistant hypotension. J Perinatol 25:114–18, 2005.

80. Seri I, Tan R, Evans J. The effect of hydrocortisone on blood pressure in preterm neonates with pressor-resistant hypotension. Pediatrics 107:1070–4, 2001.

81. Noori S, Friedlich P, Wong P, et al., Hemodynamic changes after low-dose hydrocortisone administration in vasopressor-treated preterm and term neonates. Pediatrics 118:1456–66, 2006.

82. Niijima S, Shortland DB, Levene MI, et al., Transient hyperoxia and cerebral blood flow velocity in infants born prematurely and at full term. Arch Dis Child 63:1126–30, 1988.

83. Tyszczuk L, Meek J, Elwell C, et al., Cerebral blood flow is independent of mean arterial blood pressure in preterm infants undergoing intensive care. Pediatrics 102:337–41, 1998.

84. Victor S, Appleton RE, Beirne M, et al., Effect of carbon dioxide on background cerebral electrical activity and fractional oxygen extraction in very low birth weight infants just after birth. Pediatr Res 58:579–85, 2005.

85. Murase M, Ishida A. Early hypocarbia of preterm infants: its relationship to periventricular leukomalacia and cerebral palsy, and its perinatal risk factors. Acta Paediatr 94:85–91, 2005.

86. Kaiser JR, Gauss CH, Williams DK. The effects of hypercapnia on cerebral autoregulation in ventilated very low birth weight infants. Pediatr Res 58:931–5, 2005.

87. van Alfen-van der Velden AAEM, Hopman JCW, Klaessens JHGM, et al., Effects of midazolam and morphine on cerebral oxygenation and hemodynamics in ventilated premature infants. Biol Neonate 90:197–202, 2006.

88. Roll C, Huning B, Kaunicke M, et al., Umbilical artery catheter blood sampling volume and velocity: impact on cerebral blood volume and oxygenation in very-low-birthweight infants. Acta Paediatr 95:68–73, 2006.

Chapter 3

Intraventricular Hemorrhage and White Matter Injury in the Preterm Infant

Jeffrey M. Perlman, MB, ChB

Periventricular-Intraventricular Hemorrhage

White Matter Injury in the Absence of Hemorrhage

Outcome

Gaps in Knowledge

Conclusions

CASE HISTORY

HW was a 760 g, 25-week premature male infant born to a 29-year-old G1P0 mother whose pregnancy was complicated by the onset of premature labor. The mother received a dose of betamethasone approximately 24 hours prior to a vaginal delivery. She also was placed on antibiotics and given magnesium sulfate. The infant was delivered with minimal respiratory effort and a heart rate of 80. Resuscitation included bag mask ventilation and intubation with a rapid improvement in heart rate and color. The infant was admitted to the intensive care unit and was given one dose of a surfactant preparation. The early course was complicated by a pneumothorax that required chest tube drainage, patent ductus arteriosus (PDA) initially treated with indomethacin. The infant weaned to continuous positive pressure by day of life (DOL) 8, and was briefly reintubated for the surgical ligation of the PDA and on a second occasion for a nosocomial infection. Other issues included recurrent apnea and bradycardia and frequent unprovoked desaturation episodes. He required supplemental oxygen through the 35th week of postconceptual age. He required parenteral nutrition for 3 weeks and subsequently received enteral breast milk. A cranial ultrasound scan (HUS) on DOL 5 revealed a germinal matrix hemorrhage only. Repeat scans on DOL 14, 28, and 56 revealed progressive nonhemorrhagic lateral ventriculomegaly. The infant underwent a magnetic resonance imaging evaluation on DOL 92 that revealed mild ventriculomegaly and diffuse loss of periventricular white matter. The infant was discharged on DOL 100. He has been seen and evaluated at 18 months. At that time the clinical examination was pertinent for hyperreflexia in the lower extremities, a very active toddler with minimal speech. He had recently started walking. Using the Bayley battery of tests he was found to have a mental developmental index of 75 and psychomotor developmental index of 82.

This case illustrates the typical course of a premature infant managed in the more recent era of neonatology. At this time while the premature infant, and particularly the very low birth weight (VLBW) infant (<1000 g), remains at high risk for the development of periventricular-intraventricular hemorrhage (PV-IVH) he/she is more likely to develop injury to adjacent white matter frequently in the absence of hemorrhage (1, 2). The white matter may present with cystic change or as progressive lateral ventriculomegaly in the absence of cystic change. The latter often reflects diffuse white matter injury and is best identified by magnetic resonance imaging (MRI) usually obtained close to discharge as in our case. This chapter will focus on a brief review of pathogenesis and will discuss various approaches or strategies for diagnosis and treatment as well as outcome and highlight gaps in knowledge.

PERIVENTRICULAR-INTRAVENTRICULAR HEMORRHAGE

Background

The overall occurrence of PV-IVH has declined with time although severe hemorrhage remains a significant clinical problem in the tiniest of the VLBW population (1, 3, 4). Thus, approximately 26% of infants of birth weight between 501 and 750 g and 12% between 751 and 1000 g still develop the most severe forms of hemorrhage (3). This observation is highly relevant since survival of the infants born at the cutting edge of viability continues to increase, and long-term neurocognitive deficits are more likely with severe hemorrhage. However, recent evidence points to neurocognitive deficits even with lesser grades of hemorrhage, i.e., Grade II and III IVH and even when the cranial sonogram is interpreted as being normal (5, 6) (see later). These observations are important because they point to the limitations of cranial sonography in identifying subtle white matter injury as well as injury to cortical or deep gray matter. The latter are more readily identified by MRI studies performed closer to term (7, 8) (see also Chapter 12).

Neuropathology: Relevance to Clinical Findings

The primary lesion in PV-IVH is bleeding from small vessels in the subependymal germinal matrix, a transitional gelatinous region that provides limited support for the luxurious but very immature capillary bed that courses through it (9). With maturation this matrix region becomes less prominent, and by term is essentially absent. The hemorrhage when it evolves may be confined to the germinal matrix region (Grade I IVH) or it may extend and rupture into the adjacent ventricular system (Grade II or III IVH depending on the extent of blood), or extend into the white matter (termed a Grade IV or intraparenchymal echogenicity (IPE)) (2, 10) (Fig. 3-1) The latter lesion, which is invariably unilateral, represents an area of hemorrhagic necrosis of varying size within periventricular white matter, dorsal and lateral to the external angle of the lateral ventricle (2, 11, 12) (Fig. 3-1B).

Pathogenesis

The genesis of bleeding from capillaries within the germinal matrix is complex, multifactorial, and influenced in part by intravascular, vascular, and extravascular factors. Several reasons point to a critical role for intravascular factors and specifically perturbations in blood pressure as a principal mechanism of capillary rupture and hemorrhage (see also Chapter 2). Thus, it has been shown utilizing different methods to assess cerebral blood flow (CBF) including Doppler, near-infrared spectroscopy, and xenon that the cerebral circulation of the sick infant is pressure passive, i.e., CBF varies directly with changes in systemic blood pressure (13–15). Clearly this state would be expected to increase the vulnerability of the germinal matrix capillaries to both periods of hypotension and/or hypertension. Indeed experimental studies and clinical observations support this hypothesis. Thus in a beagle puppy model,

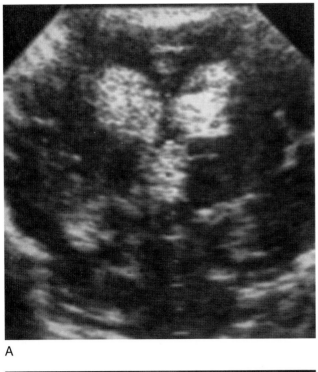

A

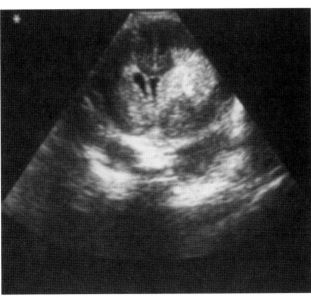

B

Figure 3-1 (A) Cranial ultrasound scan: coronal view. Note the bilateral germinal matrix and intraventricular hemorrhage (Grade III). (B) Note the large left-sided germinal matrix and intraventricular hemorrhage; note the large ipsilateral intraparenchymal echodensity involving periventricular white matter; note the less intense echogenicity suggestive of congestion within the anatomic distribution of the medullary veins.

germinal matrix hemorrhage can be produced by systemic hypertension with or without prior hypotension (16, 17). Moreover clinical temporal associations have been demonstrated between fluctuations in systemic blood pressure and simultaneous fluctuations in cerebral blood flow velocity as may occur in the ventilated premature infant with respiratory distress syndrome, increases in CBF as may occur with rapid volume expansion or a pneumothorax, and the subsequent development of PV-IVH (18–20). Conversely, decreases in CBF secondary to systemic hypotension, which may occur in utero or postnatally, may also play a prominent role in the genesis of PV-IVH in certain infants (21, 22). A presumed mechanism in this context is that of rupture upon reperfusion (1, 14). Finally, elevations in venous pressure may be an important additional intravascular mechanism of hemorrhage, and may reflect the peculiarity of the anatomy of the venous drainage of germinal matrix and the white matter (2). Thus, at the level of the head of the caudate nucleus and the foramen of Monro the terminal, choroidal, and thalamostriate veins course anteriorly to a point of confluence to form the internal cerebral vein. The blood flow then makes a U-turn at the usual site of hemorrhage raising the possibility that an elevation in venous pressure increase the potential for venous distention with obstruction of the terminal and medullary veins, and hemorrhagic infarction. Indeed simultaneous increases in venous pressure have been observed in those infants who exhibit variability in arterial blood pressure, such as occurs with respiratory distress syndrome and associated complications, e.g., pneumothorax or pulmonary interstitial emphysema, or with mechanical or high-frequency ventilation (23, 24). To summarize, it is likely that both arterial and venous perturbations contribute to the genesis of IVH. However, recent evidence suggests that these intravascular responses may be modulated by inflammation or the administration of medications to the mother such as glucocorticoids (25, 26) (see below).

In addition to the intravascular factors, vascular and extravascular influences, i.e., the poorly supported blood vessels, excessive fibrinolytic activity noted within the matrix region, and a prominent postnatal decrease in tissue pressure, may all contribute to hemorrhage (2, 27). In this regard, one potential mechanism accounting for the decrease in IVH associated with antenatal glucocorticoid administration may be via enhanced support for the blood vessels within the germinal matrix (28).

Periventricular White Matter Injury Associated with IVH

The pathogenesis of white matter injury associated with hemorrhage remains unclear, but appears to be closely linked to the adjacent bleed. Two potential pathways have been proposed to explain this intricate relationship. The first suggests a direct relationship to the PV-IVH based on several clinical observations: (a) the white matter lesion is always noted concurrent with or following a large GM and/or IVH, and is rarely if ever observed prior to the hemorrhage; (b) the white matter injury is always observed ipsilateral to the side of the larger hemorrhage when there is bilateral involvement of the ventricular system (1, 2, 12). This consistent relationship between the GM and the white matter injury may in part be explained by the venous drainage of the deep white matter (see above). A second explanation is a de novo evolution of white matter injury. Thus it is proposed that the PV-IVH and the white matter injury occur concurrently. Since both the GM and the periventricular white matter are border zone regions, the risk for ischemic injury is increased during periods of systemic hypotension, particularly in the face of a pressure-passive cerebral circulation (1, 2, 14). Hemorrhage in these regions may then occur as a secondary phenomenon, i.e., reperfusion injury. In support of this theory is the fairly consistent observation of the simultaneous detection of PV-IVH and white mater injury by cranial ultrasound imaging. Moreover elevated hypoxanthine and uric acid levels (perhaps as markers of reperfusion injury) have been observed on the first postnatal day in infants who subsequently developed white matter injury (29, 30).

The mechanism(s) contributing to periventricular white matter injury are crucial in order to prevent this lesion. Thus if the white matter injury is directly related to PV-IVH, then prevention of the latter should reduce the occurrence of the white matter injury. However, if the PV-IVH and the white matter injury occur simultaneously as a result of a primary ischemic event with the hemorrhage occurring as a

Table 3-1   Short- and Long-Term Neurologic Outcome in Infants who Received Indomethacin and Infants who Received a Placebo

Outcome	Indomethacin group (n = 574) (%)	Placebo group (n = 569) (%)	Adjusted odds ratio (95% CI)	P value
Severe IVH	9	13	0.6 (0.4–0.9)	0.02
Cerebral palsy	12	12	1.1 (0.7–1.6)	0.64
Cognitive delay (MDI < 70)	27	26	1.0 (0.8–1.4)	0.86

CI, confidence interval; IVH, intraventricular hemorrhage; MDI, mental development index.
Adapted from Schmidt B, Davis P, et al. Long-term effects of indomethacin prophylaxis in extremely low birth weight infants. N Engl J Med 344(26):1966–72, 2001.

secondary phenomenon, then prevention of the secondary hemorrhage may not affect the primary ischemic lesion. Indeed the two follow-up studies of indomethacin treatment to prevent IVH in the neonatal period are supportive of this latter concern. Thus, although the incidence of severe IVH was reduced in infants treated with indomethacin in both studies, at 18-month follow-up neurodevelopmental outcome including cerebral palsy was comparable in the indomethacin treated group when compared to controls (31, 32) (Table 3-1).

Clinical Features

In most cases, i.e., up to 70% of less severe IVH, the diagnosis is made upon a screening sonogram (2). In the earlier descriptions of PV-IVH, the majority of cases, i.e., 90%, evolved within the first 72 hours of postnatal life (33). However, the time to initial diagnosis of hemorrhage has shifted to a later onset in recent years (10). Thus, for neonates weighing less than 1000 g, the IVH diagnosis is made early, i.e., within the first 24 hours in approximately 80% of infants. However, some cases are now noted beyond the 10th postnatal day. This changing pattern may reflect the complexity of disease in the tiniest infants and the extent of supportive medical care, i.e., prolonged use of high-frequency ventilation. Infants with the more severe IVH frequently exhibit clinical signs including a bulging fontanel, seizures, a fall in hematocrit, hyperglycemia, metabolic acidosis, and pulmonary hemorrhage (1).

Complications

The two most significant complications of IVH are extension into adjacent white matter (see above) and the development of posthemorrhagic hydrocephalus (see Chapter 4).

Prevention

Perinatal

Prevention of PV-IVH and its complications continues to focus on both perinatal and postnatal strategies. Perinatal pharmacological interventions have included the administration of Phenobarbital and vitamin K without any beneficial effect (34–36). More recently a combination of aminophylline, magnesium with steroids, and ritodrine has been studied in a relatively small sample size (n = 128) with an apparent reduction in total and severe IVH (37). The antenatal administration of a single short course of glucocorticoids to augment pulmonary maturation has had the positive, unanticipated benefit of a significant reduction in the incidence of severe IVH (26, 38–45). Thus from a review of several large observational databases, the unadjusted odds ratio for severe IVH following any antenatal glucocorticoid exposure has ranged from 0.49 to 0.79 (45). The mechanism(s) whereby glucocorticoids reduces severe IVH remain unclear, but may relate to less severe respiratory distress syndrome, higher resting blood pressures, or via accelerated maturation of the germinal matrix region (27, 41, 46, 47).

One maternal medical condition associated with a lower incidence of IVH is pregnancy-induced hypertension (PIH). Thus a lower incidence of severe PV-IVH in infants born to mothers with PIH than in those without PIH, i.e., 8.2% vs. 14% with an odds ratio estimate of 0.43 (95% confidence intervals 0.30–0.61), was noted in one report (48), a finding consistent with other reports (49, 50). The mechanism(s) whereby PIH may reduce IVH remain unclear, but may relate to accelerate brain maturation in such infants, or the use of medications, specifically magnesium sulfate, to treat the mother (51–53). However, recent retrospective data suggest that magnesium sulfate is not associated with a reduction in PV-IVH (54–56). Moreover, tocolytic agents in general including magnesium sulfate are associated with an increased risk for IVH (57, 58).

Route of Delivery

There are conflicting data regarding the route of delivery and subsequent IVH (50, 59–61). Interpretation of the data is difficult since most are retrospective. This does not exclude the possibility that under certain circumstances intrapartum events may contribute to the pathogenesis of severe IVH. Thus, in some studies there is an increased risk for IVH with increasing duration of the active phase of labor, and a lower risk in those infants delivered via cesarean section prior to the active phase of labor (49, 58). Many of these studies were analyzed prior to the more frequent use of antenatal glucocorticoids (61). In a recent study in infants less than 751 g whose mothers were given steroids, vaginal delivery was a predictor for severe intraventricular hemorrhage (62). By contrast in a retrospective cohort study of extremely low birth weight infants, 401–1000 g, the influence of labor on extremely low birth weight infants who were born by cesarean delivery with reference to neonatal and neurodevelopmental outcomes was examined. The analysis revealed that labor does not appear to play a significant role in the genesis of IVH (63). Importantly any analysis that evaluates the impact of labor or route of delivery must account for an important role of placental inflammation and in particular fetal vasculitis in the genesis of IVH which may supersede the influence of the route of delivery (64). Thus in one study while vaginal delivery was associated with an increased risk of IVH by univariate analysis, the risks attributable to vaginal delivery were no longer elevated when adjustments were made in multivariate analysis for fetal vasculitis and other potential confounders (64). This issue clearly warrants further prospective study and analysis.

Postnatal Strategies to Prevent Severe IVH

Any approach to intervention should at the least consider the following: (i) the target population should be those infants who are the most likely to develop severe IVH, i.e., <1000 g (3), and (ii) the condition of the infant at delivery, which appears to be an important mediator of subsequent IVH (Table 3-2). The latter appears to be strongly influenced in part by perinatal events and in particular the administration of antenatal glucocorticoids (45) or the presence or absence of fetal vasculitis (64). The type of glucocorticoid administered to the mother may also be important. Thus antenatal exposure of dexamethasone, but not betamethasone was associated with an increased risk of white matter injury in premature infants (65).

Postnatal Factors Associated with an Increased Risk

These include decreasing gestational age, lower birth weight (<1000 g), male sex, intubation, and respiratory distress syndrome (2, 66) (Table 3-2). By contrast the

Table 3-2	Factors Associated with a Risk for the Development of Severe IVH

High risk for the development of severe IVH
Minimal intrapartum care
No glucocorticoid exposure
Chorioamnionitis/funisitis
Fetal distress
↓ Gestational age
↓ Birth weight
Respiratory distress syndrome
Respiratory morbidity, i.e., pneumothorax
Fluctuations or rapid elevations in systemic blood pressure and/or cerebral blood flow
Hypotension
Sudden and repeated increases in venous pressure
Lower risk for severe IVH in premature infants
Antenatal glucocorticoids (short course)
Medical condition, e.g., PIH
Other (IUGR)
↑ Gestation age
↑ Birth weight
Postnatal medications, e.g., indomethacin

risk for severe IVH in the nonintubated infant is low, i.e., <10% (67). For infants with respiratory distress syndrome, the risk for IVH is even greater when there are associated perturbations in arterial and venous pressures (18, 19, 23). These vascular perturbations are in part related to the infant's breathing patterns usually out of synchrony with the ventilator breath (68). The perturbations can be minimized with careful ventilator management, including the use of synchronized mechanical ventilation, assist control ventilation, sedation, or in more difficult cases with paralysis (2, 69). Interestingly enough, although surfactant administration improved respiratory ventilation it was not accompanied by a concomitant significant reduction in the incidence of IVH (70).

Postnatal Administration of Medications to Reduce Severe IVH

Medications have included the use of Phenobarbital (71–73), vitamin E (74), ethamyslate (75), and indomethacin (32, 76, 77). While there was initial enthusiasm for the use of each of these medications in the prevention of IVH, this has not been borne out over time. Noteworthy, in one study infants who received Phenobarbital exhibited a higher incidence of severe IVH when compared to controls (73). Currently, the early postnatal administration of indomethacin is of benefit in the prevention of severe hemorrhage (32, 77). Thus, two studies demonstrated a significant reduction in the incidence of severe IVH in infants who received indomethacin versus control infants. However, at long-term follow-up, the incidence of cerebral palsy was comparable between groups (30, 31) (Table 3-1). This observation coupled with the known reduction in cerebral blood flow that accompanies indomethacin administration warrants cautious use of this agent (78, 79). Perhaps it should be reserved for those infants at greatest risk (Table 3-2).

WHITE MATTER INJURY IN THE ABSENCE OF HEMORRHAGE

CASE HISTORY

PL was a 26-week appropriate for gestational age female infant born to a 38-year-old primigravida whose pregnancy was uncomplicated until the onset of preterm labor. The mother was placed on bed rest, given a course of betamethasone, treated with antibiotics, and received magnesium sulfate. However, after five days fetal distress was noted and the infant was delivered via cesarean section. Resuscitation in the delivery room included brief bag mask ventilation and the infant was placed on continuous positive airway pressure (CPAP) and triaged to the neonatal intensive care unit. The Apgar scores were 4^1, 7^5, 8^{10}, respectively. The infant rapidly weaned to room air while on CPAP. She was treated with antibiotics for seven days, in part because of the perinatal history as well as abnormal blood count indices and an elevated c reactive protein. The cultures remained negative. The clinical course was characterized by recurrent apnea and bradycardia, a coagulase *Staphylococcus epidermidis* infection, and a persistent oxygen requirement beginning in the second week that lasted through the 34 postconceptual week. A cranial sonogram performed on DOL 5 was interpreted as normal (Fig. 3-2A). Repeat sonograms done on DOL 14 and 28 were interpreted as normal. However the images obtained on DOL 42 (following the infection) and subsequently showed progressive nonhemorrhagic ventriculomegaly. An MRI close to discharge revealed mild ventriculomegaly with mild white matter changes.

This case illustrates the "new" and predominate ultrasound expression of white matter injury in the premature infant characterized by the gradual development of lateral ventriculomegaly suggestive of diffuse injury, as opposed to the more focal cystic (2, 10, 80, 81). Moreover, in previous reports cysts usually became apparent within the first 2 to 3 weeks of life. However, recent data have shown the evolution of cysts beyond the first month in an increasing numbers of cases (10, 82). The extent of injury to white matter in the premature infant when evaluated by cranial ultrasound imaging ranges from 4 to 15% (2, 66, 83, 84). However, MRI indicates that white matter injury is more prevalent than is apparent from cranial sonography (7).

Periventricular Leukomalacia

Periventricular leukomalacia (PVL) refers to necrosis of white matter adjacent to the external angles of the lateral ventricles, and has long been regarded as the principal ischemic lesion of the premature infant (2). However, more recent evidence suggests that the evolution of injury is much more complex (see below). The pathologic features of PVL include focal as well as more diffuse cerebral white matter involvement (81, 86–88). The focal periventricular necrosis is distributed commonly at the level of the occipital radiation at the trigone of the lateral ventricles, and at the level of the cerebral white matter around the foramen of Monro (2). The typical histologic changes are characterized by coagulation necrosis, microglial infiltration, astrocytic proliferation and eventual cyst formation. These cavities usually diminish in size over time secondary to gliosis. The diffuse cerebral white matter necrosis less frequently undergoes cystic change and ventricular dilation is also more prominent (Fig. 3-2B). It is more commonly noted in the smaller premature infant requiring prolonged ventilator support (81) (see above).

Pathogenesis

Experimental and clinical observations suggest two basic mechanisms, i.e., vascular and the intrinsic vulnerability of the differentiating oligodendrocyte (88–90).

Vascular Factors

Several features peculiar to the premature infant are important in this regard. The first relates to the vascular development and supply. Specifically the penetrating branches of the anterior, middle, and posterior cerebral arteries end in border zones, which are most vulnerable to decreases in CBF. It is within these border zones that the focal necrosis of PVL (as described above) typically occurs (90, 91). Furthermore, the penetrating cerebral vessels, which include long branches

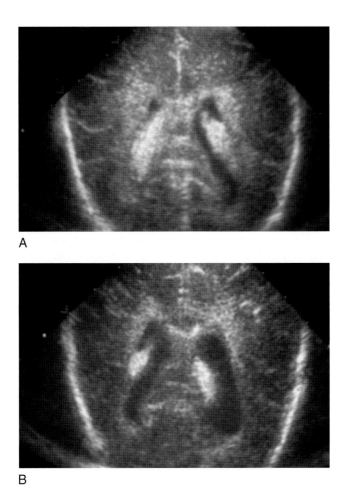

A

B

Figure 3-2 (A) Coronal ultrasound image from an infant in the first week showing normal ventricular size. (B) Coronal image from the same infant 6 weeks later demonstrating dilation of the lateral ventricles in the absence of intraventricular hemorrhage.

that terminate in the deep periventricular white matter and short branches that terminate in the subcortical white matter, vary as a function of gestational age (92). Thus early on, i.e., at approximately 24–30 weeks of gestation, the long penetrators have few side branches and limited intraparenchymal anastomosis with the short branches, resulting in border zones in white matter beyond the periventricular region. This may account for the more diffuse lesion noted in the smaller premature infant (81, 86). From 32 weeks on, there is a marked increase in vascular supply as a result of increase in vessel length and anastomosis. It is this vascular maturation that likely accounts for the uncommon presentation of this lesion in the larger infant. A second factor relates to the limited vasodilatory response of the blood vessels supplying the white matter to increases in $PaCO_2$ as compared to the vasodilatory responses of the blood vessels supplying other regions of brain, i.e., medulla or gray matter (93), as well as a persistent decrease in CBF to white matter during the phase of reperfusion following ischemia, despite recovery in all other brain areas (94). Finally, impairment of CBF autoregulation as may occur in the sick premature infant (see above) increases the risk for ischemia to the border zone regions of white matter during episodes of systemic hypotension (14, 87, 95). Clinically, loss of CBF autoregulation and/or decreases in CBF may occur in the sick infant secondary to events such as hypotension, acidosis, septic shock, hypocarbia,

PDA, recurrent apnea, bradycardia, etc., and may in part explain the association of such events and PVL (22, 96–102).

Intrinsic Vulnerability of the Differentiating Oligodendrocyte

It has been established that the early differentiating oligodendrocyte is most vulnerable to injury secondary to release of numerous factors, including free radicals, excitotoxins, cytokines, as well as a lack of growth factors. The mechanism of cell death due to these factors appears to be mediated via apoptosis (103). Moreover studies in newborn animal models subjected to hypoxia-ischemia and or infection have demonstrated apoptotic cell death in immature cerebral white matter (104, 105). In a neuropathologic study, apoptotic cell death was observed significantly more often in infants dying of white matter injury than in those infants without white matter injury (106). In the diffuse white matter injury a marked prominence of activated microglia, identified by a specific immunocytochemical marker, as well as astrocytosis has been observed. The presence of the activated microglia raises the possibility of a role for these cells in the causation of the diffuse injury to the preoligodendrocytes (see below).

Free Radical Injury

The prominence of activated microglia in the diffuse component of PVL suggests that these cells may be involved in the generation of reactive oxygen species (ROS) and reactive nitrogen species (RNS) found in the human lesion. Microglia have been shown to be activated by ischemia and to remain activated for weeks following the insult. When activated, microglia have been shown to release ROS and RNS that then result in cell death. Experimental studies have demonstrated vulnerability of the early differentiating preoligodendrocyte to free radical injury, e.g., hydrogen peroxide, hydroxyl radical (107, 108). This maturation-dependent vulnerability of preoligodendrocytes to ROS and RNS appears to be related to such factors as deficient antioxidant defenses and acquisition of iron for differentiation. Indeed specific markers have identified evidence in preoligodendrocytes for lipid peroxidation and protein nitration in the diffuse white matter injury. The role for free radical-induced damage triggering the death of the early differentiating oligodendrocyte is supported by the cryoprotection provided by free radical scavengers, i.e., superoxide dismutase, desferoxamine, and vitamin E (2, 107).

Excitotoxic Injury (Glutamate)

Glutamate can lead to the death of oligodendroglial precursors via mechanisms that involve both receptor and nonreceptor mechanisms. The nonreceptor mechanism involves glutamate intracellular entry in exchange for cystine via activation of a glutamine–cystine exchange transporter, resulting in a decrease in intracellular cystine and thereby glutathione synthesis (107). The result is glutathione depletion and free radical-mediated cell death. The latter can be totally prevented by the addition of free radical scavengers such as vitamin E (107). The receptor-mediated injury appears to be mediated via activation of AMPA/kainate type glutamate receptors. Recent data suggest that this form of cell death occurs only in developing and not mature oligodendroglia (109). It has also been shown that non-N-methyl-D-aspartate (non-NMDA) receptors are present on preoligodendrocytes that result in free radical-mediated death of these cells when activated in vitro, and in vivo lead to death of preoligodendrocytes when activated by hypoxia-ischemia in an immature animal model of diffuse white matter injury (110). The relevance of this mechanism to hypoxia ischemia-induced white matter injury has been demonstrated in an immature rat model, in which such injury is prevented by the systemic administration of the non-NMDA receptor antagonist 6-nitro-7-sulfamoylbenzo(f)quinoxaline-2,3-dione (NBQX) following termination of the insult (111).

Cytokines

Cytokines appear to be an important mechanism for preoligodendroglial cell death. It is a well established finding in animals that a paradigm of ischemia/reperfusion is accompanied by a rapid activation of microglia, secretion of cytokines, and migration of inflammatory cells (112). Moreover, cytokines and inflammatory cells are also a consistent feature of the response to infection. Within the central nervous system microglia release tumor necrosis factor (TNF)α, interleukin (IL)-1 and IL-6. Cell culture studies suggest that TNFα is toxic to oligodendroglia (113). Fairly recent evidence suggests that interferon (IFN)-γ is also toxic to oligodendroglia, an effect that is potentiated by TNFα (114). However, numerous additional cytokines, microglia, or white blood cells may be involved in this process (115). Indeed in a recent study increased levels of circulating proinflammatory cytokines during the first 72 hours of life were associated with arterial hypotension and with the development of brain damage as detected by ultrasound (116). Increases in IL-6, IL-8, and IL-10 were associated with arterial hypotension and increases in IL-6 and IL-8 were associated with severe IVH. Prolonged rupture of membranes was associated with increased postnatal levels of IFN-γ, which in turn were associated with white matter damage (116). The potential deleterious effects of cytokines may be mediated via other mechanisms, including increased permeability of the blood–brain barrier (117), vascular endothelial damage (118), and decreased cerebral blood flow to white matter following endotoxin exposure (119).

Maternal Fetal Infection and/or Inflammation and White Matter Injury

There is both experimental and clinical evidence demonstrating an association between maternal infection/inflammation of the chorion, amnion ± fetal vascular involvement, i.e., funisitis, and white matter injury. Thus, intraperitoneal injection of lipopolysaccharides into kittens and exposing pregnant rabbits to intrauterine infection induces white matter injury, similar to that observed in humans (104, 120). Several clinical studies have demonstrated an association between chorioamnionitis and PVL (85, 121). Akin to intraventricular hemorrhage, this association appears to be accentuated in the presence of funisitis (122). The link between chorioamnionitis may be mediated via cytokines. Thus high levels of cytokines (IL-6 and IL-1β) have been found in the amniotic fluid (123–125), IL-6 in cord blood (126), and elevated levels of IL-1, IL-6, and IFN in neonatal blood of preterm infants who develop PVL or cerebral palsy (116, 127–129) PVL. Finally, microglial expression of TNFα and IL-6 immunoreactivity is found twice as common in the white matter of infants with PVL than in the absence of injury to the region (130, 131). In contrast to these potential deleterious effects, in a mouse model of hypoxia ischemia lacking TNFα, focal cerebral ischemia was exacerbated (132). Injury-induced microglial activation was suppressed in the TNF-knockout mice. These latter observations point to the complex interrelationships between cytokines and white matter injury.

Clinical Factors Associated with PVL

Perinatal events associated with postnatal cystic PVL include a history of chorioamnionitis (see above), prolonged rupture of membranes, peripartum hemorrhage, severe fetal acidemia, hypovolemia, sepsis, hypocarbia, symptomatic PDA, and recurrent apnea and bradycardia (22, 96–102, 121). A common feature of many of these conditions is a reduction in systemic blood pressure. Indeed, in a recent study, chorioamnionitis was associated with increased IL-6 and IL-1β concentrations in cord blood, with increased newborn heart rate and decreased mean and diastolic blood pressures, and the cord blood IL-6 concentration correlated inversely with newborn systolic, mean, and diastolic blood pressures (25). By contrast in a study of

Table 3-3 Potential Pathways Leading to White Matter Injury

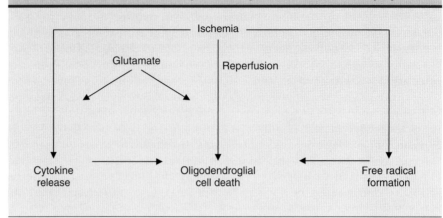

14 infants who developed PVL, only four (30%) had overt evidence of postnatal systemic hypotension and asphyxia was an uncommon finding (85). Others have also failed to demonstrate a consistent association with hypotension and PVL (133–135).

Prevention

From the preceding sections, it is likely that prevention of PVL will be difficult. First, it is relatively uncommon; second, as noted above, the pathogenesis of PVL is complex (Table 3-3); and third, the presentation is often subtle and only detected upon neuroimaging. Although there is evidence pointing to an association between perinatal infection, i.e., chorioamnionitis, and PVL (85, 121), the precise mechanism(s) linking the two remain unclear; the positive predictive value of a history of chorioamnionitis and subsequent PVL is low and approximates 10%, and many cases of infection are asymptomatic with the diagnosis only established upon histologic examination of the placenta (64). More specific potential strategies include: (i) the appropriate treatment of infants with low blood pressure for a given gestational age (see Chapter 2) with volume replacement therapy or inotropic support as clinically indicated, and (ii) the careful ventilatory management of infants with respiratory distress so as to avoid hypocarbia. However, it is important to note that the mechanism(s) of white matter injury with hypocarbia remain unclear. Thus ventilation-induced hypocarbia is often associated with higher mean airway pressures. Increases in mean airway pressure are associated with impairment of venous return, a fall in cardiac output, as well as increases in sagittal sinus pressure (24, 136). The increase in venous coupled with a concomitant decrease in CBF as may occur with hypocarbia would be expected to decrease cerebral perfusion pressure including flow to white matter. The use of antioxidant therapy to counter the free radical injury demonstrated in the experimental model is another therapeutic possibility. However, antioxidant therapy has not been uniformly successful in the treatment of other neonatal conditions presumed to be related in part to free radical injury (137).

OUTCOME

Intraventricular Hemorrhage

The infant with severe IVH is at highest risk for adverse neurodevelopmental outcome (both motor and cognitive) (see Chapter 14). This is related in part to the extent of the white matter involvement noted by cranial ultrasound imaging.

Thus, with a large IPE (>1 cm in diameter; Fig. 3-1B) the outcome is invariably poor, with major motor and cognitive defects consistently noted at follow-up (2, 12, 138). With smaller lesions (<1 cm in diameter), the outcome is less precise and a small percentage (approximately 20%) may even have a normal outcome (12).

However, as noted previously, the issue is much more complicated and even infants with a normal ultrasound scan as well as those with lesser grades of hemorrhage are at risk for motor as well as cognitive deficits. Thus in the first of these studies with normal cranial sonograms, major neurologic disability was noted in 5–10% of infants and a mental developmental index (MDI) < 70 in 25% of cases (5). In the second study of infants with lesser grades of hemorrhage (Grade I and II IVH), major neurologic disabilities were noted in 13%, and a MDI < 70 in 45% of cases (6). Moreover the comparable neurodevelopmental outcome for infants with and without IVH in the indomethacin study (Table 3-2) clearly indicates that the genesis of brain injury in the sick premature infant is much more complex than can be deduced from the neonatal neurosonographic appearance (see Chapter 13).

Periventricular Leukomalacia

Although the sonographic diagnosis of cystic PVL affects only a small percentage of preterm infants, i.e., approximately 3%, MRI performed at term shows that diffuse noncystic injury to white matter is much more common. This finding poses a significant burden in that the majority of infants have major long-term neuro-developmental problems (85, 139–142). The most commonly described long-term motor sequelae of PVL have been spastic diplegia (2). Recent reports, however, describe a more severe deficit with involvement of all four extremities as well as visual and cognitive deficits (143–147). This more severe outcome is consistent with the diffuse white matter injury noted on neuropathology in preterm infants who die with PVL as well as on MRI (81, 142). The genesis of the cognitive deficits with PVL remains unclear. It has been speculated that the injury may secondarily affect neuronal cortical organization due to injury to subplate neurons or late migrating astrocytes (2, 148). More recent data indicate substantial diffuse white matter injury identified by MRI including volumetric imaging coupled with reduced gray matter volumes in VLBW infants imaged at term (149). The latter findings may explain the substantial cognitive deficits noted at follow-up. A similar observation has been noted in adults with severe cognitive injury (150).

GAPS IN KNOWLEDGE

1. The mechanisms contributing to the motor deficits in up to 10–15% of infants and cognitive deficits in up to one-third of infants with normal sonograms and/or lesser grades of IVH remain unclear (5, 6). Along the same lines, although prophylactic indomethacin results in a reduction in the incidence of severe hemorrhage, it remains unclear why the incidence of cerebral palsy at 18 months was comparable to that observed in the control infants (32). Furthermore in both groups of infants the incidence of moderate to severe cognitive deficits in both groups was comparable and was substantially higher than the motor deficits.

2. The genesis of cognitive deficits remains unclear but critical to elucidate. Thus approximately 25 000 infants are born weighing <1000 g in the USA annually. If one assumes a 30% occurrence of moderate to severe deficits, then approximately 8000 VLBW infants will progress to moderate to severe mental retardation each year. Factors predisposing to such deficits include additional vulnerable regions, i.e., basal ganglia, hippocampus, subplate neurons, and cortical gray matter (151), medical complications of prematurity such as

chronic lung disease, necrotizing enterocolitis, nosocomial infections, hypo-glycemia, and hyperbilirubinemia, as well as medications used to treat the infants including glucocorticoids and xanthine derivatives (151). The impact of the stressful NICU environment on the developing brain and in particular the hippocampus is likely to be considerable. In addition the influence of the post discharge environment likely also plays a critical role.

3. Indomethacin appears to be the best intervention to use at the current time in the high-risk target population. However, other options need to be iden-tified given the limited impact of indomethacin at follow-up.

4. Although an association between placental inflammation and white matter has been demonstrated, it remains unclear why the majority of infants born under such circumstances do not demonstrate overt white matter injury.

5. Although there are many inherent factors that increase the vulnerability of the white matter to reductions in blood pressure and as a secondary con-sequence a reduction in CBF, it remains unclear why the majority of infants with cystic leukomalacia do not demonstrate overt evidence of postnatal hypotension. One could argue that the period of vulnerability occurs during the labor process. However, the increasing observation of late development of cystic PVL and the identification of many cases of non cystic PVL upon routine MRI points to a critical role for postnatal influences, i.e., free radi-cals, excitotoxic injury, as well as cytokines, in the genesis of preoligoden-drocyte injury.

CONCLUSIONS

PV-IVH and adjacent white matter injury remains a significant problem in the premature infant. The potential mechanisms contributing to injury are complex and involve factors related to blood flow and its regulation as well as cellular mediators including cytokines, free radical formation, and excitotoxic release. While a reduction in the occurrence of severe IVH can be achieved with indo-methacin, this has not translated into long-term neurodevelopmental benefit. This reinforces the concept of a more diffuse insidious injury to brain in sick premature infants, a concept reinforced by MRI changes identified at follow-up.

REFERENCES

1. Shalak L, Perlman JM. Hemorrhagic-ischemic cerebral injury in the preterm infant. Curr Concepts Clin Perinatol 29:745–63, 2002.
2. Volpe JJ. Neurology of the Newborn, 4th edition. Philadelphia, PA: WB Saunders, 2001.
3. Lemons JA, Bauer CR, Oh W, et al. Very low birth weight outcomes of the National Institute of Child Health and Human Development, Neonatal Research Network, January 1995 through December 1996. Pediatrics 107:e1, 2001.
4. Philips AGS, Allen WC, Tito AM, et al. Intraventricular hemorrhage in preterm infants: declining incidence in the 1980s. Pediatrics 84:797–800, 1989.
5. Laptook AR, O'Shea TM, Shankaran S, Bhaskar B. Adverse neurodevelopmental outcomes among extremely low birth weight infants with a normal head ultrasound: prevalence and antecedents. Pediatrics 115:673–80, 2005.
6. Patra K, Wilson-Costello D, Taylor HG. Grades I–II intraventricular hemorrhage in extremely low birth weight infants: effects on neurodevelopment. J Pediatr 149:169–73, 2006.
7. Inder TE, Anderson NJ, Spencer C, et al. White matter injury in the premature infant: a comparison between serial cranial sonographic and MR findings at term. Am J Neuroradiol 24:805–9, 2003.
8. Dyet LE, Kennea N, Counsell SJ. Natural history of brain lesions in extremely preterm infants studied with serial magnetic resonance imaging from birth and neurodevelopmental assessment. Pediatrics 118:536–48, 2006.
9. Hambleton G, Wiggelsworth JS. Origin of intraventricular hemorrhage in the preterm infant. Arch Dis Child 57:651–5, 1976.
10. Perlman JM, Rollins N. Surveillance protocol for the detection of intracranial abnormalities in premature neonates. Arch Pediatr Adolesc Med 154(8):822–6, 2000.

11. Gould SJ, Howard S, Hope PL, Reynold EO. Periventricular intraparenchymal cerebral hemorrhage in preterm infants: the role of venous infarction. J Pathol 151:197–202, 1987.

12. Guzzetta F, Schackelford GD, Volpe S, et al. Periventricular intraparenchymal echodensities in the premature newborn: critical determinant of neurologic outcome. Pediatrics 78:945–1006, 1986.

13. Lou CH, Lassen NA, Friis-Hansen B. Impaired autoregulation of cerebral blood flow in the distressed newborn infant. J Pediatr 94:118–25, 1979.

14. Pryds O, Griesen G, Lou H, et al. Heterogeneity of cerebral vasoreactivity in preterm infants supported by mechanical ventilation. J Pediatr 115:638–45, 1989.

15. Tsuji M, Saul JP, du Plessis A, et al. Cerebral intravascular oxygenation correlates with mean arterial pressure in critically ill premature infants. Pediatrics 106:625–32, 2000.

16. Goddard-Finegold J, Armstrong D, Zeller RS. Intraventricular hemorrhage following volume expansion after hypovolemic hypotension in the newborn beagle. J Pediatr 100:796–9, 1982.

17. Ment LR, Stewart WB, Duncan CC, et al. Beagle puppy model of intraventricular hemorrhage. J Neurosurg 57:219–23, 1982.

18. Goldberg RN, Chung D, Goldman SL, et al. The associations of rapid volume expansion and intraventricular hemorrhage in the preterm infant. J Pediatr 96:1060–3, 1980.

19. Hill A, Perlman JM, Volpe JJ. Relationship of pneumothorax to the occurrence of intraventricular hemorrhage in the premature newborn. Pediatrics 69:144–9, 1982.

20. Perlman JM, McMenamin JB, Volpe JJ. Fluctuating cerebral blood flow velocity in respiratory distress syndrome. Relation to the development of intraventricular hemorrhage. N Engl J Med 309:204–9, 1983.

21. Bada HS, Korones SB, Perry EH, et al. Mean arterial blood pressure changes in premature infants and those at risk for intraventricular hemorrhage. J Pediatr 117:607–14, 1990.

22. Miall-Allen VM, De Vries LS, Whitelaw AG. Mean arterial blood pressure and neonatal cerebral lesions. Arch Dis Child 62:1068–9, 1987.

23. Perlman JM, Volpe JJ. Are venous circulatory changes important in the pathogenesis of hemorrhagic and/or ischemic cerebral injury? Pediatrics 80:705–11, 1987.

24. Vert P, Monin P, Sibout M. Intracranial venous pressure in newborns: variations in physiologic and neurologic disorders. In Stern L, Friis-Hansen B, Kildeberg P (eds). Intensive Care of Newborns. New York: Masson, 1975, p. 185.

25. Yanowitz TD, Potter DM, Bowen A, et al. Variability in cerebral oxygen delivery is reduced in premature neonates exposed to chorioamnionitis. Pediatr Res 59:299–304, 2006.

26. Salhab W, Hyman L, Perlman JM. Partial or complete antenatal steroids treatment and neonatal outcome in extremely low birth weight infants less than or equal to 1000 grams: is there a dose dependent effect? J Perinatol 23:668–72, 2004.

27. Takashima S, Tanaka K. Microangiography and fibrilolytic activity in the matrix of the premature brain. Brain Dev 4:422–8, 1972.

28. Perlman JM, Nissen PD. Glial fibrillary acidic protein in RNA gene expression in human astroglial cells is modulated by dexamethasone. Ann Neurol 38:495, 1995 (abstract).

29. Perlman JM, Risser R. Relationship of uric acid concentrations and severe intraventricular hemorrhage/leukomalacia in the premature infant. J Pediatr 132:436–9, 1998.

30. Russell GAB, Jeffers G, Cook RWI. Plasma hypoxanthine: a marker for hypoxic-ischemic induced periventricular leukomalacia? Arch Dis Child 67:388–92, 1992.

31. Allen WC, Vohr B, Makuch RW. Antecedents of cerebral palsy in a multicenter trial of indomethacin for intraventricular hemorrhage. Arch Pediatr Adolesc Med 151:581–5, 1997.

32. Schmidt B, Davis P, et al. Long-term effects of indomethacin prophylaxis in extremely-low-birth-weight infants. N Engl J Med 344(26):1966–72, 2001.

33. Perlman JM, Volpe JJ. Intraventricular hemorrhage in the extremely small premature infant. Am J Dis Child 140:1122–4, 1986.

34. Kazzi N, Llagan NB, Liang KC, et al. Maternal administration of vitamin K does not improve the coagulation profile of preterm infants. Pediatrics 84:1045–50, 1989.

35. Pomerance JJ, Teal JG, Gogolok JF, et al. Maternally administered antenatal vitamin K: effect on neonatal prothrombin activity, partial prothrombin time and intraventricular hemorrhage. Obstet Gynecol 70:235–41, 1987.

36. Shankaran S, Papile LA, Wright LL, et al. The effect of antenatal phenobarbital therapy on neonatal intracranial hemorrhage in preterm infants. N Engl J Med 337:466–71, 1997.

37. DiRenzo G, Carlo M, Marcella G, et al. The combined maternal administration of magnesium sulfate and aminophylline reduces intraventricular hemorrhage in very preterm neonates. Am J Obstet Gynecol 192:433–8, 2005.

38. Crowley P, Chalmers I, Keirse MJNC. The effects of corticosteroid administration before preterm delivery: an overview of the evidence from clinical trials. Br J Obstet Gynecol 97:11–25, 1990.

39. Garite TJ, Rumney PJ, Briggs GC, et al. A randomized placebo controlled trial of betamethasone for the prevention of respiratory distress syndrome at 24–28 weeks gestation. Am J Obstet Gynecol 166:646–51, 1992.

40. Jobe AH, Mitchell BR, Gunkel JH. Beneficial effects of combined use of prenatal steroids and postnatal surfactant on preterm infants. Am J Obstet Gynecol 168:508–13, 1993.

41. Kari MA, Hallman M, Gronen M, et al. Prenatal dexamethasone treatment in conjunction with rescue therapy of human surfactant: a randomized placebo-controlled multicenter study. Pediatrics 93:730–6, 1994.

42. Leviton A, Dammann O, Allred EN, et al. Antenatal corticosteroids and cranial ultrasonographic abnormalities. Am J Obstet Gynecol 181(4):1007–17, 1999.

43. Maher JE, Cliver SP, Goldenberg RL, et al. March of Dimes Multicenter Study Group. The effect of glucocorticoid therapy in the very premature infant. Am J Obstet Gynecol 170:869–73, 1994.

44. Wright LL, Homar JD, Gunkel H. Evidence from multicenter networks on the current use and effectiveness of antenatal corticosteroids in low birthweight infants. Am J Obstet Gynecol 173:263–9, 1995.

45. Roberts D, Dalziel S. Antenatal corticosteroids for accelerating fetal lung maturation for women at risk for preterm birth. Cochrane Database Syst Rev 3:CD004454, 2006.

46. Demarini S, Dollberg S, Hoath SB, et al. Effects of antenatal corticosteroids on blood pressure in very low birth weight infants during the first 24 hours of life. J Perinatol 19:419–25, 1999.

47. Garland JS, Buck R, Leviton A. Effect of maternal glucocorticoid exposure on risk of severe intraventricular hemorrhage in surfactant-treated preterm infants. J Pediatr 126:272–9, 1995.

48. Perlman JM, Risser RC, Gee JB. Pregnancy induced hypertension and reduced intraventricular hemorrhage in preterm infants. Pediatr Neurol 17:29–33, 1997.

49. Kuban KCK, Leviton A, Pagano M, et al. Maternal toxemia is associated with a reduced incidence of germinal matrix hemorrhage in premature babies. J Child Neurol 7:70–6, 1992.

50. Leviton A, Pagano M, Kuban KCK, et al. The epidemiology of germinal matrix hemorrhage during the first half of life. Develop Med Child Neurol 33:138–45, 1988.

51. Gould JB, Gluck L, Kulovich MV. The relationship between accelerated pulmonary maturity and accelerated neurologic maturity in certain chronically stressed pregnancies. Am J Obstet Gynecol 127:181–6, 1997.

52. Hadi HA. Fetal cerebral maturation in hypertension disorder in pregnancy. Obstet Gynecol 63:214–19, 1984.

53. Nelson KB, Grether JK. Can magnesium sulfate reduce the risk of cerebral palsy in very low birth-weight infants? Pediatrics 95:263–9, 1995.

54. Leviton A, Paneth N, Susser MW, et al. Magnesium receipt does not appear to reduce the risk of neonatal white matter damage. Pediatrics 99:4.E2, 1997.

55. Paneth N, Jettan J, Pinto-Martron J, et al. Magnesium sulfate and risk of neonatal brain lesions and cerebral palsy in low birthweight infants. Pediatrics 99:5.1–7, 1997.

56. Canterino JC, Verma UL, Visintainer PF, et al. Maternal magnesium sulfate and the development of neonatal periventricular leucomalacia and intraventricular hemorrhage. Obstet Gynecol 93(3):396–402, 1999.

57. Atkinson MW, Goldenberg RL, Gaudier FL, et al. Maternal corticosteroid and tocolytic treatment and morbidity and mortality in very low birthweight infants. Am J Obstet Gynecol 173:299–304, 1995.

58. Groome LJ, Goldenberg RL, Cliver SP, et al. March of Dimes Multicenter Study Group. Neonatal periventricular-intraventricular hemorrhage after maternal b-sympathomimetic tocolysis. Am J Obstet Gynecol 167:873–9, 1992.

59. Anderson GD, Bada HS, Shaver BM, et al. The effect of cesarean section on intraventricular hemorrhage in the premature infant. Am J Obstet Gynecol 166:1091–101, 1992.

60. Strauss A, Kirz D, Mandalou HD, et al. Perinatal events and intraventricular/ependymal hemorrhage in the very low birthweight infant. Am J Obstet Gynecol 151:1022–7, 1985.

61. Ment LR, Oh W, Ehrenkrantz R, et al. Antenatal steroids, delivery mode and intraventricular hemorrhage in preterm infants. Am J Obstet Gynecol 172:795–800, 1995.

62. Deulofeut R, Sola A, Lee B, et al. The impact of vaginal delivery in premature infants weighing less than 1,251 grams. Obstet Gynecol 105:525–31, 2005.

63. Wadhawan R, Vohr BR, Fanaroff AA, et al. Does labor influence neonatal and neurodevelopmental outcomes of extremely-low-birth-weight infants who are born by cesarean delivery? Am J Obstet Gynecol 189:501–6, 2003.

64. Hansen A, Leviton A. The Developmental Epidemiology Network Investigators. Labor and delivery characteristics and risks of cranial ultrasonographic abnormalities among very-low-birth-weight infants. Am J Obstet Gynecol 181(4):997–1006, 1999.

65. Baud O, Foix-L'Helias L, et al. Antenatal glucocorticoid treatment and cystic periventricular leukomalacia in very premature infants. N Engl J Med 341(16):1190–6, 1999.

66. Perlman JM. White matter injury in the preterm infant: an important determinant of abnormal neurodevelopmental outcome. Early Human Dev 53:99–120, 1998.

67. Perlman JM. Intraventricular hemorrhage. Pediatrics 84:913–14, 1989.

68. Perlman JM, Thach BT. Respiratory origin of fluctuations in arterial blood pressure in premature infants with respiratory distress syndrome. Pediatrics 81:399–403, 1988.

69. Perlman JM, Goodman S, Kreusser KL, et al. Reduction of intraventricular hemorrhage by elimination of fluctuating cerebral blood flow velocity in preterm infants with respiratory distress syndrome. N Engl J Med 312:1253–7, 1985.

70. Jobe AH. Pulmonary surfactant therapy. N Engl J Med 328:861–8, 1993.

71. Bedard MP, Shankaran S, Slovis TL, et al. Effect of prophylactic phenobarbital on intraventricular hemorrhage in high risk infants. Pediatrics 73:435–9, 1984.

72. Donn S, Roloff DW, Goldstein GW. Prevention of intraventricular hemorrhage in preterm infants by phenobarbitone: a controlled trial. Lancet ii:215–17, 1981.

73. Kuban KC, Leviton A, Krishnamoorthy KS, et al. Neonatal intracranial hemorrhage and phenobarbital. Pediatrics 77:443–50, 1986.

74. Sinha S, Davis J, Tonger N, et al. Vitamin E supplementation reduces frequency of periventricular hemorrhage in very preterm infants. Lancet 11:466–71, 1987.

75. Morgan ME, Benson JT, Cooke RW. Ethamsylate reduces the incidence of periventricular haemorrhage in very low birthweight babies. Lancet 1:830–1, 1981.

76. Bada HS, Green RS, Pourcyrous M, et al. Indomethacin reduces the risk of severe intraventricular hemorrhage. J Pediatr 115:631–7, 1990.

77. Ment LR, Oh W, Ehrenkranz RA, et al. Low-dose indomethacin and prevention of intraventricular hemorrhage: a multicenter randomized trial. Pediatrics 94:543–50, 1994.

78. Edwards AD, Wyatt JS, Richardson C, et al. Effects of indomethacin on cerebral hemodynamics in very preterm infants. Lancet 335:491–5, 1990.

79. Pryds O, Griesen G, Johansen KH. Indomethacin and cerebral blood flow in preterm infants treated for patent ductus arterious. J Pediatr 147:315–16, 1988.

80. De Vries L, Wiggelsworth JS, Regev R, Dubowitz LM. Evaluation of periventricular leukomalacia during the neonatal period and infancy: correlation of imaging and postmortem findings. Early Hum Dev 17:205–19, 1988.

81. Paneth N, Rudelli R, Monte W, et al. White matter necrosis in the very low birth weight infants: neuropathologic and ultrasonographic findings in infants surviving six days or longer. J Pediatr 116:975–84, 1990.

82. De Vries LS, Regev R, Dubowitz LMS. Late onset cystic leukomalacia. Arch Dis Child 61:298–9, 1986.

83. De Vries LS, Regev R, Dubowitz LMS, et al. Perinatal risk factors for the development of extensive cystic leukomalacia. Am J Dis Child 142:732–5, 1988.

84. Leviton A, Paneth N. White matter damage in preterm newborns: an epidemiologic perspective. Early Hum Dev 24:1–22, 1990.

85. Perlman JM, Risser R, Broyles RS. Bilateral cystic periventricular leukomalacia in the premature infant: associated risk factors. Pediatrics 97:822–7, 1996.

86. Armstrong D, Norman MG. Periventricular leukomalacia in neonates: complications and sequelae. Arch Dis Child 49:367–75, 1974.

87. Banker BQ, Larroche JC. Periventricular leukomalacia of infancy: a form of neonatal anoxic encephalopathy. Arch Neurol 7:386–410, 1962.

88. De Reuck J, Chatta AS, Richardson Jr EP. Pathogenesis and evolution of periventricular leukomalacia in infancy. Arch Neurol 27:229–36, 1972.

89. De Reuck J. The human periventricular arterial blood supply and the anatomy of cerebral infarctions. Eur Neurol 5:321–34, 1971.

90. Takashima S, Tanaka K. Development of cerebrovascular architecture and its relationship to periventricular leukomalacia. Arch Neurol 35:11–16, 1978.

91. De Reuck J. Cerebral angioarchitecture and perinatal brain lesions in premature and full term infants. Acta Neurol Scand 70:391–5, 1984.

92. Rorke LB. Anatomic features of the developing brain implicated to hypoxic-ischemic injury. Brain Pathol 2:211–21, 1992.

93. Cavazzutti M, Duffy TE. Regulation of local cerebral blood flow in normal and hypoxic newborn dogs. Ann Neurol 11:247–57, 1982.

94. Szymonowicz W, Walker AM, Yu YH, et al. Regional cerebral blood flow after hemorrhagic hypotension in the preterm, near term and term lamb. Pediatr Res 28:361–70, 1990.

95. Young RSK, Hernandez MJ, Yagel SK. Selective reduction of blood flow to white matter during hypotension in newborn dogs: a possible mechanism of periventricular leukomalacia. Ann Neurol 12:445–8, 1982.

96. Faix RG, Donn SM. Association of septic shock caused by early onset Group B streptococcal sepsis and periventricular leukomalacia in the preterm infant. Pediatrics 76:415–19, 1985.

97. Fujimoto S, Togari H, Yamaguchi N, et al. Hypocarbia and cystic periventricular leukomalacia in premature infants. Arch Dis Child 71:F107–10, 1994.

98. Griesen G, Munck H, Lou H. Severe hypocarbia in preterm infants and neurodevelopmental deficit. Acta Paediatr Scand 76:401–4, 1986.

99. Low JA, Froese AF, Galbraith RS, et al. The association of fetal and newborn acidosis with severe periventricular leukomalacia in the preterm infant. Am J Obstet Gynecol 162:977–82, 1990.

100. Perlman JM, Hill A, Volpe JJ. The effect of patent ductus arteriosus on flow velocity in the anterior cerebral arteries: ductal steal in the premature newborn infant. J Pediatr 99:767–71, 1981.

101. Perlman JM, Volpe JJ. Episodes of apnea and bradycardia in the preterm newborn: impact on cerebral circulation. Pediatrics 76:333–8, 1985.

102. Wiswell TE, Graziani LJ, Kornhauser MS. Effects of hypocarbia on the development of cystic periventricular leukomalacia in premature infants treated with high frequency jet ventilation. Pediatrics 98:918–24, 1996.

103. Back SA, Volpe JJ. Cellular and molecular pathogenesis of periventricular white matter injury. MRDD Res Rev 3:96–107, 1997.

104. Yoon BH, Kim CJ, Romero CJ. Experimentally induced intrauterine infection causes fetal brain white matter lesions in rabbits. Am J Obstet Gynecol 177:797–802, 1997.

105. Yue X, Mehmet H, Penrie J, et al. Apoptosis and necrosis in the newborn piglet brain following transient cerebral hypoxia ischemia. Neuropathol Appl Neurobiol 23:16–25, 1997.

106. Chamnanvanakij S, Margraf LR, Burns D, Perlman JM. Apoptosis and white matter injury in preterm infants. Pediatr Dev Pathol 5, 2002.

107. Oka A, Belliveau MJ, Rosenberg PA, et al. Vulnerability of oligodendroglia to glutamate pharmacology, mechanisms and prevention. J Neurosci 13:1331–453, 1993.

108. Yonezawa M, Back SA, Gan X, et al. Cystine deprivation induces oligodendroglial death. Rescue by free radical scavengers and by a diffusible glial factor. J. Neurochem 67:566–73, 1996.

109. Gan XD, Back SA, Rosenberg PA, Volpe JJ. State-specific vulnerability of rat oligodendrocytes in culture to non-NMDA receptors mediated toxicity. Soc Neurosci 2:17420, 1997(abstract).

110. Yoshioka A, Bacskai B, Pleasure D. Pathophysiology of oligodendroglial excitotoxicity. J Neurosci Res 46:427, 1996.

111. Follett PL, Rosenberg RA, Volpe JJ, Jensen FG. NBQX attenuates excitotoxic injury in developing white matter. J Neurosci 20:9235–41, 2000.

112. Bona E, Andersson E, Blomgrun K, et al. Chemokines and inflammatory cell response to hypoxia ischemia in immature rats. Pediatr Res 45:500–9, 1999.

113. Selmaj K, Raine CS, Farooq M. Cytokine cytotoxicity against oliodendrocytes: apoptosis induced by lymphotoxin. J Immunol 147:1522–9, 1991.

114. Andrews T, Zhang P, Bhat NR. TNFα potentiates IFNγ-induced cell death in oligodendrocyte precursor. Neurosci Res 54:574–83, 1998.

115. Dommergues MA, Patkai J, Renauld JC, et al. Proinflammatory cytokines and interleukin 9 exacerbate excitotoxic lesions of the newborn murine neopallium. Ann Neurol 4:154–6, 2000.

116. Hansen-Pupp I, Harling S, Berg A, et al. Circulating interferon-gamma and white matter brain damage in preterm infants. Pediatr Res 58:946–52, 2005.

117. Saija A, Princi P, Lanza M, et al. Systemic cytokine administration can affect blood–brain permeability in the rat. Life Sci 56:775–84, 1995.

118. Nestlin WF, Gimbrone Jr MA. Neutrophil mediated damage to human vascular endothelium: role of cytokine activation. Am J Path 142:117–28, 1993.

119. Ando N, Takashima S, Mito M. Endotoxin, cerebral blood flow, amino acids and brain damage in young rabbits. Brain Dev 10:365–70, 1988.

120. Gilles FH, Leviton A, Kerr CS. Endotoxin leukoencephalopathy in the telencephalon of the newborn kitten. J Neurol Sci 27:183–91, 1976.

121. Zusban V, Gonzalez P, Lacaze Masmontiel T, et al. Periventricular leukomalacia: risk factors revisited. Dev Med Child Neurol 38:1066–70, 1996.

122. Leviton A, Pareth N, Reuss L, et al. Maternal infection, fetal inflammatory response and brain damage in very low birth weight infants. Pediatr Res 46:556–75, 1999.

123. Baud O, Emilie D, Pelletier E, et al. Amniotic fluid concentrations of interleukin-1beta, interleukin-6 and TNF-alpha in chorioamnionitis before 32 weeks of gestation: histological associations and neonatal outcome. Br J Obstet Gynaecol 106(1):72–7, 1999.

124. Hillier SL, Witkin SS, Krohn MA, et al. The relationship of amniotic fluid cytokines and preterm delivery, amniotic fluid infection, histologic chorioamnionitis and chorioamnion infection. Obstet Gynecol 174:330–4, 1996.

125. Saito S, Kasahara T, Kato Y, et al. Elevation of amniotic fluid interleukin-6 (IL-6), IL-8, and granulocyte stimulating factor (G-CSF) in term and preterm parturition. Cytokines 5:81–8, 1993.

126. Yoon BH, Jun JK, Romero R, et al. Interleukin-6 concentrations in umbilical cord plasma are elevated in neonates with white matter lesions associated with periventricular leukomalacia. Am J Obstet Gynecol 174:1433–40, 1996.

127. Grether JK, Nelson KD. Maternal infection and cerebral palsy in infants at normal birth weight. JAMA 278(3):207–11, 1997.

128. Grether JK, Nelson KB, Dambrosia JM, Philips TM. Interferons and cerebral palsy. J Pediatr 134:324–32, 1999.

129. Wu YW, Colford JM Jr. Chorioamnionitis as a risk factor of cerebral palsy: a meta-analysis. JAMA 284(11):1417–24, 2000 (review).

130. Deguchi K, Mizoguchi M, Takashima S. Immunohistochemical expression of tumor necrosis factor α in neonatal leukomalacia. Pediatr Neurol 14:6–13, 1996.

131. Yoon BH, Romero R, Kim CJ, et al. High expression of tumor necrosis factor α and interleukin 6 in periventricular leukomalacia. Am J Obstet Gynecol 177:406–11, 1997.

132. Bonce AJ, Boling W, Kindy MS, et al. Altered neuronal and microglial response to excitotoxic and ischemic brain injury in mice lacking TNF receptor. Nat Med 2:788–94, 1996.

133. Graziani LJ, Spitzer AR, Mitchell DG, et al. Mechanical ventilation in preterm infants: neurosonographic and developmental studies. Pediatrics 90:515–22, 1992.

134. Trounce JQ, Shaw DE, Levene MI, Rutter N. Clinical risk factors and periventricular leukomalacia. Arch Dis Child 63:17–22, 1988.

135. Weindling AM, Wilkinson AR, Cook F, et al. Perinatal events, which precede periventricular hemorrhage and leukomalacia in the newborn. Br J Obstet Gynecol 92:1218–23, 1985.

136. Mirro R, Buslta D, Green R, et al. Relationship between mean airway pressure, cardiac output and organ blood flow with normal and decreased respiratory compliance. J Pediatr 111:101–6, 1987.

137. Phelps DL, Rosenbaum AL, Isenberg SJ, et al. Tocopherol efficacy and safety for preventing retinopathy of prematurity: a randomized controlled, boule-masked trial. Pediatrics 79:489–500, 1987.

138. Stewart AL, Reynolds EOR, Hope RL, et al. Probability of neurodevelopmental disorders estimated from ultrasound appearance of brains of very preterm infants. Dev Med Child Neurol 29:3–11, 1987.

139. Fazzi E, Lanzi G, Gerardo A, et al. Neurodevelopmental outcome in very low birth weight infants with or without periventricular hemorrhage and/or leukomalacia. Acta Paediatr 81:808–11, 1992.

140. Roger B, Msall M, Owens T, et al. Cystic periventricular leukomalacia and type of cerebral palsy in preterm infants. J Pediatr 125:51–8, 1994.

141. Inder TE, Anderson NJ, Spencer C, et al. White matter injury in the premature infant: a comparison between serial cranial sonographic and MR findings at term. Am J Neuroradiol 24: 805–9, 2003.

142. Wood ward LJ, Anderson PJ, Austin NC, et al. Neonatal MRI to predict neurodevelopment outcome in preterm infants. N Engl J Med 355:685–94, 2006.

143. De Vries LS, Connell JA, Dubowitz LMS, et al. Neurological electrophysiological and MRI abnormalities in infants with extensive cystic leukomalacia. Neuropediatrics 18:61–6, 1987.

144. De Vries LS, Eken P, Groenendaal F, et al. Correlation between the degree of periventricular leukomalacia using cranial ultrasound and MRI in infancy, in children with cerebral palsy. Neuropediatrics 24:263–8, 1993.

145. Jacobson LK, Dutton GN. Periventricular leukomalacia: an important cause of visual and ocular motility dysfunction in children. Surv Ophthalmol 45(1):1–13, 2000 (review).

146. Melhem ER, Hoon AH, Ferrucci JT, et al. Periventricular leukomalacia: relationship between lateral ventricular volume on brain MR images and severity of cognitive and motor impairment. Radiology 214(1):199–204, 2000.

147. Scher MS, Dobson V, Carpenter NA, Guthrie RD. Visual and neurological outcome of infants with periventricular leukomalacia. Dev Med Child Neurol 31:353–65, 1989.

148. Volpe JJ. Encephalopathy of prematurity includes neuronal abnormalities. Pediatrics 116: 221–5, 2005.

149. Inder TE, Huppi PS, Warfield S, et al. Periventricular white matter at term is followed by reduced cerebral cortical gray matter at term. Ann Neurol 46:755–60, 1999.

150. de Groot JC, de Leeuw FE, Oudkerk M, et al. Periventricular white matter lesions predict rate of cognitive decline. Ann Neurol 52:335–41, 2002.

151. Perlman JM. Neurobehavioral deficits in premature graduates of intensive care: potential medical and environmental risk factors. Pediatrics 108:1339–48, 2001.

Chapter 4

Posthemorrhagic Hydrocephalus Management Strategies

Andrew Whitelaw, MD, FRCPCH

Question 1. What Measurements of Ventricular Size are Used in Diagnosis of PHVD?

Question 2. How Can We Distinguish Ventricular Dilatation Driven by CSF Under Pressure From Ventricular Dilatation Due to Loss of Periventricular White Matter?

Question 3. How Do We Define Excessive Head Enlargement?

Question 4. How Do We Recognize Raised Intracranial Pressure?

Question 5. What is Infant A's Prognosis?

Question 6. What is the Mechanism of PHVD?

Question 7. How Can PHVD Injure White Matter?

Question 8. What Interventions Have Been Used in PHVD and is there any Evidence of Improving Outcome?

Objectives in Treating PHVD

Current Management Strategy

Areas where Further Research is Needed

Hemorrhage into the ventricles of the brain is one of the most serious complications of premature birth despite improvements in the survival of premature infants. Large intraventricular hemorrhage (IVH) has a high risk of neurological disability and over 50% of these children go on to develop progressive ventricular dilatation (1). Increasing survival of extremely premature infants is associated with posthemorrhagic ventricular dilatation (PHVD) with high morbidity and considerable mortality (2). Overall, approximately two-thirds of these children develop cerebral palsy and about one-third have multiple impairments (3, 4). The term posthemorrhagic hydrocephalus is generally reserved for cases where PHVD is persistent and associated with excessive head enlargement. This condition still does not have a safe and effective "cure" but advances in our understanding of the pathophysiology and experience from clinical trials allow us to suggest some guidelines on assessment and management and to identify gaps in knowledge where further advances are needed.

CASE HISTORY

Infant A. A mother in her third pregnancy suffered a placental abruption at 28 weeks. The infant is male and weighed 877 g. He was intubated at birth and received surfactant prophylactically. He was ventilated at low pressures and low oxygen requirement until, on day 2, he suffered a pulmonary hemorrhage with a period of hypotension (mean arterial pressure below 25 mmHg for 2 hours) corrected by use of dopamine and blood transfusion. His respiratory status stabilized within hours. On day 3 a cranial ultrasound scan showed bilateral intraventricular hemorrhage (Figs. 4-1A and 4-1B). He progressed from minimal ventilation settings to nasal continuous positive airway pressure (CPAP). He was then scanned twice a week. Ventricular dimensions progressively enlarged until day 18 (Fig. 4-1C).

Head circumference has increased by 1.5 cm over 7 days. A lumbar puncture produced 14 mL (10 mL/kg). This reduced head circumference by 0.3 cm. Two days later, head circumference had increased by 0.5 cm from the post tap measurement. A second lumbar puncture was carried out and produced 14 mL (10 mL/kg). Head circumference decreased by 0.3 cm but then increased by 0.5 cm from the post tap measurement 2 days later. A third lumbar puncture produced only 6 mL before flow stopped. Head circumference did not decrease, the fontanel remained full, and ultrasound confirmed that the ventricles were still ballooned. A ventricular tap was carried out on the left side and 10 mL/kg removed.

As there was a need for repeated tapping of cerebrospinal fluid (CSF) and repeated lumbar puncture was becoming impractical, a ventricular access device (Ommaya reservoir) was inserted frontally in the right ventricle under general anesthesia. An amount of 15 mL (10 mL/kg) of CSF was removed at the time of insertion. In order to be sure of avoiding raised pressure and resultant CSF leak with a risk of infection, the reservoir was tapped at 10 mL/kg daily for 5 days. Following this, the reservoir was tapped as required to control excessive expansion or suspected pressure symptoms. Head circumference enlargement necessitated tapping 10 mL/kg every 1–2 days. When he was weaned from nasal CPAP to nasal catheter oxygen, apneas increased at the time of head expansion and decreased following tapping. Pressure measurement at the start of tapping typically showed a pressure of 6–7 mmHg. After 10 mL/kg had been removed, pressure had fallen to 3 mmHg.

This regime of tapping as required was reviewed every 7 days to confirm that head enlargement in 1 week had not been excessive. CSF protein was initially 4.1 g/L. Tapping the reservoir continued to be necessary for 6 weeks and, on a few days, it was obvious that 10 mL/kg had been insufficient to control head enlargement and the subsequent tap had been increased to 15 mL/kg. CSF protein continued to remain high (1.8–2.0 g/L) and tapping was continued for a further 2 weeks, by which time CSF protein had decreased to 1.45 g/L and the baby's weight had increased to nearly 2500 g. Nasal catheter oxygen was no longer required. A ventriculoperitoneal low-pressure shunt was inserted under general anesthesia when the infant reached full term. Postoperatively there was no pulmonary problem, CSF leak, or infection but the infant needed to be on a considerable head-up tilt to facilitate adequate shunt function and control of head circumference. Although control of head circumference and suspected pressure had been maintained, the ventricles remained large.

QUESTION 1. WHAT MEASUREMENTS OF VENTRICULAR SIZE ARE USED IN DIAGNOSIS OF PHVD?

The chances of progressive ventricular dilatation increase with the amount of blood visible in the ventricles. With a small IVH (grade 2 on the Papile scale (5) or 2a on

De Vries's grading (6)), measurement of ventricular size once a week for 4 weeks and then at discharge is appropriate but with a large IVH (grade 3 Papile (5) or 2b on De Vries's grading (6)), twice weekly ultrasound dilatation is likely and may be rapid. Although large balloon-shaped ventricles are obvious without formal measurements, quantitative documentation is essential if serial scans are being done by different ultrasonographers and in epidemiological studies and clinical trials. Reference ranges for measurement of the width (midline to lateral border) of the lateral ventricles at the mid-coronal level (Fig. 4-1C) were first published in 1981 (7). Since 1984, an action line 4 mm above the 97th centile for age has been used as a definition of serious PHVD in therapeutic trials (3, 4) and as a secondary outcome in randomized trials of neonatal intensive care interventions (Fig. 4-2A).

This measurement has the advantage that it is highly reproducible between observers since it is relatively unaffected by angulation of the scan head anteriorly or posteriorly as the lateral wall of the ventricle in this orientation runs fairly parallel

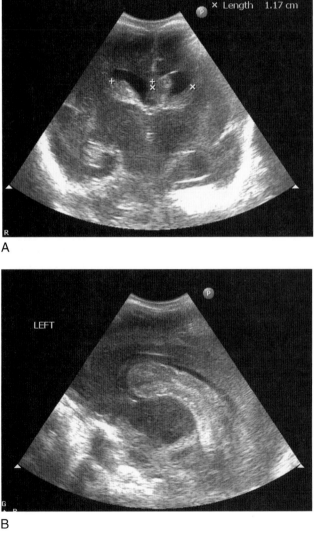

A

B

Figure 4-1 (A) Infant A. Cranial ultrasound, mid-coronal view, on day 3, showing hemorrhage in both lateral ventricles. (B) Infant A. Cranial ultrasound, left parasagittal view, on day 3 showing extensive blood clot within the left lateral ventricle.

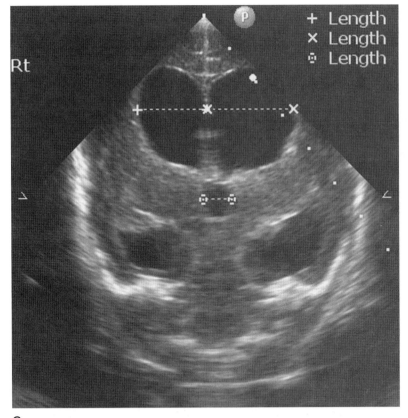

C

Figure 4-1. cont'd, (C) Infant A. Cranial ultrasound, mid-coronal view, on day 18, showing enlargement of both lateral ventricles and the third ventricle.

to the midline. The frequency of PHVD using this definition is 1 in 2500 to 1 in 3000 births among residents of Bristol, UK. However, ventricular enlargement is not always sideways and sometimes the most marked changes are enlargement posteriorly or a change from thin slit to round balloon. With this in mind, Davies et al. (8) published reference ranges for anterior horn width (to capture the change in shape to balloon; 97th centile approximately 3 mm) (Fig. 4-2B), thalamo-occipital (to capture posterior enlargement; 97th centile approximately 25 mm) (Fig. 4-2C), third ventricular width (97th centile approximately 2 mm)

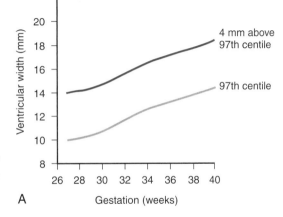

Figure 4-2 (A) 97th centile for ventricular width with the 97th centile + 4 mm line as criterion for diagnosis of PHVD. (Modified from Levene M. Measurement of the growth of the lateral ventricles in preterm infants with real-time ultrasound. Arch Dis Child 56:900–4, 1981.)

A

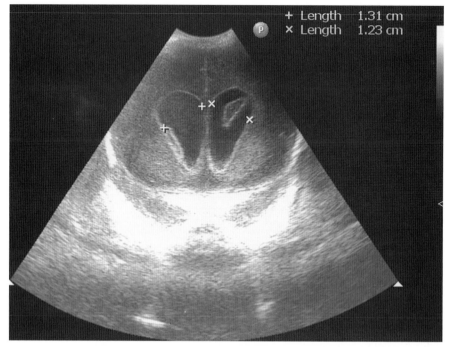

B

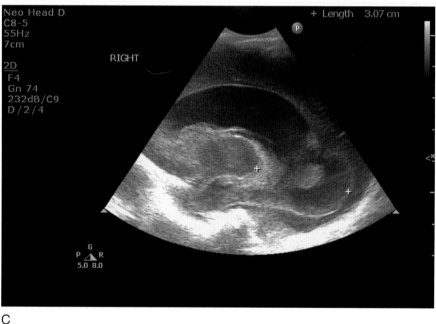

C

Figure 4-2. cont'd, (B) Infant A. Cranial ultrasound coronal view frontally on day 18 showing the anterior horn width marked with calipers (×). (C) Infant A. Cranial ultrasound right parasagittal view on day 18 showing the thalamo-occipital dimension with calipers (×).

(Fig. 4-1C), and fourth ventricular width. We have found the anterior horn width, thalamo-occipital, and third ventricular width to be practical and useful but with greater interobserver variation. We have used all three measurements since 2003 requiring all three measurements (bilaterally) to be 1 mm over the 97th centile as criteria for PHVD. Fourth ventricular width we have found too challenging to achieve reproducible measurements and we do not use this routinely.

QUESTION 2. HOW CAN WE DISTINGUISH VENTRICULAR DILATATION DRIVEN BY CSF UNDER PRESSURE FROM VENTRICULAR DILATATION DUE TO LOSS OF PERIVENTRICULAR WHITE MATTER?

This distinction is important as removing fluid which has accumulated as a replacement for dead brain is unlikely to improve outcome.

CSF-driven ventricular enlargement can be slow or rapid, is characterized by balloon-shaped lateral ventricles, and, if CSF pressure is measured, it is raised or near the upper limit of normal (mean 3 mmHg, upper limit 6 mmHg (9)). Furthermore, head circumference growth over time will be accelerated although this may lag behind ventricular enlargement by 1–2 weeks. In contrast, ventricular enlargement from atrophy is always slow, is more irregular in outline rather than balloon shaped, and, if CSF pressure is measured, it is not raised. Head circumference velocity is either normal or slow but is not accelerated. Nonprogressive mild ventricular dilatation at term is widely recognized as a marker of periventricular leukomalacia.

QUESTION 3. HOW DO WE DEFINE EXCESSIVE HEAD ENLARGEMENT?

Head circumference enlarges by approximately 1 mm per day between 26 weeks of gestation and 32 weeks, and about 0.7 mm per day between 32 and 40 weeks (9). We regard a persistent increase of 2 mm per day as excessive. Measuring head circumference accurately, although low-tech, is not as easy as it sounds. The relevant measurement is the maximum fronto-occipital circumference. Detecting a difference of 1 mm from day to day is difficult and we do not react to a difference of 2 mm from one day to the next unless there is other evidence of raised intracranial pressure. However, an increase of 4 mm over 2 days is more likely to be real and an increase of 14 mm over 7 days is definitely excessive.

QUESTION 4. HOW DO WE RECOGNIZE RAISED INTRACRANIAL PRESSURE?

We may detect a change in palpation of the fontanel from concave to bulging and, as described above, we can document excessive head enlargement. The preterm skull is very compliant and can easily accommodate an increase in CSF by expanding with separation of the sutures. When CSF pressure was measured with an electronic transducer in infants expanding their ventricles after IVH, the mean CSF pressure was approximately 9 mmHg, three times the mean in normal infants (9). There was a considerable range, with some infants expanding their ventricles and heads at a pressure of 5–6 mmHg and a small number with CSF pressure around 15 mmHg. A CSF pressure of 9 mmHg does not necessarily produce clinical signs but may be associated with an increase in apnea or vomiting, hypotinia, hypertonia, or decreased alertness. A structured neurological examination of the newborn such as that published by Dubowitz et al. (11) is recommended.

Serial Doppler resistance index (RI) on the anterior cerebral artery is a useful and practical way of detecting impairment of cerebral perfusion by raised intracranial pressure and can easily be done during ultrasound imaging. Resistance index is systolic velocity − diastolic velocity/systolic velocity. This measurement is independent of the angle of insonation. If intracranial pressure rises to a level exceeding the infant's compensation, end-diastolic velocity tends to decrease, eventually becoming zero (RI is then 1.0) (Fig. 4-3).

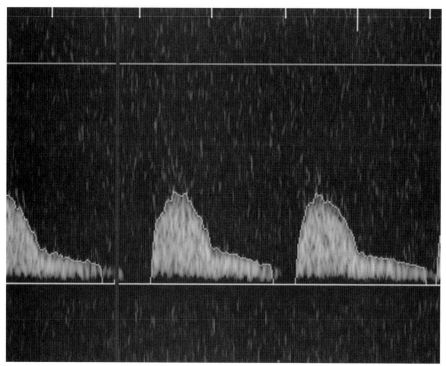

Figure 4-3 Cerebral blood flow velocity Doppler spectra from an infant with PHVD and intracranial pressure of 15 mmHg. There is loss of end-diastolic velocities. When the pressure was reduced to 6 mmHg, end-diastolic velocities returned.

A serial increase in RI while the ventricles are rapidly expanding would be evidence that pressure was rising (12). This assumes that the infant does not have a significant left-to-right shunt at ductal level or that pCO_2 has not decreased recently as both these physiological changes can increase RI. Severe intracranial hypertension may cause reversed end-diastolic velocities. The sensitivity of RI can be increased by applying pressure to the fontanel during the examination. An infant who is close to the limit of cranial compliance responds by a large decrease in end-diastolic velocities, i.e., an increase in RI (13).

Other physiological changes with rising intracranial pressure are somatosensory evoked potentials (14). However, there are very few neonatal units where serial evoked potentials are a practical investigation after IVH.

QUESTION 5. WHAT IS INFANT A'S PROGNOSIS?

The prognosis at diagnosis of PHVD using the above criteria is influenced by the presence of identifiable parenchymal lesions. The Ventriculomegaly and PHVD Drug Trial used the 4 mm + 97th centile definition of PHVD and had standardized follow-up. If careful ultrasound examination shows no persistent echodensities or echolucencies (cysts), then approximately 40% of the children will develop cerebral palsy and about 25% will have multiple impairments (3, 4).

The presence of extensive haemorrhagic parenchymal infarction (Fig. 4-4), in addition to PHVD, increases risk of cerebral palsy from around 40% to 80–90% (3, 4) and large amounts of blood clot within the ventricles after IVH increase the risk of later shunt dependence.

Cerebral magnetic resonance imaging (MRI) at term is increasingly used to assess infants with PHVD as this technique can reveal parenchymal injury that

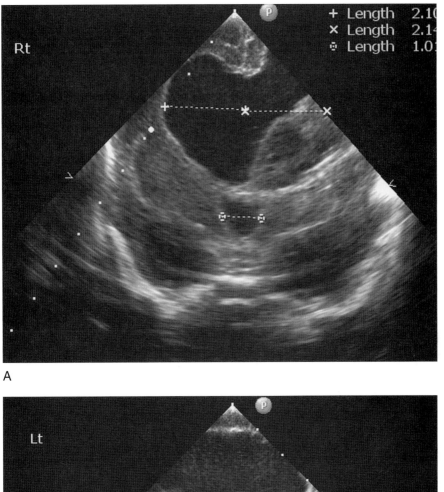

A

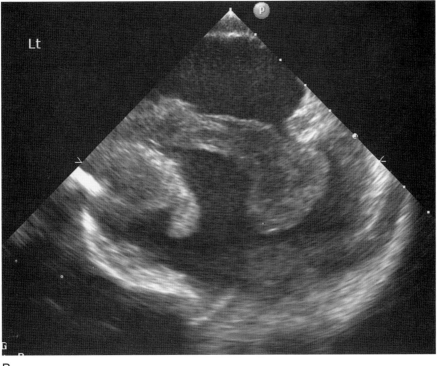

B

Figure 4-4 Cranial ultrasound, coronal view (A) and left parasagittal (B) of an infant with PHVD showing a large amount of clot within the left ventricle and a parenchymal infarction communicating with the left ventricle.

cannot be easily demonstrated with ultrasound (15). These lesions include abnormal signal in the white matter without cyst formation, gray matter abnormality, and cerebellar secondary atrophy.

QUESTION 6. WHAT IS THE MECHANISM OF PHVD?

Following a large IVH, multiple blood clots can obstruct the ventricular system or channels of reabsorption initially leading to an initial phase of CSF accumulation. Although tissue plasminogen activator can be demonstrated in posthemorrhagic CSF, fibrinolysis is very inefficient in the CSF, due to low levels of plasminogen and high levels of plasminogen activator inhibitor (16, 17). This potentially reversible obstruction by thrombi may lead to a chronic obliterative, fibrosing arachnoiditis, and subependymal gliosis (18) involving deposition of extracellular matrix proteins in the foramina of the fourth ventricle and the subarachnoid space (19). Figure 4-5A shows the brainstem and cerebellum of an infant with PHVD who died aged 2 months. A layer of collagenous connective tissue surrounds the brainstem. Figure 4-5B shows perivascular deposition of the extracellular matrix protein laminin in the subependymal region in another infant with PHVD who died aged 2 months.

Heep et al. (20) found that levels of the carboxyterminal propeptide of type I procollagen were significantly higher in the CSF of neonates with PHVD, 3 to 4 weeks after IVH, than in those with congenital hydrocephalus that was not due to ventricular hemorrhage.

Transforming growth factor beta (TGFβ) is likely to be a key mediator of this process as TGFβ is involved in the initiation of wound healing and fibrosis (21). TGFβ elevates the expression of genes encoding fibronectin, various types of collagen (22, 23), and other extracellular matrix components (24), and is involved in a number of serious diseases involving excessive deposition of collagen and extracellular matrix, including diabetic nephropathy (24) and cirrhosis (25). TGFβ has three isoforms, TGFβ1, -β2, and -β3. TGFβ1 is stored in platelets. Thus IVH by definition provides a store of TGFβ1 for many weeks in the CSF. TGFβ is elevated in the CSF of adults with hydrocephalus after subarachnoid hemorrhage and intrathecal administration of TGFβ to mice resulted in hydrocephalus (26, 27). We have demonstrated that CSF from infants with PHVD has TGFβ1 and -β2 concentrations which are 10 to 20 times those of nonhemorrhagic CSFs and that the concentration of TGFβ in CSF is predictive of later shunt surgery (28). Heep et al. have confirmed elevated TGFβ1 in posthemorrhagic hydrocephalus CSF and also demonstrated that a product of TGFβ, aminoterminal propeptide of type 1 collagen, was elevated (29). Chow et al. demonstrated elevation of TGFβ2 and nitrated chondroitin sulfate proteoglycans (an extracellular matrix protein) in posthemorrhagic hydrocephalus CSF (30).

We have recently used a rat pup model of PHVD to look at the possible role of TGFβ in PHVD (31). Very little TGFβ1, -β2, or β3 is immunohistochemically demonstrable in the brain of 21-day-old normal rats. In contrast, in 21-day-old rats that had received intraventricular injections of blood on day 7 and 8, immunoreactivity for all three isoforms of TGFβ was significantly elevated. TGFβ1 was present in the periventricular white matter, TGFβ2 in neurones and periventricular oligodendrocytes, and TGFβ3 in oligodendrocytes and reactive microglia. TGFβ1 and -β2 levels were elevated in injected animals and TGFβ1 was significantly related to the severity of hydrocephalus. The increase in TGFβ was accompanied by an increase in phosphorylated p44/42 MAP kinases (P-Erk1/2) – downstream intracellular mediators of several of the effects of TGFβ – in a distribution similar to that of TGFβ1 and -β2, and by deposition of the extracellular matrix proteins fibronectin, laminin, and vitronectin (32).

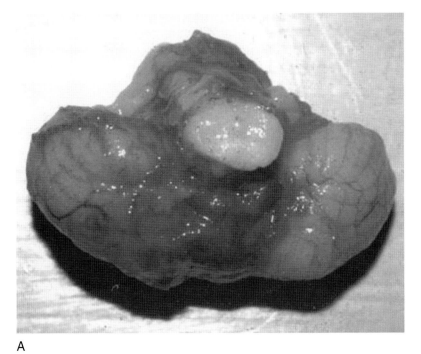

A

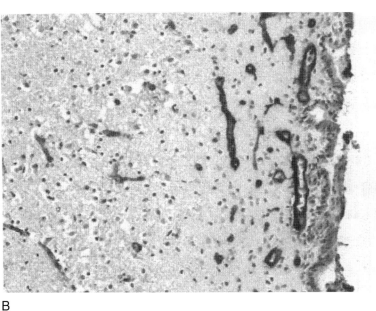

B

Figure 4-5 (A) Brainstem and cerebellum of an infant with PHVD who died aged 2 months. In addition to the brown staining from old blood, there are gray strands of connective tissue wrapped around the brainstem. (B) Subependymal region of the brain of an infant with PHVD who died aged 2 months. Immunostaining shows increased perivascular deposition of the extracellular matrix protein laminin.

Transgenic mice which overexpress TGFβ1 in the central nervous system are born with hydrocephalus (33). Thus there is a strong possibility of a role for TGFβ in the development and/or maintenance of hydrocephalus after ventricular hemorrhage. However, the time course is not fully understood and we do not know whether interventions that interfere with the production and/or actions of TGFβ prevent PHVD.

QUESTION 7. HOW CAN PHVD INJURE WHITE MATTER?

Damage to periventricular white matter is probably exacerbated by ischemia due to raised intracranial pressure and parenchymal compression, by oxidative stress due to the generation of free radicals, and by the actions of inflammatory cytokines.

Raised Intracranial Pressure, Parenchymal Compression, and Ischemia

PHVD raises CSF pressure to, on average, three times the normal (10). Figure 4-3 shows that an intracranial pressure of 15 mmHg was high enough to prevent cerebral blood flow during diastole. Cerebral perfusion was restored when the pressure was reduced to 6 mmHg. Clearly, a reduction of perfusion of this magnitude substantially increases the risk of ischemic injury. There is also evidence that distortion of periventricular axons due to ventricular dilatation may cause injury independently of ischemia (34).

Free Radical-Mediated Injury

Nonprotein-bound iron is readily detectable in the CSF of neonates with PHVD (35). Hemoglobin that enters the CSF as a result of IVH releases large amounts of iron, which is likely to exceed the protein-binding capacity of the CSF and lead to the generation of hydroxyl free radicals from hydrogen peroxide via the Fenton reaction. Inder et al. (36) demonstrated products of lipid peroxidation in the CSF of infants with periventricular leukomalacia. Whether these are also present in PHVD has not yet been investigated. Further evidence of potential oxidative stress comes from the finding of raised concentrations of hypoxanthine in the CSF of infants with PHVD (37). Normally, xanthine and hypoxanthine are oxidized by xanthine dehydrogenase to form uric acid, with NAD^+ as the electron acceptor. However, under conditions of ischemia, xanthine dehydrogenase is modified to form xanthine oxidase, which uses oxygen as the electron acceptor (38). On restoration of cerebral perfusion, xanthine oxidase-mediated oxidation of xanthine and hypoxanthine generates superoxide and hydrogen peroxide, which cause oxidative damage. Oligodendrocyte progenitors are relatively abundant in the periventricular white matter of premature infants and are highly susceptible to oxidative damage (39).

Proinflammatory Cytokines

Clinical evidence suggests that inflammation causes damage to immature white matter (40). The concentrations of tumor necrosis factor-α, interleukin-1β, interleukin-6, interleukin-8, and interferon-γ are significantly elevated in the CSF of infants with PHVD (41). Tumor necrosis factor-α and interleukin-1β have both been implicated in the development of periventricular leukomalacia (42), and it seems likely that these proinflammatory cytokines also contribute to white matter damage in PHVD.

Loss of White and Gray Matter

In the rat model of PHVD, there is a significant negative correlation between the extent of ventricular dilatation and both the thickness of the corpus callosum and that of the frontal cortex (43). The development of hydrocephalus is associated with a mean reduction in the thickness of the corpus callosum of 48%, and of the frontal cortex of 31%. Loss of white matter is also marked in the lateral periventricular region, where we have shown that loss of myelin and axons is associated with a reduced density of oligodendrocytes (43).

QUESTION 8. WHAT INTERVENTIONS HAVE BEEN USED IN PHVD AND IS THERE ANY EVIDENCE OF IMPROVING OUTCOME?

Ventriculoperitoneal shunt surgery

Ventriculoperitoneal (VP) shunt surgery is the conventional approach for other types of established hydrocephalus (Fig. 4-6). Treatment of PHVD is more difficult than other types of hydrocephalus because the large amount of blood in the ventricles combined with the small size and instability of the patient make an early VP shunt operation impossible. In one series of 19 infants with PHVD requiring shunt surgery, there were 29 shunt blockages and 12 infections (44). The risk of shunt blockage was increased if the CSF protein was over 1.5 g/L at the time of shunt insertion. In a series of 36 infants shunt-operated for PHVD, shunt blockage and infection occurred only in those operated before 35 days of age (45). There is a considerable complication rate throughout the child's life from such surgery and the child is permanently dependent on the shunt system.

A VP shunt is a treatment but not a cure and the child is vulnerable to shunt dysfunction. Shunt blockage after the cranial sutures have fused can rapidly raise intracranial pressure with permanent cerebral damage resulting. Cases of sudden blindness and death have been recorded in such circumstances. Repeated shunt revisions are associated with a worsening of neurologic outcome (46). Shunt infection is another complication which can further injure the developing brain.

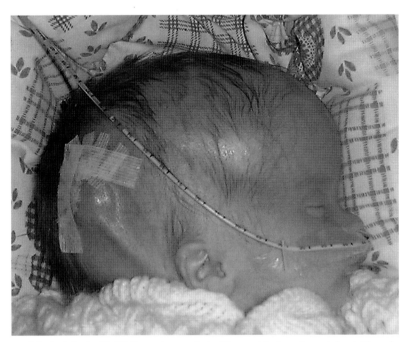

Figure 4-6 An infant with PHVD newly operated with a ventriculoperitoneal shunt. The valve and catheter are visible under the skin.

Table 4-1	Therapeutic Interventions which have been Used in Infants with PHVD

Repeated early lumbar punctures/ventricular taps
Diuretic drugs to reduce CSF production
Intraventricular fibrinolytic therapy
External ventricular drain
Ventricular reservoir and repeated taps
Third ventriculostomy
Choroid plexus coagulation
Ventriculoperitoneal shunt after CSF clears and protein <1.5 g/L
Drainage, irrigation, and fibrinolytic therapy
None are both safe and effective

OBJECTIVES IN TREATING PHVD

1. To minimize the need for VP shunt.
2. To reduce secondary injury to the brain from pressure, distortion, free radical, and inflammation during the period of up to 3 months before a VP shunt becomes technically feasible and unavoidable.
3. To minimize iatrogenic injury from interventions, especially in those infants where PHVD resolves after a period of weeks.

Some therapeutic interventions that have been used in infants with PHVD are listed in Table 4-1.

Repeated Lumbar Punctures or Ventricular Taps

Repeated lumbar punctures (LP) were suggested as a way of controlling pressure, preventing progressive ventricular enlargement, and removing some of the red cells and protein from the CSF. Kressuer et al. showed that a minimum of 10 mL/kg needed to be removed in order to have a significant effect on ventricular size (47). In contrast to older children and adults, "coning" after lumbar puncture in the presence of raised intracranial pressure is extremely rare in neonates. This is probably due to the pressure being only mildly raised in infants with open fontanels and sutures. Having done hundreds of lumbar punctures in infants with slightly raised pressure, I have not seen any infant with PHVD cone. It is, however, wise to limit the volume of CSF removed to a maximum of 20 mL/kg and larger volumes removed faster than 1 mL/kg/min may be followed by apnea, bradycardia, and desaturation. In our experience, only a minority of infants with PHVD have consistently communicating PHVD with a sufficient yield of CSF. Tapping of ventricular CSF has therefore to be considered. A policy of repeated early tapping lumbar or ventricular CSF for PHVD has been tested in four controlled clinical trials (48). Overall there was no evidence that this approach reduced VP shunt surgery or disability and there was 7% infection among the infants who had repeated tapping in the ventriculomegaly trial (4).

Drug Treatment to Reduce CSF Production

Faced with this lack of effect and risk of infection from invasive procedures, pharmacologic treatment to reduce CSF production seemed an excellent approach. Acetazolamide had been in clinical use for benign intracranial hypertension and appeared to have acceptable adverse effects as long as electrolyte and acid–base were monitored. Uncontrolled reports were positive about the effect of acetazolamide in PHVD. Further work showed that acetazolamide produced an initial increase in cerebral blood flow mediated by an increase in tissue CO_2 and inhibition of respiratory elimination of CO_2 (49). Clinical investigation of infants with chronic lung disease of prematurity showed that acetazolamide produced an increase in pCO_2 (50). Eventually a large multicenter randomized trial of acetazolamide combined with furosemide (which also reduces CSF production) was carried out. Not only was there no clinical benefit but, to many neonatologists' surprise, the group receiving the combined drug treatment had significantly worse outcome in terms of shunt surgery and death or disability (51).

Intraventricular Fibrinolytic Therapy

The idea of injecting a fibrinolytic agent intraventricularly grew out of: (i) Pang's PHVD model in which blood was injected intraventricularly into dogs, where 80% developed hydrocephalus but if urokinase was injected intraventricularly, only 10% became hydrocephalic (52); (ii) our own laboratory work showing that there was weak endogenous fibrinolytic activity in posthemorrhagic CSF (16, 17); and (iii) the relative safety and effectiveness of low-dose fibrinolyic therapy administered locally. A number of small nonrandomized trials of intraventricular streptokinase, urokinase, and tissue plasminogen activator (TPA), as well as one small randomized trial, have collectively shown that there is no reduction in VP shunt surgery and there is a risk of secondary intraventricular bleeding (53). This finding can be understood in terms of the TGFβ hypothesis. As TGFβ is stored in platelets, lysing thrombi will release TGFβ more rapidly into the CSF (28); if the released TGFβ is not removed or drained, this will assist the production of extracellular matrix proteins which "glue up" the channels of reabsorption of CSF.

External Ventricular Drain

The insertion of an external ventricular drain is a logical way of providing continuous relief from raised pressure, preventing distortion from ventricular enlargement and removing protein and red cells. This approach has certainly been used in a small number of centers but to our knowledge this has not been tested in a randomized trial (54). This is a neurosurgical procedure and a concern among neurosurgeons has been the risk of infection from prolonged presence of a ventricular drain.

Tapping CSF via an Ommaya Reservoir

The most widely used approach we have encountered in neonatal units that see a considerable number of infants with PHVD is the insertion of a ventricular access device, an Ommaya reservoir, in those cases where repeated tapping is necessary to control excessive head enlargement and suspected raised pressure (Fig. 4-7). This approximates the conservative arm of the Ventriculomegaly and PHVD Drug Trials and, in our, view, should be regarded as standard treatment now (55). Not all infants with PHVD demonstrate excessive head enlargement or signs of raised pressure so this is a selective approach. Once it becomes obvious that repeated CSF tapping is necessary, the surgically inserted reservoir enables this to be done whenever the need arises and can be done in a small peripheral neonatal unit without neurosurgical staff or neonatologists familiar with ventricular tapping (55). It is clear that in units with sufficient volume of patients, a ventricular access device can be inserted into extremely small infants (e.g., 700 g) with a very low complication rate. In Bristol, UK, a total of 50 such procedures have been carried out in preterm infants with no cases of peroperative mortality or infection. There is currently a trial of this approach in the Netherlands comparing two different entry criteria, one being ventricular width over the 97th centile and the other being 4 mm over the 97th centile.

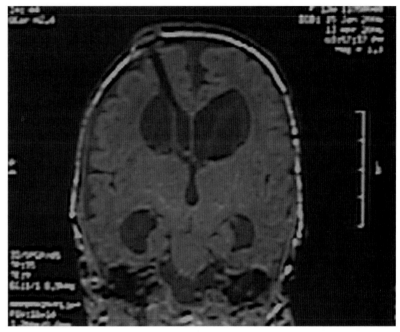

Figure 4-7 MRI scan (T1 weighted) coronal view showing ventricular dilatation with a subcutaneous Ommaya reservoir and catheter to the right lateral ventricle.

Third Ventriculostomy

Third ventriculostomy is carried out endoscopically and can be a good treatment for other types of hydrocephalus, especially aqueduct stenosis. The endoscope is inserted into the ventricular system and then into the third ventricle. A hole is made in the midline of the floor of the third ventricle, carefully avoiding the arteries on either side. This communication between the third ventricle and the subarachnoid space allows CSF to bypass obstruction in the aqueduct and foramina of the fourth ventricle. However, in PHVD, the problem is reabsorption of CSF and is not usually restricted to the aqueduct and fourth ventricle. Experience with third ventriculostomy in PHVD has been limited and disappointing (56).

Choroid Plexus Coagulation

Choroid plexus coagulation is carried out endoscopically and is based on the fact that most CSF production comes from the choroid plexus within the lateral ventricles and third ventricle. As the problem with PHVD is primarily failed reabsorption and not overproduction of CSF, it would seem unlikely that this approach would be successful in PHVD. Choroid plexus coagulation has never been subjected to a controlled trial in PHVD (57).

Drainage, Irrigation, and Fibrinolytic Therapy

Drainage, irrigation, and fibrinolytic therapy (DRIFT) is an approach that grew out of the unsatisfactory results of the above treatments and the emerging evidence that permanent hydrocephalus develops partly as a cytokine response to intraventricular blood over several weeks. The objective is to remove as much as possible of the intraventricular blood before hydrocephalus becomes irreversible.

The procedure involves insertion of right frontal and left occipital ventricular catheters. TPA is injected intraventricularly at a dose that is insufficient to produce a systemic effect and this is left for approximately 8 hours. Artificial CSF (Torbay Pharmaceutical, Paignton, UK) is then pumped into the frontal ventricular catheter at 20 mL/h with continuous intracranial pressure monitoring. The occipital ventricular catheter is connected to a sterile close ventricular drainage system and the height of the drainage reservoir adjusted to maintain intracranial pressure below 7 mmHg. The drainage fluid initially looks like cola but gradually clears to look like white wine, at which point irrigation is stopped and the catheters removed. This commonly takes 72 hours but can be up to 7 days. Figure 4-8 shows MRI documenting the removal of intraventricular debris with this procedure.

A pilot study at Southmead Hospital, Bristol, UK, recruited 25 infants with the same criteria for PHVD as in the Ventriculomegaly Trial and PHVD Drug Trial, i.e., ventricular width 4 mm over the 97th centile (58). Only one infant died and 6 of 24 survivors required a shunt. This rate of shunt or death (28%) was considerably lower than in the two previous two large trials with the same entry criteria. DRIFT is now being tested in a multicenter randomized clinical trial and preliminary results indicate that involving a larger number of surgeons, neonatologists, and nurses is associated with a higher rate of secondary hemorrhage and a higher rate of shunt or death than in the pilot study. An important endpoint of this trial is neurodevelopmental assessment at 2 years past term and pending the results from that, DRIFT has to be regarded as a highly invasive intervention which has not been shown to be better than standard therapy.

CURRENT MANAGEMENT STRATEGY

1. Document PHVD using recognized quantitative criteria.
2. Make sure the ventricular enlargement is CSF-driven and not due to atrophy.
3. Evaluate the infant for signs of raised intracranial pressure.
4. If there is evidence of raised pressure, lumbar puncture 10 mL/kg.
5. Document the CSF protein concentration.
6. If lumbar puncture fails to produce 10 mL/kg and there is evidence of pressure, ventricular tap 10 mL/kg.
7. If there is no evidence of raised pressure, measure head circumference daily and ultrasound scan at least twice a week.
8. If there is excessive head enlargement, then lumbar puncture 10 mL/kg. Repeat as necessary according to head enlargement or signs of pressure.
9. If more than two lumbar punctures or more than one ventricular tap become necessary, consider insertion of a ventricular access device to facilitate tapping.
10. Following surgical insertion of a ventricular reservoir (Ommaya reservoir) it has been our experience that it is important to avoid raised pressure in the early postoperative period as this may lead to leakage from the suture line and subsequent infection. Thus we suggest carrying out daily taps of 10 mL/kg from the ventricular reservoir for the first 5 days postinsertion.
11. Subsequently, tap the ventricular access device if there is excessive head enlargement or evidence of pressure. Increase the volume of tapping to 15 or 20 mL/kg as required to control head enlargement. If more than 20 mL/kg requires to be removed, increase the frequency of tapping to twice a day.
12. Ventriculoperitoneal shunting is carried out if there is persistent need for tapping to maintain normal head growth or if there is persistent excessive head enlargement. If an infant has had a reservoir inserted and is having repeated taps to maintain normal head growth this is continued until CSF protein <1.5 g/L and the infant is free from infection with an acceptable weight. (This is usually 2.5 kg in Bristol but could be lower in individual cases.) When these conditions are met, tapping stops and the head

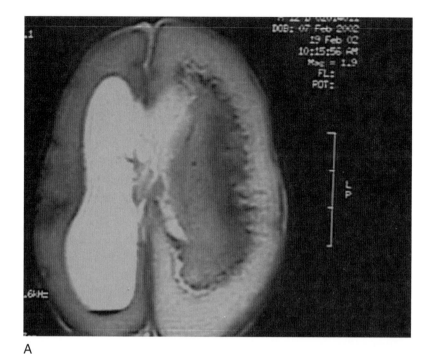

A

B

Figure 4-8 (A) MRI scan (T2 weighted) of an infant with PHVD showing extensive intraventricular debris. Parenchymal injury and edema of the left ventricle and gravitation of blood to the occipital pole of the right ventricle. (B) MRI scan (T2 weighted) of the same infant after DRIFT, showing removal of the intraventricular debris and reduced hemispheric edema.

circumference is measured daily. If the head circumference increases by 2 mm/day ultrasound is used to confirm that the increase is CSF and not brain growth. Insertion of a VP shunt is indicated if the excessive growth persists over several days in the above circumstances. Occasionally, infants demonstrate raised intra-cranial pressure without expanding the head at 2 mm/day and shunting is required. Similarly, some infants grow at a rate just below 2 mm/day but do so persistently and cross all the centiles, eventually developing an inappropriately large head for the body. If there is some intra-abdominal pathology such as necrotizing enterocolitis which contraindicates a VP shunt, tapping the reservoir continues until the abdomen normalizes. Different neurosurgeons will have different limits for CSF protein and weight at which they will consider shunt surgery can be done but the general principle is that the lower the CSF protein and the greater the weight, the better.

13. With all of the above invasive techniques careful attention to prevention of infection is crucial as the host defenses are minimal and infection in the brain worsens prognosis.

AREAS WHERE FURTHER RESEARCH IS NEEDED

1. Although IVH has been greatly reduced, especially by prenatal corticosteroids, further research on prevention of IVH is needed.
2. The mechanisms of PHVD are still not fully understood and interventions aimed at a molecular rather than a mechanical level have not reached clinical trials.
3. Further research into the mechanisms of white matter injury in PHVD is needed in order to improve neurodevelopmental outcome.

REFERENCES

1. Volpe JJ. Neurology of the Newborn, 4th edition. Philadelphia, PA: WB Saunders, 2001, pp. 428–93.
2. Murphy BP, Inder TE, Rooks, et al. Posthemorrhagic ventricular dilatation in the premature infant: natural history and predictors of outcome. Arch Dis Child 87:F37–41, 2002.
3. Ventriculomegaly Trial Group. Randomised trial of early tapping in neonatal posthaemorrhagic ventricular dilatation. Arch Dis Child 65:3–10, 1990.
4. International PHVD Drug Trial Group. International randomised trial of acetazolamide and furosemide in posthaemorrhagic ventricular dilatation. Lancet 352:433–40, 1998.
5. Papile LA, Burstein J, Burstein R, et al. Incidence and evolution of subependymal and intraventricular hemorrhage: a study of infants with birth weights less than 1,500 gm. J Pediatr 92(4):529–34, 1978.
6. De Vries LS, Dubowitz LM, Dubowitz V, et al. Predictive value of cranial ultrasound in the newborn baby: a reappraisal. Lancet 2(8447):137–40, 1985.
7. Levene M. Measurement of the growth of the lateral ventricles in preterm infants with real-time ultrasound. Arch Dis Child 56:900–4, 1981.
8. Davies MW, Swaminathan M, Chuang SL, et al. Reference ranges for linear dimensions of intracranial ventricles in preterm neonates. Arch Dis Child 82:F218–23, 2000.
9. Fenton TR. A new growth chart for preterm babies: Babson and Benda's chart updated with recent data and a new format. BMC Pediatr 3:13, 2003.
10. Kaiser A, Whitelaw A. Cerebrospinal fluid pressure during posthemorrhagic ventricular dilatation in newborn infants. Arch Dis Child 60:920–3, 1985.
11. Dubovitz L, Dubowitz V, Mercuri E. The Neurological Assessment of the Preterm and Full-term Newborn Infant, 2nd edition. London: Mac Keith Press, 2000.
12. Quinn MW, Ando Y, Levene MI. Cerebral arterial and venous flow-velocity measurements in posthaemorrhagic ventricular dilatation. Dev Med Child Neurol 34:863–9, 1992.
13. Taylor GA, Madsen JR. Neonatal hydrocephalus: hemodynamic response to fontanelle compression: correlation with intracranial pressure and need for shunt placement. Radiology 201:685–9, 1996.
14. De Vries LS, Pierrat V, Minami T, et al. The role of short latency somatosensory evoked responses in infants with rapidly progressive ventricular dilatation. Neuropediatrics 21:136–9, 1990.
15. Inder TE, Wells SJ, Mogridge NB, et al. Defining the nature of the cerebral abnormalities in the premature infant: a qualitative magnetic resonance imaging study. J Pediatr 143(2):171–9, 2003.
16. Whitelaw A, Mowinckel MC, Abildgaard U. Low levels of plasminogen in cerebrospinal fluid after intraventricular haemorrhage: a limiting factor for clot lysis? Acta Paediatr 84:933–6, 1995.
17. Hansen A, Whitelaw A, Lapp C, et al. Cerebrospinal fluid plasminogen activator inhibitor-1: a prognostic factor in posthaemorrhagic hydrocephalus. Acta Paediatr 86:995–8, 1997.
18. Hill A, Shackelford GD, Volpe JJ. A potential mechanism of pathogenesis for early post-hemorrhagic hydrocephalus in the premature newborn. Pediatrics 73:19–21, 1984.
19. Larroche JC. Posthemorrhagic hydrocephalus in infancy. Biol Neonate 20:287–99, 1972.

20. Heep A, Stoffel-Wagner B, Soditt V, et al. Procollagen I C-propeptide in the cerebrospinal fluid of neonates with posthaemorrhagic hydrocephalus. Arch Dis Child Fetal Neonatal Ed 87:F34–6, 2002.

21. Beck LS, Chen TL, Amman AJ, et al. Accelerated healing of ulcer wounds in the rabbit ear by recombinant human transforming growth factor beta-1. Growth Factors 2:273–82, 1990.

22. Ignotz RA, Massague J. Transforming growth factor beta stimulates the expression of fibronectin and collagen and their incorporation into the extracellular matrix. J Biol Chem 261:4337–45, 1986.

23. Roberts AB, Sporn MB, Assoian RK, et al. Transforming growth factor type β rapid induction of fibrosis and angiogenesis in vivo and stimulation of collagen formation in vitro. Proc Natl Acad Sci USA 83:4167–71, 1986.

24. Border WA, Ruoslahti E. Transforming growth factor-beta 1 induces extracellular matrix formation in glomerulonephritis. Cell Differ Dev 32:425–31, 1990.

25. Castilla A, Prieto J, Fausto N. Transforming growth factors beta 1 and alpha in chronic liver disease. Effects of interferon alfa therapy. N Engl J Med 324:933–40, 1991.

26. Kitazawa K, Tada T. Elevation of transforming growth factor beta-1 level in cerebrospinal fluid of patients with communicating hydrocephalus after subarachnoid hemorrhage. Stroke 25:1400–4, 1994.

27. Tada T, Kanaji M, Kobayashi S. Induction of communicating hydrocephalus in mice by intrathecal injection of human recombinant transforming growth factor beta-1. J Neuroimmunol 50:153–8, 1994.

28. Whitelaw A, Christie S, Pople I. Transforming growth factor β-1: a possible signal molecule for post-hemorrhagic hydrocephalus? Pediatr Res 46:576–80, 1999.

29. Heep A, Bartmann P, Stoffel-Wagner B, et al. Cerebrospinal fluid obstruction and malabsorption in human neonatal hydrocephaly. Childs Nerv Syst 22:1249–55, 2006.

30. Chow LC, Soliman A, Zandian M, et al. Accumulation of transforming growth factor-beta2 and nitrated chondroitin sulfate proteoglycans in cerebrospinal fluid correlates with poor neurologic outcome in preterm hydrocephalus. Biol Neonate 88(1):1–11, 2005.

31. Cherian SS, Love S, Silver IA, et al. Posthemorrhagic ventricular dilation in the neonate: development and characterization of a rat model. J Neuropathol Exp Neurol 62(3):292–303, 2003.

32. Cherian S, Thoresen M, Silver IA, et al. Transforming growth factor-betas in a rat model of neonatal posthaemorrhagic hydrocephalus. Neuropathol Appl Neurobiol 30(6):585–600, 2004.

33. Wyss-Coray T, Feng L, Masliah E, et al. Increased central nervous system production of extracellular matrix components and development of hydrocephalus in transgenic mice overexpressing transforming growth factor-beta 1. Am J Pathol 147:53–67, 1995.

34. Del Bigio MR. Neuropathological changes caused by hydrocephalus. Acta Neuropathol 85:573–85, 1993.

35. Savman K, Nilsson UA, Blennow M, et al. Non-protein-bound iron is elevated in cerebrospinal fluid from preterm infants with posthemorrhagic ventricular dilatation. Pediatr Res 49:208–12, 2001.

36. Inder T, Mocatta T, Darlow B, et al. Elevated free radical products in the cerebrospinal fluid of VLBW infants with cerebral white matter injury. Pediatr Res 52:213–18, 2002.

37. Bejar R, Saugstad OD, James H, et al. Increased hypoxanthine concentrations in cerebrospinal fluid of infants with hydrocephalus. J Pediatr 103:44–8, 1983.

38. Nishino T, Tamura I. The mechanism of conversion of xanthine dehydrogenase to oxidase and the role of the enzyme in reperfusion injury. Adv Exp Med Biol 309A:327–33, 1991.

39. Back SA, Luo NL, Borenstein NS, et al. Late oligodendrocyte progenitors coincide with the developmental window of vulnerability for human perinatal white matter injury. J Neurosci 21:1302–12, 2001.

40. Leviton A, Paneth N, Reuss ML, et al. Maternal infection, fetal inflammatory response, and brain damage in very low birth weight infants. Pediatr Res 46:566–75, 1999.

41. Savman K, Blennow M, Hagberg H, et al. Cytokine responses in cerebrospinal fluid from preterm infants with posthaemorrhagic ventricular dilatation. Acta Paediatr 91:1357–63, 2002.

42. Kadhim H, Tabarki B, Verellen G, et al. Inflammatory cytokines in the pathogenesis of periventricular leukomalacia. Neurology 56:1278–84, 2001.

43. Cherian S, Whitelaw A, Thoresen M, et al. The pathogenesis of neonatal post-hemorrhagic hydrocephalus. Brain Pathol 14:305–11, 2004.

44. Hislop JE, Dubowitz LM, Kaiser AM, et al. Outcome of infants shunted for post-haemorrhagic ventricular dilatation. Dev Med Child Neurol 30:451–6, 1988.

45. Taylor AG, Peter JC. Advantages of delayed VP shunting in post-haemorrhagic hydrocephalus seen in low-birth-weight infants. Childs Nerv Syst 17(6):328–33, 2001.

46. Tuli S. Risk factors for repeated cerebrospinal shunt failures in pediatric patients with hydrocephalus. J Neurosurg 92(1):31–8, 2000.

47. Kreusser KL, Tarby TJ, Kovnar E, et al. Serial lumbar punctures for at least temporary amelioration of neonatal posthemorrhagic hydrocephalus. Pediatrics 75(4):719–24, 1985.

48. Whitelaw A. Repeated lumbar or ventricular punctures in newborns with intraventricular hemorrhage. Cochrane Database Syst Rev 1:CD000216, 2001.

49. Thoresen M, Whitelaw A. Effect of acetazolamide on cerebral blood flow velocity and CO_2 elimination in normotensive and hypotensive newborn piglets. Biol Neonate 58(4):200–7, 1990.

50. Cowan F, Whitelaw A. Acute effects of acetazolamide on cerebral blood flow velocity and pCO_2 in the newborn infant. Acta Paediatr Scand 80(1):22–7, 1991.

51. Whitelaw A, Kennedy CR, Brion LP. Diuretic therapy for newborn infants with posthemorrhagic ventricular dilatation. Cochrane Database Syst Rev 2:CD002270, 2001.

52. Pang D, Sclabassi RJ, Horton JA. Lysis of intraventricular blood clot with urokinase in a canine model: 3.Effects of intraventricular urokinase on clot lysis and posthemorrhagic hydrocephalus. Neurosurgery 19(4):553–72, 1986.

53. Whitelaw A. Intraventricular streptokinase after intraventricular hemorrhage in newborn infants. Cochrane Database Syst Rev 1:CD000498, 2001.

54. Berger A, Weninger M, Reinprecht A, et al. Long-term experience with subcutaneously tunneled external ventricular drainage in preterm infants. Childs Nerv Syst 16(2):103–9, 2000.

55. de Vries LS, Liem KD, van Dijk K, et al. Dutch Working Group of Neonatal Neurology. Early versus late treatment of posthaemorrhagic ventricular dilatation: results of a retrospective study from five neonatal intensive care units in The Netherlands. Acta Paediatr 91(2):212–17, 2002.

56. Buxton N, Macarthur D, Mallucci C, et al. Neuroendoscopic third ventriculostomy in patients less than 1 year old. Pediatr Neurosurg 29(2):73–6, 1998.

57. Pople IK, Edwards RJ, Aquilina K. Endoscopic methods of hydrocephalus treatment. Neurosurg Clin N Am 12(4):719–35, 2001.

58. Whitelaw A, Pople I, Cherian S, et al. Phase 1 trial of prevention of hydrocephalus after intraventricular hemorrhage in newborn infants by drainage, irrigation, and fibrinolytic therapy. Pediatrics 111:759–65, 2003.

Chapter 5

Brain Cooling for Neonatal Encephalopathy: Potential Indications for Use

Abbot R. Laptook, MD

Encephalopathy and Hypoxia-Ischemia

Pathogenesis of Hypoxic-Ischemic Brain Injury

Diagnosis of Neonatal HIE

Outcome Following Neonatal HIE

Potential Therapies for Neonatal HIE

Clinical Experience with Brain Cooling for HIE

Clinical Application of Brain Cooling

This chapter addresses important concepts in the diagnosis, management, and treatment for newborns with hypoxic-ischemic encephalopathy (HIE). The past 30 years has seen a steady shift in the investigative focus of HIE in the near-term and term newborn. From 1970 to the late 1980s, the focus was on defining perinatal hypoxia-ischemia and understanding its relationship to early childhood neurodevelopment. Over the past 15 years, the focus has shifted to understanding the pathogenesis of tissue damage following perinatal hypoxia-ischemia, and examining potential therapies that are mechanistically driven. At present the most contentious issue regarding newborn encephalopathy is the application of hypothermia as a treatment for the subset of infants in whom hypoxia-ischemia is a critical component.

The following case presentation is provided to illustrate a number of important issues confronting clinicians when providing care for an infant with HIE. Specific points relevant to the case that are pertinent to diagnosis, management, and treatment of newborns with HIE will be discussed throughout this chapter.

CASE HISTORY

The mother was a 29-year-old Gravida 1 now Para 1 who presented to a level II hospital in spontaneous labor at term. Antepartum laboratory evaluation and the pregnancy were unremarkable. Rupture of membranes occurred spontaneously at 19 hours prior to delivery. The mother developed a low-grade temperature in labor and was started on antibiotics. The fetus was noted to have fetal tachycardia near the end of labor (fetal heart rate ∼ 200 bpm). The mother progressed to a spontaneous vertex vaginal delivery and meconium stained amniotic fluid was noted with delivery of the head. The infant was noted to be limp at delivery with no respiratory effort and was intubated to suction the trachea for meconium. No meconium was retrieved and positive pressure ventilation was initiated after the infant did not respond to tactile stimulation. The heart rate was always greater than 100 bpm, and due to persistent poor respiratory effort (it is not clear when spontaneous breathing was initiated) and hypotonia, the infant was intubated between 10 and 15 minutes following birth and was moved to the nursery. Apgar scores were assigned as 2, 4, 4, 4, and 5 at 1, 5, 10, 15, and 20 minutes, respectively. The cord blood gas was a pH of 7.01, pCO_2 of 62 mmHg, pO_2 of 22 mmHg, and base excess of -15.8 mEq/L. The infant was stabilized with mechanical ventilation, volume expansion for poor peripheral perfusion, and sodium bicarbonate for metabolic acidosis. Blood pressure was normotensive (mean 44 mmHg), initial blood glucose concentration was 113 mg/dL, and the temperature was 38.6°C, although the time of acquisition of the temperature is unclear. Initial arterial blood gas in the nursery on ventilator support and 100% O_2 was a pH of 7.13, pCO_2 of 22 mmHg, pO_2 of 442 mmHg, and base excess of -20.1 mEq/L.

The infant was transferred to a level III neonatal intensive care unit (NICU) at 4 hours of age. During transport the infant was noted to have occasional rhythmic jerks of the left leg and occasional extension of the right arm. On arrival in the NICU at 4½ hours of age the neurological evaluation consisted of lethargy, decreased spontaneous activity, diffusely increased tone peripherally with hypotonia centrally, suck present, incomplete Moro reflex, and normal size pupils and response to light. The infant was also noted to have prominent molding, caput, and bruising of the head.

The case description is typical of the type of data available to clinicians caring for newborns with encephalopathy. Further information may be desirable but not available; for example, fetal heart rate tracing, site used to acquire the cord blood gas (artery, vein, or mixed sample), and etiology of the maternal fever.

ENCEPHALOPATHY AND HYPOXIA-ISCHEMIA

Encephalopathy is a clinically defined condition in which there is difficulty initiating and maintaining respirations, a subnormal level of consciousness, and associated depression of tone, reflexes, and possibly seizures (1). Encephalopathy manifests at birth or shortly thereafter and may evolve over the first days following birth.

The case description is a nice illustration of an infant with definite encephalopathy as evidenced by a lethargic sensorium, decreased activity, need for ventilation at delivery, and diffuse hypotonia.

For many years healthcare providers assumed that the primary etiology of newborn encephalopathy was hypoxia-ischemia or asphyxia in origin. It is now understood that encephalopathy is a nonspecific response of the brain to injury which may occur via multiple causal pathways (2). Hypoxia-ischemia represents one of these paths and HIE is therefore a subset of encephalopathy. Hypoxia-ischemia and asphyxia are terms that are often used interchangeably but they are not physiologically equivalent. Pure ischemia or hypoxia-ischemia is rare in newborn medicine and some combination of hypoxia, ischemia, and hypercapnia is more common. Is it important to establish the presence or absence of hypoxia-ischemia given that HIE represents a potentially modifiable condition in contrast to other etiologies of encephalopathy such as brain malformations, toxic exposures, genetic disorders, and metabolic defects. The potential number of infants affected by HIE in the USA can be derived from the following assumptions: 4 million births per year, approximately 92% greater than or equal to 36 weeks gestation, 2–4 infants with encephalopathy per 1000 births (3), and a 30% fraction of encephalopathy attributable to hypoxia-ischemia (2). This leads to a possible target cohort of 2200 to 4400 infants per year in whom the potential for adverse long-term neurodevelopmental disability and associated greater healthcare needs justifies attempts to improve outcome.

PATHOGENESIS OF HYPOXIC-ISCHEMIC BRAIN INJURY

Hypoxia-ischemia is associated with two phases of pathologic events that culminate in brain injury. These phases are primary and secondary energy failure based on characteristics of the cerebral energy state used to describe the temporal sequence in newborn animals (4). Primary energy failure is characterized by reductions in cerebral blood flow and O_2/substrates (4, 5). High-energy phosphorylated compounds such as ATP and phosphocreatine are reduced and tissue acidosis is prominent. This phase is an essential prerequisite for all deleterious events that follow. Primary energy failure is associated with acute intracellular derangements such as loss of membrane ionic homeostasis, release/blocked reuptake of excitatory neurotransmitters, defective osmoregulation, and inhibition of protein synthesis (6). Excessive stimulation of neurotransmitter receptors and loss of ionic homeostasis mediate an increase in intracellular calcium and osmotic dysregulation. Elevation in intracellular calcium triggers a number of destructive pathways by activating lipases, proteases, and endonucleases (7).

Resolution of hypoxia-ischemia within a specific time interval reverses the fall in high-energy phosphorylated metabolites and intracellular pH, and promotes recycling of neurotransmitters (Fig. 5-1). The duration of time for hypoxia-ischemia to be successfully reversed and promote recovery will be affected by maturation, preconditioning events, substrate availability, body temperature, and simultaneous disease processes. Although recovery of the cerebral energy state may occur following primary energy failure, a second interval of energy failure may occur at a time remote from the initiating event. Secondary energy failure differs from primary energy failure in that declines in phosphocreatine and ATP are not accompanied by brain acidosis (4). The presence and severity of secondary energy failure depends on the extent of primary energy failure. The pathogenesis of secondary energy failure is not as well understood as that of primary energy failure, but likely involves multiple pathophysiologic processes including excessive

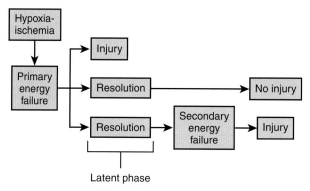

Latent phase

Figure 5-1 Different sequences may occur following hypoxia-ischemia. Hypoxia-ischemia leads to primary energy failure which can be so severe that injury occurs as a direct result of the initial insult. Alternatively, resuscitation may be successful and no injury occurs. Finally, primary energy failure may resolve and be followed by secondary energy failure at a time remote from the insult. Secondary energy failure is almost always followed by tissue injury. The latent phase represents a potential therapeutic window to successfully initiate brain protective strategies.

excitatory neurotransimitters, oxidative injury, apoptosis, inflammation, and altered growth factors and protein synthesis (8–12).

The interval between primary and secondary energy failure represents a latent phase that corresponds to a therapeutic window. Initiation of therapies during the latent phase in perinatal animals has been successful in reducing brain damage and substantiates the presence of a therapeutic window (13–15). The duration of the therapeutic window is approximately 6 hours in near-term fetal sheep based on the neuroprotection associated with brain cooling initiated at varying intervals following brain ischemia (13–15). The duration of the therapeutic window can be modified depending on characteristics of the hypothermic regimen, e.g., time of initiation, duration of treatment, and extent of hypothermia (16–18).

The clinical presentation of the case description does not help providers know if the infant has resolved the brain biochemical alterations of primary energy failure, or if the patient has entered into the latent phase. Furthermore at present there are no clinically available neurophysiologic markers that are known to correlate with the cerebral energy state.

DIAGNOSIS OF NEONATAL HIE

Establishing diagnostic criteria for encephalopathy that indicate hypoxia-ischemia as the etiologic factor is challenging for two reasons. First, the clinical presentation of an encephalopathic infant can be viewed as a phenotype that is common to many causes of encephalopathy. Second, translating the physiological consequences of hypoxia-ischemia into clinical criteria is often not straightforward even if hypoxia-ischemia is truly present. Diagnostic criteria need to be robust and signify a high likelihood of developing brain injury yet exclude other etiologies for the encephalopathy. Some publications advocate diagnostic criteria that define hypoxia-ischemia based on whether it is sufficient to result in cerebral palsy (19). This type of retrospective diagnosis is of limited value to the practitioner who is caring for an infant with encephalopathy and the outcome is uncertain. Of greater utility are data that support a sequence of events (20, 21), including pertinent obstetric history (e.g., uterine rupture, abruption placenta) (20), measures of impaired placental gas exchange (e.g., umbilical artery pH in the cord blood) (22), poor adaptation at birth and need for resuscitation (e.g., low Apgar scores), presence or development of an encephalopathy, and evidence of other organ system dysfunction (e.g., renal dysfunction) (23). Much of this sequence is embodied in the criteria put forth in prior publications of the American Academy of Pediatrics for proper use of the term asphyxia (profound fetal academia, pH < 7.0, Apgar 0–3 beyond 5 minutes, neurological dysfunction, and multisystem dysfunction) (24). Of equal importance is a rapid determination to exclude other causes of encephalopathy.

The case description highlights some of the controversy regarding the ability of the above criteria to identify all infants in whom hypoxia-ischemia contributes to the encephalopathy. There is objective evidence supporting hypoxia-ischemia at birth based on the metabolic acidosis in the cord blood gas with further confirmation on the first blood gas in the nursery. The clinical presentation could be consistent with hypoxia-ischemia (poor respiratory effort and probable secondary apnea, need for resuscitation, and hypotonia). However, other diagnostic possibilities need to be considered. The use of antibiotics in the mother raises the possibility that infection may be contributing to this infant's clinical presentation. Sepsis can lead to a systemic inflammatory response which may alter the neurologic examination (25, 26). Meningitis obviously can lead to encephalopathy but is rare shortly after birth and many infants will not be subjected to lumbar puncture due to frequently encountered cardiovascular or pulmonary instability. The head was noted to be bruised and caput was prominent. Intracranial hemorrhage is not common at term but occurs in low frequency and can lead to encephalopathy. Imaging the brain can be done rapidly with ultrasonography or computed tomography scans but most NICUs do not have this ability in the early morning hours when this infant was transported (3 a.m.).

The intent of any set of diagnostic criteria is to identify infants with acute hypoxia-ischemia proximate to the time of birth; distinguishing the infant with acute from acute superimposed on chronic events remains a concern (2). The neurological evaluation at 4½ hours of age was notable for diffusely increased tone peripherally with central hypotonia. The increased tone is somewhat atypical since tone is usually hypotonic both peripherally and centrally following acute hypoxia-ischemia around the time of birth. Hypertonia could signify an event remote from delivery (hours, days, or even weeks) with superimposed hypoxia-ischemia at the time of birth (the double hit hypothesis) (2). Alternatively the increased tone could signify underlying seizure activity secondary to a central nervous system etiology especially in view of the observations on transport (occasional rhythmic jerks of the left lower extremity and extension of the right upper extremity). This is an extremely challenging area for clinicians since there may not be a single diagnosis in each patient and the brain may become more vulnerable to hypoxia-ischemia in the presence of other conditions (27, 28).

OUTCOME FOLLOWING NEONATAL HIE

The relationship between obstetric risk factors, perinatal events, neonatal signs, and long-term outcome has been extensively investigated. The most complete analyses are data from the National Collaborative Peri-Natal Project with follow-up to 7 years of age. These analyses established that perinatal hypoxia-ischemia can cause brain injury such as cerebral palsy. The pathway from perinatal events to permanent brain injury must progress through neonatal encephalopathy if there is to be an etiologic link between perinatal events and brain damage (20, 21). Specifically a sequence of events and signs need to be present during labor, delivery, and the neonatal period to support this link. However, the presence of neonatal HIE should not be equated with the development of permanent brain injury. Follow-up of infant cohorts with presumed neonatal HIE demonstrate that the presence and extent of brain injury varies as a function of the severity of encephalopathy (29, 30). Early childhood (3.5 years) and school age outcome of 226 term infants with presumed HIE was correlated with the most severe stage of encephalopathy documented in the first week of life for a cohort from Canada. The prognosis following the extremes of encephalopathy was uniformly favorable after mild involvement and uniformly poor (death or disability) after severe involvement. Infants with a moderate encephalopathy had a variable outcome making accurate prognosis difficult.

What is the prognosis for the infant in the case description? It is difficult to extrapolate from the Canadian cohort even though the diagnosis of HIE was ascertained within hours of birth since outcome was correlated with the most severe stage of encephalopathy in the first week of life. In view of the development of potential specific interventions for HIE (see below), there has been intense interest in identifying clinical markers either alone or with laboratory and/or neurophysiologic variables to predict outcome shortly after birth (31–37). The case description is of an infant with a moderate encephalopathy, possibly complicated by seizures, and with the extent of metabolic acidosis would be viewed as high risk for an adverse outcome (death or disability) by some of these publications. In spite of the work in this area, identification of the infant at risk for serious morbidity or death following perinatal hypoxia-ischemia remains an important area of investigation.

POTENTIAL THERAPIES FOR NEONATAL HIE

The management of neonates with HIE has been limited to supportive intensive care. The latter includes correction of hemodynamic and pulmonary disturbances (hypotension, metabolic acidosis, and hypoventilation), correction of metabolic disturbances (glucose, calcium, magnesium, and electrolytes), treatment of seizures if present, and monitoring for other organ system dysfunction. This management approach does not target any component of the pathophysiologic sequence leading to hypoxic-ischemic brain injury and is directed at avoiding injury from secondary events associated with hypoxia-ischemia.

Over the past 15 years brain-specific therapies have been developed with the specific intent to block or attenuate one or more components of the cascade of events triggered by hypoxia-ischemia and contributing to brain injury. Potential therapies that are being investigated include brain cooling, allopurinol, magnesium, minocycline, erythropoietin, insulin-like growth factor, MK-801, BAF (boc-aspartyl[OMe]-fluoromethylketone), and stem cells (38–40). Each of these therapies addresses one or more mechanisms involved in the multiple pathways contributing to brain injury as cited above. Of all of these potential therapies, brain cooling has the most experimental support. Brain hypothermia is the prototypical example of a nonspecific neuroprotective therapy signifying that it affects multiple processes in the events leading to brain injury. A relatively small reduction in brain temperature (1–6°C) of neonatal animals is associated with better maintenance of the cerebral energy state during and immediately following ischemia (41), attenuation of the release of excitatory neurotransmitters (42), and decreased caspase-3 activation and morphologic evidence of apoptosis (43, 44). Other neuroprotective effects of cerebral hypothermia have been demonstrated in adult animals and include normalization of the decrease in protein synthesis (45), reduction of free radicals (46), and modulation of microglial activation and cytokine production (47). The net effect of modest hypothermia on multiple pathways is an attenuation of secondary energy failure (48) and histopathologic evidence of neuroprotection (13, 14, 16–18, 49, 50). The efficacy of modest hypothermia as a neuroprotective regimen in adult animals is influenced by the time of initiation and duration and depth of hypothermia (16–18). Neuroprotection associated with modest brain cooling is present among newborns of multiple species (rodents, swine, sheep), can be demonstrated across the developmental span from fetus to adult (51), and can be achieved when cooling is initiated at an interval up to 5.5 hours following an hypoxic-ischemic event (14).

CLINICAL EXPERIENCE WITH BRAIN COOLING FOR HIE

The encouraging laboratory results of neuroprotection associated with modest brain cooling have provided the foundation to investigate this therapy in near-term and term infants with HIE. Multiple pilot studies involving small numbers of newborn humans (less than 25 in each pilot) have been performed and established feasibility of patient identification, enrollment, and initiation of therapy within 6 hours of birth (52–56). Each pilot study used different criteria for identification of infants with HIE but all included a correlate of impaired placental gas exchange and neurologic abnormalities on examination. Pilot studies used body cooling or a combination of head and body cooling. Cooling was not associated with any greater risk than infants maintained under routine temperature control but these conclusions are limited since the numbers of infants in each pilot was small.

In a larger multicenter pilot study of brain cooling, Eicher et al. evaluated measures of efficacy and safety (57, 58). Infants with presumed HIE were randomized to either whole-body cooling (33°C rectal, $n = 32$) for 48 hours initiated within 6 hours of birth or normothermia (37°C rectal, $n = 33$) (57). In this study 77% of the infants were classified as a severe stage of encephalopathy on enrollment (Sarnat III) and 75% of the infants were out-born. Cooling was initiated with plastic bags filled with ice wrapped in a washcloth and applied to both head and body for 2 hours and then placed on a cooling blanket (Cincinnati Sub-Zero Blanketrol) with servo control of rectal temperature. Outcome at 12 months was available in 76 and 84% of normothermic and cooled groups, respectively. Death or severely abnormal motor scores (Bayley Psychomotor Development Index < 70) was less frequent in the cooled group (52%) compared to the normothermic group (84%, $p = 0.019$). There were no differences in severely abnormal cognitive scores. Adverse events (longer dependence on pressors, higher prothrombin time, lower platelet counts, and seizures) were more frequent in the hypothermia group but were not severe enough to stop cooling (58). The reports by Eicher et al. (57, 58) provide further support for the feasibility and safety of the intervention, and suggest benefit, but results are limited by sample size.

These encouraging results have been followed by two large multicenter clinical trials to test the effectiveness and safety of different modes of brain cooling for infants with encephalopathy of presumed hypoxic-ischemic origin. The CoolCap trial compared selective head cooling with mild systemic hypothermia or conventional care (59). Eligible infants needed to meet all components of a stepwise approach for study entry using clinical evidence of hypoxia-ischemia, followed by evidence of moderate or severe encephalopathy (modified Sarnat assessment), and an abnormal amplitude-integrated EEG (aEEG). The cooling regimen ($n = 116$) is summarized in Table 5-1. Conventional care ($n = 118$) was characterized by servo control of the abdominal skin temperature using a radiant warmer to maintain rectal temperature between 36.8 and 37.2°C. The primary outcome was death or severe disability (any one of the following: Bayley Mental Development Index < 70, Gross Motor Function Level of 3–5, or bilateral cortical visual impairment) was available in 93% of infants and occurred in 66% and 55% of control and cooled infants, respectively (odds ratio (OR) 0.61, 95% confidence interval (CI) 0.34–1.09, $p = 0.1$). When adjusted for aEEG severity and age at randomization there was a strong trend for reduction in adverse outcome associated with cooling (OR 0.57, CI 0.32–1.01, $p = 0.05$). In a subgroup analysis a reduction in the primary outcome was found with head cooling for infants with less severe abnormalities of the aEEG (OR 0.47, 95% CI 0.26–0.87, $p = 0.02$) but not in those with severe abnormalities of the aEEG (OR 1.8, CI 0.49–6.4, $p = 0.5$).

The NICHD Neonatal Research Network enrolled 208 near-term and term infants with moderate and severe encephalopathy to compare whole body cooling

Table 5-1   Brain Cooling Trials: Cooling Regimens

	CoolCap (59)	Body cooling (60)
Mode of cooling	Head and systemic	Systemic
Equipment	Cooling cap and radiant warmer	CSZ Blanketrol[a]
Target core: temperature	34–35°C	33.5°C
Target core: site	Rectum	Esophagus
Temperature control of core site	Servo control of abdominal skin[b]	Servo control of esophagus
Age of initiation	<6 h	5 ± 1.1 h
Time to target core temperature following initiation of cooling	2 h	~1.5 h[c]
Duration of cooling	72 h	72 h
Rate of rewarming	0.5°C/h	0.5°C/h

[a]CSZ: Cincinnati Sub-Zero Hyper-hypothermia system.
[b]Temperature control of the cooling cap was via manual control.
[c]96% of infants in the body cool trial had achieved the target esophageal temperature by 1.5 h.

($n = 102$) with a control group ($n = 106$) (60). The cooling regimen is summarized in Table 5-1. The control group was cared for on overhead radiant warmers with servo control of abdominal skin temperature; temperature control was per usual care guidelines of each center. The esophageal temperature was recorded but not used for management of infants in the control group. The primary outcome was death or moderate/severe disability and was available in 98% of the infants. Severe disability was defined similar to the CoolCap study but with the addition of hearing loss requiring amplification. Moderate disability was defined as the combination of a Bayley Mental Development Index between 70 and 84 combined with any of the following: Gross Motor Function Level of 2, persistent seizure disorder, or hearing impairment not requiring amplification. The primary outcome occurred in 44% in the hypothermic group and 62% in the control group resulting in a relative risk of 0.72 (95% CI 0.54–0.95, $p = 0.01$) for hypothermia compared to control after adjusting for center. This result persisted after adjustment for both center and level of encephalopathy at randomization. The secondary outcome of death or moderate/severe disability among infants with moderate encephalopathy at randomization occurred in 32% in the hypothermic group and 48% in the control group (relative risk 0.69, CI 0.44–1.07, $p = 0.09$). Among infants with severe encephalopathy at randomization death or moderate/severe disability occurred in 72% in the hypothermic group and 85% in the control group (relative risk 0.85, CI 0.64–1.13, $p = 0.24$).

CLINICAL APPLICATION OF BRAIN COOLING

Should the Infant in Our Case Description Be Offered Cooling?

Whether clinicians adopt the use of brain cooling primarily depends on how the strength of the evidence is viewed. At present there are two large multicentered trials that were well planned and rigorously performed (59, 60). Each study had a well-defined hypothesis and primary outcome, clearly defined entry criteria, randomization among treatment and comparison groups, predetermined sample size, and analytic plan for the results. The interventions could not be blinded but the outcomes were ascertained without knowledge of the intervention.

There are important differences between the CoolCap and body cooling trials. Each study attempted to enroll patients with a high risk of an adverse outcome and provide a suitable group in which benefits can be detected. Characteristics of infants at the time of randomization in each trial are summarized in Table 5-2. The two trials used different entry criteria that were distinguished primarily by the use of the aEEG in the CoolCap trial. There are multiple reports demonstrating the predictive value of an early aEEG for the outcome of full-term infants with HIE (61–63). The available data regarding prediction of outcome using the combination of an aEEG with the neurological assessment are limited to short-term outcome (64). The use of the aEEG and any other laboratory/neurophysiologic marker remains an important area of ongoing research for future investigations of neuroprotective interventions. The mode of cooling used in each trial was different and it is unknown if one cooling regimen is superior to the other. It is well established that body and head cooling lead to different thermal characteristics within the brain (65, 66). Given that there are regions of the brain that are more vulnerable to injury from HIE (67), the mode of brain cooling may have an important effect on efficacy of the intervention. Novel means of regional brain temperature maps using magnetic resonance spectroscopy may provide key insights into the optimal use of brain cooling (68). The primary outcome differs between the two trials. The outcome is broader in the body cooling trial since it includes hearing loss as part of severe disabilities and also includes moderate disabilities. Although it is difficult to directly compare the primary outcomes due to these differences, components of the primary outcome can be compared (Figs. 5-2 and 5-3).

Table 5-2 Brain Cooling Trials: Characteristics at Randomization

	CoolCap		Body cooling	
	Control, $n = 118$	Cool, $n = 116$	Control, $n = 106$	Cool, $n = 102$
Gestational age (wks)	39 ± 1[a]	39 ± 2	39 ± 2	39 ± 2
Birth weight (kg)	3.5 ± 0.6	3.4 ± 0.7	3.4 ± 0.6	3.4 ± 0.7
Head circumference (cm)	35 ± 2	35 ± 2	34 ± 2	34 ± 2
Female (%)	51	45	37	50
Out-born (%)	–	–	42	47
Emergent C/S (%)	69	64	75	71
10 minute Apgar <6 (%)[b]	27	17	–	–
10 minute Apgar <5 (%)	–	–	77	84
pH[c]	6.9 ± 0.2	6.9 ± 0.2	6.8 ± 0.2	6.9 ± 0.2
Encephalopathy (%)				
Moderate	–	–	62	68
Severe	–	–	38	32
aEEG (%)				
Moderate abnormal	64	54	–	–
Severe abnormal	27	36	–	–
Seizures (%)				
Clinical	–	–	48	43
aEEG	64	59	–	–
Postnatal age (h)	4.8	4.7	4.3	4.3

[a]Data are mean ± s.d.
[b]Apgar scores were only reported for 166 infants.
[c]pH values represent cord blood or within the first hour following birth.

Both studies demonstrate benefit with brain cooling; in the body cooling trial there is a difference in the primary outcome and in the CoolCap trial the unadjusted analysis shows a strong direction of effect towards benefit (CI 0.34–1.09). The adjusted analysis for differences in aEEG severity upon randomization in the CoolCap trial (CI 0.32–1.01) provides greater assurance of a benefit from cooling. Since the primary outcome of each trial was a combined endpoint of death or disability, it is important to ascertain that the therapy did not salvage infants

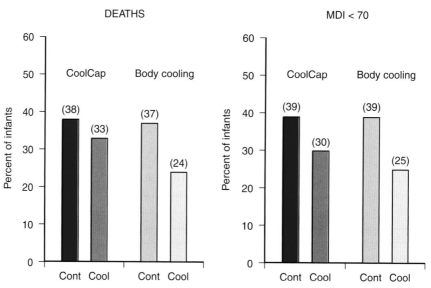

Figure 5-2 Comparison of the percentage of infants who died and survivors with a Mental Development Index (MDI, Bayley scores) < 70 at 18–22 months in the CoolCap and body cooling trials. The numbers over each column represent the actual percentage. Cont and Cool represent the control and cooled groups, respectively.

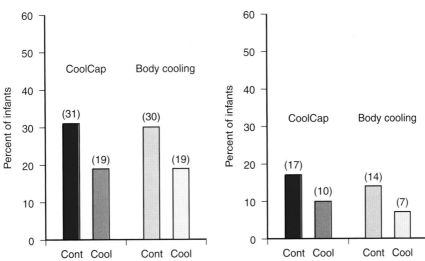

Figure 5-3 Comparison of the percentage of infants with disabling cerebral palsy (CP) and visual impairment (blindness) at 18–22 months in the CoolCap and body cooling trials. Disabling CP is based upon a Gross Motor Performance Score of 3–5 in the body cooling trial and a classification of neuromotor disability in the CoolCap trial. The numbers over each column represent the actual percentage. Cont and Cool represent the control and cooled groups, respectively.

with severe disability who would have otherwise died in the absence of the intervention. The results plotted in Figures 5-2 and 5-3 provide assurance that this did not happen. These results were obtained in spite of all the unknown variables contributing to each infant's presentation at enrollment in either trial.

In the infant in the case description we do not know the specific "event" that resulted in the altered neurologic state. It is not evident when this event occurred and whether this was a single or repetitive event. At the time of randomization, it is not known if there are other etiologies for the clinical presentation. There is no information regarding the in utero environment which may have preconditioned the infant. These unknown variables are not only concerns for investigations of brain cooling, but also are applicable to any trial of neuroprotective therapies.

Should this infant be offered brain cooling? The data from both trials support its use. The similarity among the results of these two trials (Figs. 5-2 and 5-3) using two different modes of brain cooling and possibly targeting groups of infants with different risks for adverse outcome provides additional comfort in accepting the efficacy of this intervention. The results of these trials certainly do not establish brain cooling as a panacea for HIE. The number needed to treat is 6 based on the body cooling trial and there are few therapies that are as effective. However, this also means that most infants undergoing cooling will not benefit. The primary outcome of death or disability in the infants undergoing hypothermia in the body cooling and CoolCap trials were 44 and 55%, respectively, indicating that there is ample room for improvement in outcome. There is no information that the hypothermia regimens tested are optimal conditions to improve outcome. The hypothermia regimens evaluated were extrapolated from animal studies and for the most part are not based on experiments designed to optimize the therapy. Whether outcome can be improved by altering the cooling regimens or by the addition of other neuroprotective therapies should be addressed in future investigations.

If brain cooling is to be performed, where should it be done and by whom? There are well-delineated recommendations regarding this therapy in an Executive Summary of the NICHD Workshop on Hypothermia and Perinatal Asphyxia (69). Brain cooling merits special consideration as a therapy since both regimens of the two

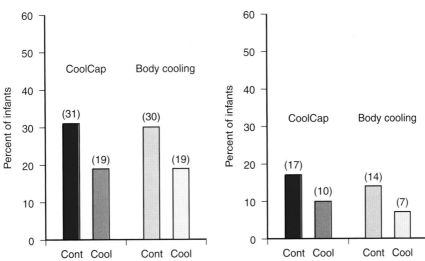

large multicenter trials represent treatments that clinicians are not trained to perform. Even if individual medical providers are trained to use the therapy, the complete implementation of brain cooling goes far beyond the skill of an individual or group of providers. To implement brain cooling a published protocol (body cooling or CoolCap) should be strictly adhered to, appropriate personnel need to be available day and night, and there should be collection of appropriate data and assurance of follow-up after discharge to ascertain outcome. Providers must be highly experienced in evaluating treatment candidates, knowledgeable in the techniques to administer hypothermia, and have a comprehensive follow-up program to determine neurodevelopmental outcome. These criteria are best accomplished by large centers which have an existing infrastructure to meet the above stipulations needed to offer this therapy. Given that more than 40% of the patients in the body cooling trial were outborn, large regional referral centers will be critical for providing this intervention. At present centers that participated in the NICHD Neonatal Network trial and many US centers involved in the CoolCap trial continue to use hypothermia as an emergency therapy for infants at high risk for death or disability.

REFERENCES

1. American College of Obstetricians and Gynecologists and American Academy of Pediatrics. Background. In Neonatal Encephalopathy and Cerebral Palsy: Defining the Pathogenesis and Pathophysiology. Washington. DC: American College of Obstetricians and Genecologists Distribution Center, 2003, pp. 1–11.
2. Badawi N, Kurinczuk JJ, Keogh JM, et al. Intrapartum risk factors for newborn encephalopathy: the Western Australian case-control study. BMJ 317:1554–8, 1998.
3. Badawi N, Kurinczuk JJ, Keogh JM, et al. Antepartum risk factors for newborn encephalopathy: the Western Australian case-control study. BMJ 317:1549–53, 1998.
4. Lorek A, Takei Y, Cady EB, et al. Delayed ("secondary") cerebral energy failure after acute hypoxia-ischemia in the newborn piglet: continuous 48-hour studies by phosphorus magnetic resonance spectroscopy. Pediatr Res 36:699–706, 1994.
5. Laptook AR, Corbett RJ, Arencibia-Mireles O, et al. Glucose-associated alterations in ischemic brain metabolism of neonatal piglets. Stroke 23:1504–11, 1992.
6. Johnston MV, Trescher WH, Ishida A, et al. Neurobiology of hypoxic-ischemic injury in the developing brain. Pediatr Res 49:735–41, 2001.
7. Siesjo BK, Bengtsson F. Calcium fluxes, calcium antagonists, and calcium-related pathology in brain ischemia, hypoglycemia, and spreading depression: a unifying hypothesis. J Cereb Blood Flow Metab 9:127–40, 1989.
8. Fellman V, Raivio KO. Reperfusion injury as the mechanism of brain damage after perinatal asphyxia. Pediatr Res 41:599–606, 1997.
9. Liu XH, Kwon D, Schielke GP, et al. Mice deficient in interleukin-1 converting enzyme are resistant to neonatal hypoxic-ischemic brain damage. J Cereb Blood Flow Metab 19:1099–108, 1999.
10. Mehmet H, Yue X, Squier MV, et al. Increased apoptosis in the cingulate sulcus of newborn piglets following transient hypoxia-ischaemia is related to the degree of high energy phosphate depletion during the insult. Neurosci Lett 181:121–5, 1994.
11. Tan WK, Williams CE, During MJ, et al. Accumulation of cytotoxins during the development of seizures and edema after hypoxic-ischemic injury in late gestation fetal sheep. Pediatr Res 39:791–7, 1996.
12. Gluckman PD, Guan J, Williams C, et al. Asphyxial brain injury: the role of the IGF system. Mol Cell Endocrinol 140:95–9, 1998.
13. Gunn AJ, Gunn TR, de Haan HH, et al. Dramatic neuronal rescue with prolonged selective head cooling after ischemia in fetal lambs. J Clin Invest 99:248–56, 1997.
14. Gunn AJ, Gunn TR, Gunning MI, et al. Neuroprotection with prolonged head cooling started before postischemic seizures in fetal sheep. Pediatrics 102:1098–106, 1998.
15. Gunn AJ, Bennet L, Gunning MI, et al. Cerebral hypothermia is not neuroprotective when started after postischemic seizures in fetal sheep. Pediatr Res 46:274–80, 1999.
16. Carroll M, Beek O. Protection against hippocampal CA1 cell loss by post-ischemic hypothermia is dependent on delay of initiation and duration. Metab Brain Dis 7:45–50, 1992.
17. Colbourne F, Corbett D. Delayed and prolonged post-ischemic hypothermia is neuroprotective in the gerbil. Brain Res 654:265–72, 1994.
18. Colbourne F, Corbett D. Delayed postischemic hypothermia: a six month survival study using behavioral and histological assessments of neuroprotection. J Neurosci 15:7250–60, 1995.
19. Hankins GD, Speer M. Defining the pathogenesis and pathophysiology of neonatal encephalopathy and cerebral palsy. Obstet Gynecol 102:628–36, 2003.
20. Nelson KB, Ellenberg JH. The asymptomatic newborn and risk of cerebral palsy. Am J Dis Child 141:1333–5, 1987.

21. Freeman JM, Nelson KB. Intrapartum asphyxia and cerebral palsy. Pediatrics 82:240–9, 1988.

22. Goldaber KG, Gilstrap LC, 3rd, Leveno KJ, et al. Pathologic fetal acidemia. Obstet Gynecol 78:1103–7, 1991.

23. Perlman JM, Tack ED. Renal injury in the asphyxiated newborn infant: relationship to neurologic outcome. J Pediatr 113:875–9, 1988.

24. American Academy of Pediatrics and American College of Obstetricians and Gynecologists. Care of the neonate. In Guidelines for Perinatal Care, 5th edition. Elk Grove Village, IL: American Academy of Pediatrics, 2002, pp. 187–235.

25. Grether JK, Nelson KB. Maternal infection and cerebral palsy in infants of normal birth weight. JAMA 278:207–11, 1997.

26. Gomez R, Romero R, Ghezzi F, et al. The fetal inflammatory response syndrome. Am J Obstet Gynecol 179:194–202, 1998.

27. Shalak LF, Laptook AR, Jafri HS, et al. Clinical chorioamnionitis, elevated cytokines, and brain injury in term infants. Pediatrics 110:673–80, 2002.

28. Kendall G, Peebles D. Acute fetal hypoxia: the modulating effect of infection. Early Hum Dev 81:27–34, 2005.

29. Robertson C, Finer N. Term infants with hypoxic-ischemic encephalopathy: outcome at 3.5 years. Dev Med Child Neurol 27:473–84, 1985.

30. Robertson CH, Finer NN, Grace MG. School performance of neonatal encephalopathy associated with birth asphyxia at term. J Pediatr 114:753–60, 1989.

31. Perlman JM, Risser R. Can asphyxiated infants at risk for neonatal seizures be rapidly identified by current high-risk markers? Pediatrics 97:456–62, 1996.

32. Ekert P, Perlman M, Steinlin M, et al. Predicting the outcome of postasphyxial hypoxic-ischemic encephalopathy within 4 hours of birth. J Pediatr 131:613–17, 1997.

33. Carter BS, McNabb F, Merenstein GB. Prospective validation of a scoring system for predicting neonatal morbidity after acute perinatal asphyxia. J Pediatr 132:619–23, 1998.

34. Patel J and Edwards AD. Prediction of outcome after perinatal asphyxia. Curr Opin Pediatr 9:128–32, 1997.

35. Groenendaal F, de Vries LS. Selection of babies for intervention after birth asphyxia. Semin Neonatol 5:17–32, 2000.

36. Nagdyman N, Komen W, Ko HK, et al. Early biochemical indicators of hypoxic-ischemic encephalopathy after birth asphyxia. Pediatr Res 49:502–6, 2001.

37. Huang CC, Wang ST, Chang YC, et al. Measurement of the urinary lactate:creatinine ratio for the early identification of newborn infants at risk for hypoxic-ischemic encephalopathy. N Engl J Med 341:328–35, 1999.

38. Vannucci RC, Perlman JM. Interventions for perinatal hypoxic-ischemic encephalopathy. Pediatrics 100:1004–14, 1997.

39. Peeters C, van Bel F. Pharmacotherapeutical reduction of post-hypoxic-ischemic brain injury in the newborn. Biol Neonate 79:274–80, 2001.

40. Gluckman PD, Pinal CS, Gunn AJ. Hypoxic-ischemic brain injury in the newborn: pathophysiology and potential strategies for intervention. Semin Neonatol 6:109–20, 2001.

41. Laptook AR, Corbett RJ, Sterett R, et al. Quantitative relationship between brain temperature and energy utilization rate measured in vivo using 31P and 1H magnetic resonance spectroscopy. Pediatr Res 38:919–25, 1995.

42. Thoresen M, Satas S, Puka-Sundvall M, et al. Post-hypoxic hypothermia reduces cerebrocortical release of NO and excitotoxins. Neuroreport 8:3359–62, 1997.

43. Edwards AD, Yue X, Squier MV, et al. Specific inhibition of apoptosis after cerebral hypoxia-ischaemia by moderate post-insult hypothermia. Biochem Biophys Res Commun 217:1193–9, 1995.

44. Fukuda H, Tomimatsu T, Watanabe N, et al. Post-ischemic hypothermia blocks caspase-3 activation in the newborn rat brain after hypoxia-ischemia. Brain Res 910:187–91, 2001.

45. Bergstedt K, Hu BR, Wieloch T. Postischaemic changes in protein synthesis in the rat brain: effects of hypothermia. Exp Brain Res 95:91–9, 1993.

46. Globus MY, Busto R, Lin B, et al. Detection of free radical activity during transient global ischemia and recirculation: effects of intraischemic brain temperature modulation. J Neurochem 65:1250–6, 1995.

47. Goss JR, Styren SD, Miller PD, et al. Hypothermia attenuates the normal increase in interleukin 1 beta RNA and nerve growth factor following traumatic brain injury in the rat. J Neurotrauma 12:159–67, 1995.

48. Thoresen M, Penrice J, Lorek A, et al. Mild hypothermia after severe transient hypoxia-ischemia ameliorates delayed cerebral energy failure in the newborn piglet. Pediatr Res 37:667–70, 1995.

49. Wagner BP, Nedelcu J, Martin E. Delayed postischemic hypothermia improves long-term behavioral outcome after cerebral hypoxia-ischemia in neonatal rats. Pediatr Res 51:354–60, 2002.

50. Taylor DL, Mehmet H, Cady EB, et al. Improved neuroprotection with hypothermia delayed by 6 hours following cerebral hypoxia-ischemia in the 14-day-old rat. Pediatr Res 51:13–19, 2002.

51. Laptook AR, Corbett RJ. The effects of temperature on hypoxic-ischemic brain injury. Clin Perinatol 29:623–49, 2002.

52. Gunn AJ, Gluckman PD, Gunn TR. Selective head cooling in newborn infants after perinatal asphyxia: a safety study. Pediatrics 102:885–92, 1998.

53. Azzopardi D, Robertson NJ, Cowan FM, et al. Pilot study of treatment with whole body hypothermia for neonatal encephalopathy. Pediatrics 106:684–94, 2000.

54. Thoresen M, Whitelaw A. Cardiovascular changes during mild therapeutic hypothermia and rewarming in infants with hypoxic-ischemic encephalopathy. Pediatrics 106:92–9, 2000.
55. Shankaran S, Laptook A, Wright LL, et al. Whole-body hypothermia for neonatal encephalopathy: animal observations as a basis for a randomized, controlled pilot study in term infants. Pediatrics 110:377–85, 2002.
56. Debillon T, Daoud P, Durand P, et al. Whole-body cooling after perinatal asphyxia: a pilot study in term neonates. Dev Med Child Neurol 45:17–23, 2003.
57. Eicher DJ, Wagner CL, Katikaneni LP, et al. Moderate hypothermia in neonatal encephalopathy: efficacy outcomes. Pediatr Neurol 32:11–17, 2005.
58. Eicher DJ, Wagner CL, Katikaneni LP, et al. Moderate hypothermia in neonatal encephalopathy: safety outcomes. Pediatr Neurol 32:18–24, 2005.
59. Gluckman PD, Wyatt JS, Azzopardi D, et al. Selective head cooling with mild systemic hypothermia after neonatal encephalopathy: multicentre randomised trial. Lancet 365:663–70, 2005.
60. Shankaran S, Laptook AR, Ehrenkranz RA, et al. Whole-body hypothermia for neonates with hypoxic-ischemic encephalopathy. N Engl J Med 353:1574–84, 2005.
61. Toet MC, Hellstrom-Westas L, Groenendaal F, et al. Amplitude integrated EEG 3 and 6 hours after birth in full term neonates with hypoxic-ischaemic encephalopathy. Arch Dis Child Fetal Neonatal Ed 81:F19–23, 1999.
62. Hellstrom-Westas L, Rosen I, Svenningsen NW. Predictive value of early continuous amplitude integrated EEG recordings on outcome after severe birth asphyxia in full term infants. Arch Dis Child Fetal Neonatal Ed 72:F34–8, 1995.
63. al Naqeeb N, Edwards AD, Cowan FM, et al. Assessment of neonatal encephalopathy by amplitude-integrated electroencephalography. Pediatrics 103:1263–71, 1999.
64. Shalak LF, Laptook AR, Velaphi SC, et al. Amplitude-integrated electroencephalography coupled with an early neurologic examination enhances prediction of term infants at risk for persistent encephalopathy. Pediatrics 111:351–7, 2003.
65. Laptook AR, Shalak L, Corbett RJ. Differences in brain temperature and cerebral blood flow during selective head versus whole-body cooling. Pediatrics 108:1103–10, 2001.
66. Thoresen M, Simmonds M, Satas S, et al. Effective selective head cooling during posthypoxic hypothermia in newborn piglets. Pediatr Res 49:594–9, 2001.
67. Miller SP, Ramaswamy V, Michelson D, et al. Patterns of brain injury in term neonatal encephalopathy. J Pediatr 146:453–60, 2005.
68. Thornton JS, Cady EB, Shanmugalingam S, et al. Cerebral temperature mapping by magnetic resonance spectroscopy in a model of total body and selective head cooling. Pediatr Res (abstract 57), 2005.
69. Higgins RD, Raju TN, Perlman J, et al. Hypothermia and perinatal asphyxia: executive summary of the National Institute of Child Health and Human Development workshop. J Pediatr 148:170–5, 2006.

Chapter 6

General Supportive Management of the Term Infant with Neonatal Encephalopathy Following Intrapartum Hypoxia-Ischemia

Jeffrey M. Perlman, MB, ChB

Delivery Room Management
Early Identification of Infants at Highest Risk of Developing
    Hypoxic-Ischemic Brain Injury
Supportive Care
Gaps in Knowledge

CASE HISTORY

HI was a 3200 g, 38 week male infant born to a 28-year-old G2 P1 mother following an uncomplicated pregnancy. Labor was complicated by a maternal temperature of 38.5°C (mother was treated with antibiotics), prolonged second stage associated with variable decelerations, and a bradycardic episode that resulted in an emergent cesarean section. Meconium staining of the amniotic fluid was noted. The infant was delivered floppy and with no respiratory effort. Resuscitation included intubation for meconium that was negative, reintubation and positive pressure ventilation (PPV). The initial heart rate was 50 beats per minute (BPM) but increased rapidly to >100 BPM within 30 seconds of PPV. The infant's color improved and he took a first gasp at 4 minutes and first respiratory effort at 8 minutes. A rectal temperature in the delivery room was 38.2°C. The Apgar scores were 1^1, 4^5, 7^{10}. The infant was transferred to the neonatal intensive care unit for further management. The cord arterial blood gas revealed a pCO_2 of 101 mmHg, pH of 6.78, and base deficit of −23 mEq/L. The initial arterial blood gas at 30 minutes revealed a PaO_2 of 146 mmHg (on 50% oxygen), pCO_2 of 30 mmHg, and pH of 7.12. Initial blood glucose was 32 mg/dL. This was treated with a 2 cc/kg bolus of D10 water with subsequent glucose of 84 mg/dL. The initial clinical assessment revealed a lethargic infant with a low-level sensory response. The anterior fontanel was soft. The capillary refill time was approximately 2 seconds. The cardiovascular examination was pertinent for a heart rate of 134, blood pressure 44/24 mmHg with a mean of 34 mmHg. He was intubated and on modest ventilator support with equal but coarse breath sounds. The abdomen was soft and without masses. The central nervous examination revealed pupils that were 3 mm and reactive. There was a weak gag and suck, central hyponia with proximal weakness. The reflexes were present and symmetric. The encephalopathy at this stage was categorized as Sarnat Stage 2 encephalopathy. Because of the history and clinical examination, the infant underwent an amplitude-integrated EGG examination that revealed a moderately suppressed pattern without seizure activity. The infant met criteria for cooling. After obtaining informed consent at 4 hours of age, the infant was enrolled into the control group of an ongoing hypothermia study. At approximately 12 hours of age the infant began to exhibit subtle seizure activity with blinking of the eyes, mouth smacking, and horizontal eye deviation associated with desaturation episodes. A clinical diagnosis of seizures was made and the infant was loaded with Phenobarbital (40 mg/kg). The seizures persisted over the next 12 hours and the infant was in addition loaded with phosphenytoin and also received additional Phenobarbital and ativan before there was control of the clinical as well as the electrographic seizures. The encephalopathy peaked on day of life (DOL) 2 and the infant remained in Sarnat Stage 2 encephalopathy. The supportive management included initial fluid restriction; the initial urine output was less than 1 cc/kg/hour for the first 24 hours but increase thereafter and by DOL 3 the infant was in a diuretic phase. The initial sodium was 136 mEq/L that reached a nadir of 128 on DOL 3 but corrected over the next 36 hours. The initial serum bicarbonate level was 18 with an anion gap of 16. Both resolved spontaneously by DOL 2. The infant received assisted ventilation until DOL 3 and the pCO_2 values ranged between 40 and 50 mmHg. Additional abnormalities included a low calcium and magnesium (DOL 2) and mildly elevated liver enzymes. The infant was started on low-dose dopamine for approximately 24 hours for a low mean blood pressure. The infant was treated with antibiotics for 7 days for presumed sepsis although the blood cultures and spinal fluid remained negative. Parenteral nutrition was initiated on DOL 3, tube feedings were started on DOL 4, and the infant was able to achieve full nipple feedings on DOL 14. The neurologic examination improved although was still abnormal, i.e., central hypotonia and increased deep tendon reflexes at the time of discharge. Magnetic resonance imaging (MRI) on DOL 2 revealed marked striking hyperintensities in the diffusion-weighted images within the putamen and thalamus bilaterally. A repeat MRI on DOL 10 revealed hyperintensities in the same distribution as well as perirolandic involvement on the T2-weighted images. A repeat EEG was pertinent for mild backgrounds slowing. Finally, the placental pathology was consistent with acute chorioamnionitis. The infant was discharged on DOL 16.

This case illustrates typical evolving neonatal encephalopathy following intrapartum hypoxia-ischemia against the background of placental infection/inflammation. The brain injury that develops is an evolving process initiated during the insult and extends into a recovery period, the latter referred to as the "reperfusion phase" of injury (1–3). Management of such an infant should be initiated in the delivery room with effective resuscitation and continued through the evolving process. This comprises identification of the infant at high risk for developing evolving brain injury, supportive therapy to facilitate adequate perfusion and nutrients to the brain, and neuroprotective strategies, i.e., therapeutic hypothermia to ameliorate the processes of ongoing brain injury (see Chapter 5). These are briefly discussed in the following.

DELIVERY ROOM MANAGEMENT

Resuscitation of the depressed neonate is aimed at restoring blood flow and oxygen delivery to the tissues. It has long been recommended that resuscitation of such infants be initiated with 100% oxygen. However, there is an increasing body of experimental and clinical evidence that has questioned the value of oxygen over room air in the resuscitation of the newborn infant (4). A Cochrane Review of clinical studies ($n = 5$) was pertinent for a significant reduction in the relative risk of death at latest follow-up in favor of infants resuscitated with room air (odds ratio 0.71, 95% confidence interval 0.54–0.94), although no individual study reached this conclusion (5). The only study with follow-up to 18 months (albeit with a high drop-out rate) showed no differences in neurologic handicap (6). Experimental studies raise some concerns with regard to the benefit of room air over oxygen as it relates to the brain. Thus resuscitation with 100% oxygen is associated with significantly more rapid restoration of hypoxia-depressed cerebral blood flow (CBF), improved cerebral perfusion, and significantly lower levels of excitatory amino acid levels in striatum as well as more favorable short as well as long term outcome in surviving adult mice (7, 8). Based on these observations it may be prudent to continue to utilize supplemental oxygen in the depressed term infant as described in this case, in order to facilitate restoration of CBF and oxygen delivery, until there are sufficient evidence-based data to suggest otherwise.

EARLY IDENTIFICATION OF INFANTS AT HIGHEST RISK OF DEVELOPING HYPOXIC-ISCHEMIC BRAIN INJURY

The initial step in management is early identification of those infants at greatest risk for evolving to the syndrome of hypoxic-ischemic encephalopathy (HIE). This is a highly relevant issue because the therapeutic window, i.e., the time interval following hypoxia-ischemia during which interventions might be efficacious in reducing the severity of ultimate brain injury, is likely to be short. Based on experimental studies it is estimated to vary from 2 to 6 hours. Given this presumed short window of opportunity, infants must be identified as soon as possible following delivery in order to facilitate the implementation of early interventions as in the case presented above. What placed this infant at high risk? There was clinical evidence to suggest chorioamnionitis, there was fetal bradycardia prior to delivery, the infant was severely depressed, there was the need for resuscitation in the delivery room (i.e., intubation and positive pressure ventilation), and there was evidence of severe fetal acidemia (9), followed by evidence of an early abnormal neurologic examination and an abnormal assessment of cerebral function, i.e., integrated EEG (10–12). Indeed the infant progressed to stage 2 encephalopathy with seizures.

SUPPORTIVE CARE

A summary of supportive management is given in Table 6-1.

Ventilation

Assessment of adequate respiratory function is critical in the infant with HIE. Inadequate ventilation and frequent apnea episodes are not uncommon in severely affected infants necessitating assisted ventilation. Changes in $PaCO_2$ can affect CBF

Table 6-1	A Guide to the Supportive Management of an Infant at Risk for Hypoxic-Ischemic Cerebral Injury
Delivery room	Resuscitation of the depressed infant ± supplemental oxygen
Ventilation	Maintain $PaCO_2$ within a normal range
Perfusion	Promptly treat hypotension
	Avoid hypertension
Fluid status	Initial fluid restriction
	Follow serum sodium and daily weights
Blood glucose	Maintain blood glucose within a normal range
	Avoid hypoglycemia
Seizures	Treat clinical seizures, particularly with an electrographic correlate
	Potential role of prophylactic Phenobarbital
Electrolyte imbalance	Monitor serum electrolytes, calcium and magnesium

such that hypercarbia increases and hypocarbia decreases blood flow (13). Hypocarbia has been associated with hearing loss in term infants and with periventricular leukomalacia (PVL) in premature infants. Thus careful monitoring of the arterial blood gases and level of $PaCO_2$ is of particular importance. Experimental studies suggest that modest elevation in pCO_2 (50–55 mmHg) at the time of hypoxia-ischemia is associated with better outcome than when the $PaCO_2$ is within the normal or in the mid 30 range (14). However, this is a complex issue in that progressive hypercarbia in ventilated premature infants is associated with loss of autoregulation (15). In patients with head trauma, hyperventilation has been used as a strategy to lower intracranial pressure. However, when hyperventilation with associated hypocarbia has been used for the treatment of term infants with pulmonary hypertension there has been associated hearing loss. Moreover in the management of preterm infants with respiratory distress syndrome (RDS), the presence of hypocarbia has been associated with PVL (see Chapter 3). Because of the divergent experimental and clinical data, it is recommended that the $PaCO_2$ be maintained in the normal range in mechanically ventilated infants at risk for HIE.

Maintenance of Adequate Perfusion

Given a high likelihood of a pressure-passive circulation (16), the management strategy should be to maintain the arterial blood pressure within a normal range for age and gestation. It is not uncommon for infants with hypoxia-ischemia to exhibit hypotension as in our case. The hypotension may be related to myocardial dysfunction, endothelial cell damage, and, rarely, volume loss. The treatment should be directed towards the cause, i.e., volume for isotropic support for myocardial dysfunction or volume replacement for intravascular depletion (17). On rare occasions infants may be hypertensive; this is usually observed in association with seizures.

Fluid Status

Hypoxic-ischemic infants often progress to a fluid overload state. This may be related to renal failure secondary to acute tubular necrosis or to inappropriate antidiuretic hormone release (SIADH). Clinically such infants present with an increase in weight, low urine output, and hyponatremia. The management is fluid restriction. Indeed in our case all these findings were present. The treatment comprised fluid restriction and the gradual introduction of sodium supplementation on DOL 2. Others have taken a different approach to treat the oliguria based on the following presumed mechanism. Thus after hypoxia-ischemia adenosine acts as a vasoconstrictive metabolite that contributes to the decreased glomerular filtration rate. This vasoconstriction can be blocked by theophylline. In two randomized controlled studies "asphyxiated" infants received a single dose of theophylline (8 mg/kg) within in the first hour. Theophylline was associated with a decrease in serum creatinine and urinary b2-microglobulin as well as enhanced creatinine clearance (18, 19).

Control of Blood Glucose Concentration

In the context of cerebral hypoxia-ischemia, experimental studies suggest that both hyperglycemia and hypoglycemia may accentuate brain damage. In adult experimental models as well as in humans, hyperglycemia accentuates brain damage, whereas in immature animals subjected to cerebral hypoxia-ischemia, hyperglycemia to a blood glucose concentration of 600 mg/dL entirely prevents the occurrence of brain damage (20, 21). Conversely the effects of hypoglycemia in experimental neonatal models vary as do the mechanisms of the hypoglycemia. Thus, insulin-induced hypoglycemia is detrimental to immature rat brain subjected to hypoxia-ischemia. However, if fasting induces hypoglycemia, a high degree of protection is noted (21). This protective effect is presumed to be secondary to the increased concentrations of ketone bodies, which presumably serve as alternative substrates to the immature brain. In the clinical situation hypoglycemia when associated with hypoxia-ischemia is detrimental to the brain. Thus term infants delivered in the presence of severe fetal acidemia (umbilical arterial pH < 7.0) and who presented with an initial blood sugar <40 mg/dL were 18 times more likely to progress to moderate to severe encephalopathy as compared to infants with a blood sugar >40 mg/dL. This was another risk factor in our case because the infant presented with an initial blood glucose of 32 mg/dL. Thus, in the ongoing management of hypoxia-ischemia, a glucose level should be screened shortly after birth and monitored closely (22). If the blood glucose is low it should be promptly corrected.

Seizures

Hypoxic-ischemic cerebral injury is the most common cause of early-onset neonatal seizures. Although seizures are a consequence of the underlying brain injury, seizure activity in itself may contribute to ongoing injury. Experimental evidence strongly suggests that repetitive seizures disturb brain growth and development as well as increase the risk for subsequent epilepsy (23, 24). Despite the potential adverse effects of seizures, the question of which infants should be treated remains controversial. This is in part related to the observation that not all clinical seizures have an electrographic correlate (25, 26) (see also Chapter 8). Clinical seizures are treated with an anticonvulsant, usually Phenobarbital, and treatment is continued if seizures persist until the anticonvulsant therapy (e.g., Phenobarbital, phosphenytoin, or Lorazepam) has been maximized, particularly when the seizures are associated with systemic signs, i.e., hypertension, bradycardia, and/or desaturations. The optimal management of electrographic seizures in the absence of clinical seizures in the nonparalyzed infant remains unclear. Most are usually not treated because they are generally brief in nature and require excessive anticonvulsants for controlling the seizure activity. However, others prefer to eliminate all seizure activity.

Prophylactic Phenobarbital

Experimental data indicate that barbiturate pretreatment and even early post-treatment in adult animals subjected to cerebral hypoxia-ischemia reduces the severity of ultimate brain damage. The prophylactic administration of "high-dose" barbiturates to infants at highest risk for evolving to HIE has been evaluated in two small studies with conflicting results. In the first randomized study, the administration of Thiopental initiated within 2 hours and infused for 24 hours did not alter the frequency of seizures, intracranial pressure, or short-term neurodevelopmental outcome at 12 months (27). Of importance was the observation that systemic hypotension occurred significantly more often in the treated group. In the second randomized study, Phenobarbital 40 mg per kg body weight administered intravenously between 1 and 6 hours to asphyxiated infants was associated with subsequent neuroprotection (28). Although there was no difference in the frequency of seizures between the two groups in the neonatal period, 73% of the pretreated infants compared to 18% of the control group ($p < 0.05$) revealed normal neurodevelopmental outcome at 3-year follow-up. No adverse effect of Phenobarbital administration was observed in this study. Thus, the role of prophylactic barbiturates in high-risk infants remains unclear at the current time.

Cerebral Edema and Increased Intracranial Pressure

Based on an understanding of the mechanisms of brain injury, it is not surprising that cytotoxic edema complicates the clinical course of infants with HIE. In severe cases, cerebral edema is accompanied by the elevation of intracranial pressure which impairs tissue perfusion. Strategies that have been considered in the treatment of this complication include hyperventilation, glucocorticosteroids, and mannitol. At the current time, there is no known effective strategy available for clinicians to lower intracranial pressure following hypoxia-ischemia in neonates. Neuroprotective strategies such as therapeutic hypothermia are more appropriate in this regard (see Chapter 5).

Potential Neuroprotective Strategies Aimed at Ameliorating Secondary Brain Injury

In addition to hypothermia (see Chapter 5) there are additional potential neuroprotective strategies being considered.

Oxygen Free Radical Inhibitors and Scavengers

One therapeutic approach for the destruction of oxygen free radicals generated during and following hypoxia-ischemia is the administration of specific enzymes known to degrade highly reactive radicals to a nonreactive component. Superoxide dismutase and catalase are antioxidant enzymes conjugated to polyethylene glycol that prolongs their circulatory half-life and facilitates penetration across the blood–brain barrier (1). Because of their large molecular sizes, they are restricted to the vascular space. Thus, the positive effects of these conjugated compounds are presumably from within cerebral vasculature by improving CBF (1). In newborn animals, neuroprotection has only been shown when these agents have been administered several hours prior to the hypoxic-ischemic insult (29).

A second group of free radical inhibitors that have been shown to be effective in experimental animals are agents that inhibit specific reactions in the production of xanthines. Thus, both allopurinol and oxypurinol, xanthine oxidase inhibitors, protected immature rats from hypoxic-ischemic brain damage when the drugs were administered early during the recovery phase following resuscitation (1). In experiments and a clinical study, allopurinol administered to asphyxiated infants reduced blood concentrations of oxygen free radicals when compared to control infants (30, 31).

A third group of free radical inhibitors has targeted the formation of free radicals, specifically hydroxyl radical, from free iron during reperfusion (1). Thus, deferoxamine, a chelating agent, prevents the formation of free radicals from iron, reduces the severity of brain injury, and improves cerebral metabolism in animal models of hypoxia-ischemia when given during reperfusion (31).

Excitatory Amino Acid Antagonists

Given the important role of excessive stimulation of neuronal surface receptors by glutamate in promoting a cascade of events leading to cellular death (1), it has been logical to identify pharmacologic agents that would either inhibit glutamate release or block its postsynaptic action. Glutamate receptor antagonists (i.e., N-methyl-D-aspartate (NMDA) subtypes) have been extensively investigated in experimental animals. Noncompetitive antagonists provided a reduction in brain damage in adult animals even when administered up to 24 hours after the insult. The available NMDA antagonists include dizocilpine (MK-801), magnesium, phencyclidine (PCP), dextrometrophan, and ketamine (1).

Potential Role of Magnesium

Magnesium is an NMDA antagonist blocking neuronal influx of Ca^{2+} within the ion channel. The effect of magnesium also appears to be dependent on the maturation of the glutamate receptor system. Thus, in a developmental study in mice, excitotoxic neuronal death was limited by magnesium which was effective only after development of several aspects of the excitotoxic cascade, including the coupling of the calcium influx following NMDA over stimulation, and the presence of magnesium-dependent calcium channels (32).

The potential neuroprotective effect of magnesium has revealed conflicting data in experimental neonatal studies. Thus, when administered shortly following an intracerebral injection of NMDA, magnesium sulfate reduced brain injury in newborn rats. However, other neonatal studies have failed to demonstrate neuroprotection. In a piglet model of asphyxia, magnesium sulfate administered 1 hour following resuscitation failed to decrease the severity of delayed energy failure. In addition, in a near-term fetal lamb model, magnesium sulfate administered before and during umbilical cord occlusion did not influence the electrophysiologic responses or neuronal loss (1, 33, 34).

Magnesium sulfate is an attractive agent because of its frequent use in the USA. It is often administered to mothers as a tocolytic agent or to prevent seizures in mothers with pregnancy-induced hypertension. Retrospective observation in premature infants noted a reduced incidence of cerebral palsy at 3 years in those exposed to antenatal magnesium sulfate (35). A small randomized clinical study showed some subtle benefits, i.e., on computed tomography imaging from magnesium infusion (36). Clearly, future research is necessary in order to determine the potential neuroprotective role of magnesium potentially in combination with therapeutic hypothermia.

Calcium Channel Blocks

The elevation of cytosolic calcium during hypoxic-ischemic injury makes the reduction of intracellular accumulation a highly desirable therapy. One strategy of preventing calcium toxicity is to inhibit Ca^{2+} influx into neurons by using calcium channel blocks (e.g., flunarizine, nimodipine, nicardipine). Flunarizine has been studied in fetus and newborn animals and the neuroprotective effect has only been demonstrated when given prophylactically but not following hypoxic-ischemic insults (1). Nicardipine was tested in four severely asphyxiated infants but the positive effect was counteracted by the adverse effects of significant hemodynamic disturbance (37). Indeed, current calcium channel blocks are in general contraindicated in the neonate and young infant in the USA because of significant adverse cardiovascular effects.

Other Studied Therapies in Immature Animals

Other avenues of potential neuroprotection include platelet-activating factor antagonists (38), adenosinergic agents (39), monosialoganglioside GM_1 (40), growth factors, e.g., nerve growth factor (NGF) (41), insulin growth factor-1 (42), and blocking the apoptotic pathways, i.e., minocycline (43), erythropoietin, etc. (44, 45).

GAPS IN KNOWLEDGE

1. The role of oxygen versus room air in the delivery room management of the depressed infant is critical to resolve.
2. Is there a critical mean blood pressure below which cerebral perfusion becomes compromised?

3. Is there a benefit to prophylactic anticonvulsant therapy in the high-risk infant given that up to 50% of infants enrolled in the hypothermia studies presented with early seizures (46, 47)?
4. Can aggressive glucose management modulate outcome in high-risk infants?
5. Developing additional neuroprotective strategies.

REFERENCES

1. Volpe JJ. Hypoxic-ischemic encephalopathy. In Volpe JJ (ed.). Neurology of the Newborn. Philadelphia, PA: WB Saunders, 2001.
2. Shalak L, Perlman JM. Hypoxic ischemic cerebral injury. Curr Concepts Early Hum Dev 80: 125–41, 2004.
3. Perlman JM. Intervention strategies for neonatal hypoxic-ischemic cerebral injury. Clin Therapeut 28:1353–65, 2006.
4. Richmond S, Goldsmith JP. Air or 100% oxygen in neonatal resuscitation. Clin Perinatol 33: 11–27, 2006.
5. Tan A, Schulze A, O'Donnell CPF, Davis PG. Air versus oxygen for resuscitation of infants at birth (Cochrane Review). Cochrane Library, Issue 3. Chichester: John Wiley, 2004.
6. Saugstad OD, Ramji S, Irani SF, et al. Resuscitation of newborn infants with 21% or 100% oxygen: follow-up at 18 to 24 months. Ann Pediatr (Barc) 112:296–300, 2003.
7. Presti AL, Kishkurno SV, Slinko SK, et al. Reoxygenation with 100% oxygen versus room air: late neuroanatomical and neurofunctional outcome in neonatal mice with hypoxic-ischemic brain injury. Pediatr Res 60:55–9, 2006.
8. Solas AB, Kutzche S, Vinje M, Saugstad OD. Cerebral hypoxemia-ischemia and reoxygenation with 21% or 100% oxygen in newborn piglets: effects on extracellular levels of excitatory amino acids and microcirculation. Pediatr Crit Care Med 2:340–5, 2001.
9. Perlman JM, Risser R. Can asphyxiated infants at risk for neonatal seizures be rapidly identified by current high-risk markers? Pediatrics 97:456–62, 1996.
10. Hellstrom-Westas L, Rosen I, Svenningsen NW. Predictive value of early continuous amplitude integrated EEG recordings on outcome after severe birth asphyxia in full term infants. Arch Dis Child 72:F34–8, 1995.
11. al Naqeeb N, Edwards AD, Cowan FM, Azzopardi D. Assessment of neonatal encephalopathy by amplitude-integrated electroencephalography. Pediatrics 103;1263–9, 1999.
12. Shalak L, Corbett R, Laptook AR, Perlman JM. Amplitude-integrated electroencephalography coupled with an early neurologic examination enhances prediction of term infants at risk for persistent encephalopathy. Pediatrics 111:351–7, 2003.
13. Rosenberg AA, Jones MD Jr, Traystman RJ, et al. Response of cerebral blood flow to changes in $PaCO_2$ in fetal, newborn and adult sheep. Am J Physiol 242:H862, 1982.
14. Vannucci RC, Brucklacher RM, Vannucci SJ. Effect of carbon dioxide on cerebral metabolism during hypoxia-ischemia in the immature rat. Pediatr Res 42:24–9, 1997.
15. Kaiser JR, Gauss CH, Williams DK. The effects of hypercapnia on cerebral autoregulation in ventilated very low birth weight infants. Pediatr Res 58:931–5, 2005.
16. Pryds O, Greisen G, Lou H, Friis-Hansen B. Vasoparalysis associated with brain damage in asphyxiated term infants. J Pediatr 117:119–25, 1990.
17. Wyckoff MH, Perlman JM, Laptook AR. Use of volume expansion during delivery room resuscitation in near term and term infants. Pediatrics 115:950–5, 2005.
18. Jenik AG, Ceriani Cernades JM, Gorenstein A, et al. A randomized double blind placebo control of the effects of theophylline on renal function in term infants with perinatal asphyxia. Pediatrics 105:e45, 2000.
19. Bhat MA, Shah ZA, Makhadoomi MS, Mufti MH. Theophylline for renal function in term infants with perinatal asphyxia: a randomized placebo controlled study. J Pediatr 149:180–4, 2006.
20. Vannucci RC, Mujsce DJ. Effect of glucose on perinatal hypoxic-ischemic brain damage. Biol Neonate 62:215–24, 1992.
21. Yager JY. Hypoglycemic injury to the immature brain. Clin Perinatol 29:651–74, 2002.
22. Salhab W, Wyckoff M, Laptook AR, Perlman JM. Initial hypoglycemia and neonatal brain injury in term infants with severe fetal acidemia. Pediatrics 114:361–6, 2004.
23. Dzhala V, Ben-Ari Y, Khazipov R. Seizures accelerate anoxia-induced neurona death in the neonatal rat hippocampus. Ann Neurol 48:632–40, 2000.
24. Holmes GL, Gairsa JL, Chevassus AL, Ben-Ari Y. Consequences of neonatal seizures in the rat: morphological and behavioral effects. Ann Neurol 44:845–57, 1998.
25. Mizrahi EM. Consensus and controversy in the clinical management of neonatal seizures. Clin Perinatol 16:485–500, 1989.
26. Scher MS, Aso K, Beggerly ME, et al. Electrographic seizures in preterm and fullterm infants neonates: clinical correlates associated brain lesions and risk for neurologic sequelae. Pediatrics 91:128–34, 1993.
27. Goldberg RN, Moscoso P, Bauer CR, et al. Use of barbiturate therapy in severe perinatal asphyxia: a randomized controlled trial. J Pediatr 109:851–6, 1986.

28. Hall RT, Hall FK, Daily DK. High-dose Phenobarbital therapy in term newborn infants with severe perinatal asphyxia: a randomized prospective study with three-year follow-up. J Pediatr 132:345–8, 1998.

29. Shimizu K, Rajapakse N, Horiguchi T, et al. Neuroprotection against hypoxia-ischemia in neonatal rat brain by novel superoxide dismutase mimetics. Neurosci Lett 346:41–4, 2003.

30. Van Bel F, Shadid M, Moison RM, et al. Effect of allopurinol on postasphyxial free radical formation, cerebral hemodynamics and electrical brain activity. Pediatrics 101:185–93, 1998.

31. Peeters-Scholte C, Braun K, Koster J, et al. Effects of allopurinol and deferoxamine on reperfusion injury of the brain in newborn piglets after neonatal hypoxia-ischemia. Pediatr Res 54:516–22, 2003.

32. Marret S, Gressens P, Gadisseux JF, Evrard P. Prevention by magnesium of excitotoxic neuronal death in the developing brain: an animal model of clinical intervention studies. Dev Med Child Neurol 37:473–84, 1995.

33. Penrice J, Amess PN, Punwani S, et al. Magnesium sulfate after transient hypoxia-ischemia fails to prevent delayed cerebral energy failure in the newborn piglet. Pediatr Res 41:443–7, 1997.

34. de Haan HH, Gunn AJ, Williams CE, et al. Magnesium sulfate therapy during asphyxia in near-term fetal lambs does not compromise the fetus but does not reduce cerebral injury. Am J Obstet Gynecol 176:18–27, 1997.

35. Nelson KB, Grether JK. Can magnesium sulfate reduce the risk of cerebral palsy in very low birth-weight infants? Pediatrics 95:263–9, 1995.

36. Ischiba H. Randomized controlled trial of magnesium sulfate infusion for severe birth asphyxia. Pediatr Int 44:505–9, 2002.

37. Levene MI, Gibson NA, Fenton AC, et al. The use of a calcium-channel blocker, nicardipine, for severely asphyxiated newborn infants. Dev Med Child Neurol 32:567–74, 1990.

38. Liu XH, Eun BL, Silverstein FS, Barks JD. The platelet-activating factor antagonist BN 52021 attenuates hypoxic-ischemic brain injury in the immature rat. Pediatr Res 40:797–803, 1996.

39. Halle JN, Kasper CE, Gidday JM, Koos BJ. Enhancing adenosine A1 receptor binding reduces hypoxic-ischemic brain injury in newborn rats. Brain Res 759:309–12, 1997.

40. Tan WK, Williams CE, Mallard CE, Gluckman PD. Monosialoganglioside GM1 treatment after a hypoxic-ischemic episode reduces the vulnerability of the fetal sheep brain to subsequent injuries. Am J Obstet Gynecol 170:663–9, 1994.

41. Holtzman DM, Sheldon RA, Jaffe W, et al. Nerve growth factor protects the neonatal brain against hypoxic-ischemic injury. Ann Neurol 39:114–22, 1996.

42. Johnston BM, Mallard EC, Williams CE, Gluckman PD. Insulin-like growth factor-1 is a potent neuronal rescue agent after hypoxic-ischemic injury in fetal lambs. J Clin Invest 97:300–8, 1996.

43. Arvin KL, Han BH, Du Y, et al. Minocycline markedly protects the neonatal brain against hypoxic-ischemic injury. Ann Neurol 52:54–61, 2002.

44. Aydin A, Genc K, Akhisaroglu M, et al. Erythropoietin exerts neuroprotective effect in neonatal rat model of hypoxic-ischemic brain injury. Brain Dev 25:494–8, 2003.

45. Kumral A, Ozer E, Yilmaz O, et al. Neuroprotective effect of erythropoietin on hypoxic-ischemic brain injury in neonatal rats. Biol Neonate 83:224–8, 2003.

46. Gluckman PD, Wyatt JS, Azzopardi D, et al. Selective head cooling with mild systemic hypothermia after neonatal encephalopathy: multicentre randomized trial. Lancet 365:663–70, 2005.

47. Shankaran S, Laptook AR, Ehrenkranz RA, et al., for the National Institute of Child Health and Human Development Neonatal Research Network. Whole-body hypothermia for neonates with hypoxic-ischemic encephalopathy. N Engl J Med 353:1574–84, 2005.

Chapter 7

Stroke in the Fetus and Neonate

Koray Özduman, MD • Gabrielle de Veber, MD
• Laura R. Ment, MD

The emergence of sophisticated neuroimaging techniques has permitted the diagnosis of stroke in the developing brain in utero. These strategies have provided an ever growing body of information on both intrauterine and neonatal stroke and necessitated a reconsideration of the descriptions of vascular events occurring in pregnancy and after birth. Stroke in the fetus is a rare event, while the incidence of neonatal stroke is reported to be 2–9 per 1000 live term births. The diagnosis of stroke has included hemorrhagic, ischemic, and thrombotic events in the fetus and term neonate, and most authors have tended to include infants with onset of stroke during the third trimester as well as those with peripartum and neonatal events in series investigating the etiology and outcome of "neonatal" stroke.

Review of risk factors and genetic studies suggests that, like many other human diseases, stroke in the developing brain is a complex disorder. Differences in clinical presentation and outcome are reported between those cases occurring in utero and those which happen during or after birth. Furthermore, recent laboratory advances have also suggested a difference between infants who experience stroke in the fetal and neonatal time periods. Defining the timing, environmental risk factors, and molecular susceptibilities will aid in the diagnosis, prevention, and possible treatment of this important injury to the developing brain.

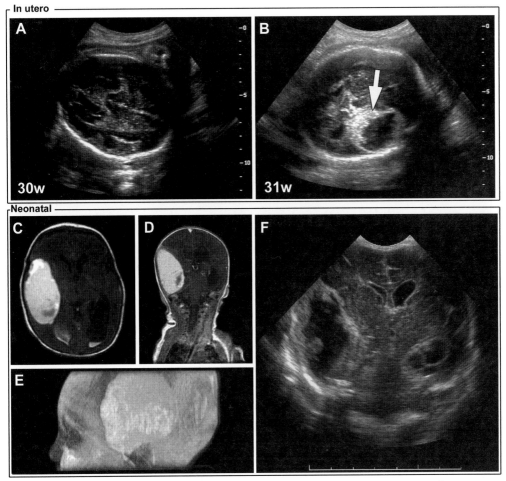

Figure 7-1 Pre- and postnatal imaging findings in the patient with alloimmune thrombocytopenia and resultant fetal stroke. Intrauterine ultrasound images (A, B) show the hemorrhage in the temporal lobe at 31 weeks (arrow). Axial and coronal T1-weighted MRI images (C, D) show the intraparenchymal hematoma in the right temporal lobe as well as ventriculomegaly and intraventricular blood. (E) Three-dimensional reconstruction of the MRI images. (F) A postnatal ultrasound image in the coronal plane.

CASE HISTORIES

Patient 1

The patient was the 1.57 kg product of a 32-week gestation born by caesarian section to a G2 P1 31-year-old female. The gestation was significant for alloimmune thrombocytopenia, class A1 diabetes, fetal intracranial hemorrhage at 31 weeks (Figs. 7-1A and 7-1B), and the onset of preterm labor. Apgar scores were 9 at 1 minute and 9 at 5 minutes, and the infant's platelet count was 13 000. She was treated with fresh frozen plasma, IVIG, and platelet transfusions, with resolution of her thrombocytopenia.

Computed tomography (CT) and subsequent magnetic resonance imaging (MRI) demonstrated a large right frontotemporal-parietal hemorrhage with shift of the midline and ventriculomegaly (Figs. 7-1C–F). Subsequent hospital course was complicated by the development of obstructive hydrocephalus, surgery for clot removal, hyperbilirubinemia treated with phototherapy, sepsis treated with antibiotics, and neonatal seizures well controlled on Phenobarbital. Phenobarbital was discontinued prior to hospital discharge and seizures have not recurred.

The child was evaluated at age 12 months and was found to have a nonfocal neurologic examination and developmental milestones appropriate for age.

Patient 2

The patient was the 3.25 kg product of a 39-week gestation complicated by systemic lupus erythematosus (SLE) to a G2 P 0 AB1 39-year-old female. The patient's mother was blood type A-positive, antibody screen negative, rubella immune, and group-B streptococcus negative; she was treated briefly with prednisone for her SLE during the first trimester.

On the day prior to delivery, she presented for routine obstetric visit in labor; routine fetal ultrasound from the previous week was unremarkable. Labor was augmented by pitocin, but delivery was accomplished by caesarean section secondary to failure to progress. Apgar scores were 5 at 1 minute and 9 at 5 minutes, and the child was noted to have petechiae on her abdomen.

In the newborn intensive care unit, the infant was stable and her platelet count was 28 000. Later on the first day of life, the infant developed focal seizures and was treated with Phenobarbital. A cranial ultrasound was unremarkable on the first day of life, but a CT scan the following day and subsequent MRI study demonstrated left frontal, parietal, and occipital as well as right parietal hemorrhage with subarachnoid hemorrhage (Figs. 7-2A–E). EEG was unremarkable.

Evaluation for hemorrhagic neonatal stroke demonstrated platelet-specific maternal antibodies with incompatibility at the HPA-1A locus. All other testing, including that for protein C, protein S, antithrombin III, Factor V Leiden, prothrombin mutation, MTHFRC mutation, total homocysteine level, and lipoprotein a, was unremarkable.

At age 6 months, neurodevelopmental examination was unremarkable, and follow-up MRI demonstrated resolution of hemorrhage with focal encephalomalacia (Figs. 7-2F and 7-2G).

DEFINITIONS

Definitions for fetal and neonatal stroke are presented in Table 7-1.

Stroke in the developing brain of the fetus and neonate may be caused by a wide variety of pathological conditions. Although pre- and perinatal events are increasingly recognized, more thoroughly investigated, and better analyzed, current evidence and knowledge are still limited. A lack of consensus on the terminology of cerebrovascular events in the fetal or neonatal period further complicates knowledge of this important spectrum of injuries to the developing brain.

The National Institute of Neurological Disorders and Stroke defines *perinatal cerebral infarction* as that which occurs between 28 weeks of gestation and 28 days of life (1). This definition groups perinatal, peripartum, and neonatal events and suggests common pathophysiologies for stroke at different points in time. However, numerous reports lack data on the timing of stroke and published classification schemes include both fetal and neonatal cases in etiologic and

Table 7-1	Definitions
Term	**Definition**
Fetal stoke	Focal ischemic, thrombotic and/or hemorrhagic event occurring between 14 weeks of gestation and the onset of labor (or beginning of the cesarean section for patients without labor) resulting in delivery
Neonatal stroke	Focal ischemic, thrombotic and/or hemorrhagic event occurring between labor resulting in delivery and 28 days of life. For those patients without labor, between delivery and 28 days

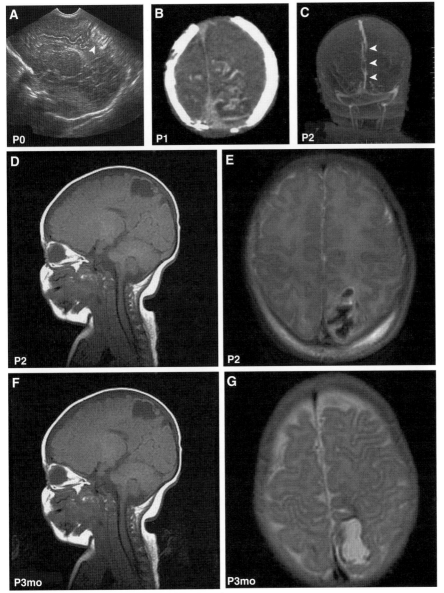

Figure 7-2 Imaging findings of the patient with neonatal stroke secondary to maternal antiplate-let antibodies. Early neonatal imaging with ultrasound study (A) at the day of birth, CT study (B) on day 1 and MRI study (C–E) on day 2 of life. Note the parenchymal hemorrhagic stroke in the parasaggital location. The MRI confirms the findings and showing intact venous flow in the sinuses (arrows) excludes the diagnosis of a venous sinus thrombosis (C). (F, G) The follow-up MRI with T1W image in the sagittal plane and T2W image in the axial plane, showing resolution of the hemorrhage with focal encephalomalacia.

descriptive classification schemes. This has been in large measure attributable to the lack of sophisticated fetal diagnostic modalities and routine fetal imaging strategies.

Cerebrovascular events may occur in utero and it is likely that these cases are characterized by different risk factors and outcome when compared to stroke occurring in neonates, infants, or children (2). The hypervascularity, alterations in microvascular morphology, and lack of autoregulation make the fetal germinal matrix susceptible to hemorrhage following ischemic events (3, 4). Furthermore, when we analyzed 128 cases of fetal stroke either reported in the literature or our cases we did not find any difference in etiology and outcome of stroke when the

Table 7-2   Fetal Stroke Diagnosed Before and After 28 Weeks of Gestation

	Total sample	Dx at <28 weeks	Dx at ≥28 weeks	p (chi square)
Cases	128	44	84	
Hemorrhagic	105 (82%)	35 (80%)	70 (83%)	≤1
Intraparenchymal hemorrhage	39 (30%)	17 (39%)	24 (29%)	≤1
Subependymal hemorrhage	15 (12%)	6 (14%)	9 (11%)	≤1
Intraventricular hemorrhage	62 (48%)	17 (39%)	45 (54%)	<0.2
Pure infarct	4 (3%)	0	4 (5%)	<0.2
Ventriculomegaly	79 (62%)	26 (60%)	53 (63%)	p≤1
Porencephaly	28 (22%)	11 (25%)	17 (20%)	≤1
Calcifications	5 (4%)	4 (9%)	1 (1%)	<0.05*
Known etiology	68 (53%)	29 (66%)	39 (46%)	<0.05*
Known outcome	118 (92%)	39 (89%)	79 (94%)	≤1
Adverse outcome	103/118 (88%)	33/39 (85%)	70/79 (89%)	≤1

diagnosis of stroke was made before or after 28 weeks of gestation (Table 7-2). These data suggest that a clear distinction between ischemic and hemorrhagic stroke in the fetus is often not possible; furthermore, they offer no reason to differentiate strokes prior to the onset of 28 weeks of gestation with those diagnosed in the third trimester.

For the purposes of this chapter, we propose that *fetal stroke* is defined as *a focal ischemic, thrombotic, and/or hemorrhagic event occurring between 14 weeks of gestation and the onset of labor resulting in delivery* (5). For those patients without labor the period is between 14 weeks and start of the cesarean delivery. Ischemic/hemorrhagic events which occur earlier in pregnancy may present in the form of other pathological pictures such as hydranencephaly (2). These pathologies of uncertain cause are excluded from the definition of fetal stroke.

Similarly, *neonatal stroke* is defined as *a focal ischemic or thrombotic and/or hemorrhagic event occurring between labor resulting in delivery and 28 days of life.* For those patients without labor this period is between delivery and 28 days. Stroke in the term newborn brain may present in the form of arterial ischemic infarction, venous sinus thrombosis, hemorrhage due to underlying vascular or neoplastic lesion, or primary hemorrhage. These lesions are commonly symptomatic in the neonatal period. In contrast earlier fetal events are less readily recognized and may become manifest in utero, postnatally, or not at all.

ETIOLOGY: RISK FACTORS

Etiology and Risk Factors for Fetal Stroke

In our review of 128 fetal stroke cases from the literature we identified a possible predisposing condition in 68 (53%) pregnancies (Tables 7-3 and 7-4). Similarly, Ghi et al. (54) in their extensive review of fetal subdural, intraparenchymal, and intraventricular hemorrhages reported that a predisposing condition could be identified or suspected in 47% of the cases diagnosed in utero. Most cases of fetal stoke are attributed to hematological disorders and maternal trauma. No obvious risk factor was identified in a significant subset of patients. Few have undergone a comprehensive investigation to identify possible genetic or environmental etiologies (5, 55). A list of causative conditions and their time of presentation is presented in Table 7-3.

The most common causes of fetal stroke were complicated *twin pregnancies* (in 11 cases; 9.7% of all fetal cases, 19% of fetal cases with identified cause) and

Table 7-3   Possible Causative Factors Relative to the Timing of Diagnosis[a]

	Gestational age at diagnosis																											Relative frequency among cases with a diagnosis (%)
	14	15	16	17	18	19	20	21	22	23	24	25	26	27	28	29	30	31	32	33	34	35	36	37	38	39	40	
Maternal conditions																												
Maternal diabetes									1							1		1			1							7
Maternal JRA											1																	2
ITP																		1										2
Maternal warfarin use																1			1									3
Maternal epilepsy																		2	1									3
Maternal antiepileptic use																		1										2
Maternal gastroenteritis with fever					1	1																						2
Maternal hypercoagulability															1	1		1	1		1							7
Maternal trauma															1	1				2				1				8
Pregnancy disorders																												
Placental hemorrhage												1			1			1										2
Placental thromboses												1	2		1													3
Preeclampsia/hypertension												1	2		1								1					5
Placental abruption													2															3
Polyhydramnios									1						1				1									5
In utero growth retardation										1								1	1		1		1					7
Oligohydramnios									1		1							1	1		1		1					5
Complicated twin pregnancy	1									1	2	2		1	2	1	1	1										21
Hydrops of unknown cause															2									1				2
Fetal disorders																												
TORCH infection							1									1												2
Pyruvate carboxylase def.					1				1																			3
Carnitine palmitoyl trsf. def					1	1			1							1												3
Suspected genetic cause				1					1																			3
Rh isoimmunization								2			1																	5
Alloimmune thrombocytopenia						2									1			1	1		2/1	2						15
Von Willebrandt disease																		1	1	1								2
Protein C deficiency																							1					2
Total per week	1			2	3	3		7	3	5	3	5	1	6	6		3	10	3	9	3	1	2	1				

[a]For each gestational age the number of cases diagnosed at this age are indicated. Hemorrhagic cases are indicated in red and non-hemorrhagic cases indicated in black.

alloimmune thrombocytopenia (in 7 cases; 6.2% of all fetal cases, 12% of fetal cases with identified cause) followed by *maternal trauma, maternal diabetes,* and *in utero growth retardation* (in 4 cases each; each 4% of all fetal cases and 7% of fetal cases with an identified cause). The vast majority of events (97%) occurred after 20 weeks of gestation, which corresponds to a period of development when the fetal brain can mount up an astrocytic reaction to the presumed hemorrhagic injury.

For descriptive purposes, the etiologies of fetal stroke may be grouped into *maternal conditions, pregnancy disorders,* and *fetal conditions. Maternal medical conditions* such as diabetes, epilepsy, and juvenile rheumatoid arthritis are significant causes of fetal stroke and are present in 20% of fetal cases with an identifiable cause (11).

Maternal coagulation disorders have also been reported as causes of fetal stroke. These include maternal hypercoagulability, anticoagulation with warfarin, and immune thrombocytopenic purpura (ITP) (9, 13, 18). In two of the four cases of maternal hypercoagulability cases fetal stroke was the sole clinical manifestation, while the other two cases had other systemic evidence of coagulopathy. In addition, there were two cases related to *maternal epilepsy* and one case attributed to *maternal antiepileptic drug use* (14).

The most commonly encountered *pregnancy-related condition* was a complicated multiple gestation. In our analysis 13 (10%) of the fetuses were products of complicated twin pregnancies and they made up 19% of the cases with an identifiable cause. The incidence of ischemic brain injury in *multiple gestations* is reported to be relatively high and is estimated to be 30% for monochorionic twins and 3% for dichorionic twins (56, 57). The risk is particularly increased upon the death of a twin and this creates an indication for fetal MRI imaging. Unfortunately neither the ultrasound nor MRI can exclude brain damage in the surviving twin with absolute certainty (58). Ischemic injury has been postulated as a major mechanism in cases of significant maternal trauma, placental hemorrhage, or placental abruption. Maternal trauma can affect the fetus through multiple mechanisms, including direct fetal brain trauma, maternal hypotension, and placental injury. In our analysis trauma was associated with fetal stroke in 5 (7%) of the cases with a cause. Evidence for placental hemorrhage was observed in one pregnancy and placental abruption was documented before fetal stroke in two cases.

Fetal conditions were thought to be causative in 17 cases (29%) of fetal stroke. Among cases with an identifiable cause *alloimmune thrombocytopenia* was the most common cause in our analysis (7 cases, 12% of cases with a diagnosis). Alloimmune thrombocytopenia is estimated to occur in 1 in 2000–5000 pregnancies (59). Stroke is the most significant complication and reported to occur in 10–30% of cases (60). One-fourth to half of these hemorrhages are known to occur in utero (60). *Inborn errors of metabolism* were commonly identified as causative factors. Although it is very uncommon for an inborn error of metabolism to present as fetal stroke, their incidence among cases with an identifiable cause was 6.8% in our analysis. Pyruvate carboxylase and carnitine-palmitoyl transferase deficiencies are thought to act through different mechanisms but both conditions were associated with hemorrhagic lesions in the fetus (35, 38, 39, 61, 62). It has been postulated that chronic ischemia secondary to metabolic depletion in the germinal matrix tissues may be the cause of stroke in patients with pyruvate carboxylase deficiency as the germinal matrix has been demonstrated to have a high metabolic rate during the period of neurogenesis/gliogenesis (35, 61, 62). Both cases of pyruvate carboxylase had subependymal hemorrhages (5, 35). In contrast, long-chain fatty acid oxidation is not required for the energy metabolism of the brain in animal models, which makes energy depletion an unlikely mechanism for stroke in these cases (39). Both cases of carnitine-palmitoyl transfericency were associated with intraparenchymal calcifications (38, 39). Hereditary thrombophilias are commonly reported in cases of neonatal stroke; however, only two cases were present in our analysis of 113 (29, 32). Finally, there was only one case attributable to congenital infection (41).

Etiology and Risk Factors for Neonatal Stroke

Etiological factors of stroke in the neonate can also be grouped into *maternal, pregnancy/labor-related,* and *fetal* conditions (Table 7-4). Among the maternal causes, Lee et al. (7) found *infertility* as an independent risk factor for perinatal stroke. An association with *diabetes* has been found both for fetal and neonatal stroke (8).

Pregnancy/labor complications are reported in more than half of cases with neonatal stroke (7, 34). *Prolonged rupture of membranes* or *prolonged second stage of labor* are associated with an increased risk of neonatal stroke. *Perinatal asphyxia* has been associated with border-zone cerebral ischemia and an association with focal cerebral ischemia is debated (22). Govaert et al. (22) reported this in 3% of neontal cases, which makes it a rare cause of focal arterial infarction. *Birth trauma* may result in thrombosis of the middle cerebral artery (MCA) (23). Cardiac abnormalities are a common cause of stroke in the childhood and both *congenital cardiac defects* and *corrective surgery* may result in neonatal stroke (47, 48). Iatrogenic causes of neonatal stroke have also been reported, which included *catheterization* of the umbilical vein (52) or the temporal vein (51) or the use of *extracorporeal membrane oxygenation* (ECMO) (50). *Sepsis* or *bacterial meningitis* in the neonatal period may result in neonatal stroke (40).

Among fetal causes of neonatal stroke *thrombophilias* deserve a special consideration. Several groups have reported a high incidence of thrombophilias in cases of neonatal stroke but their role is more likely permissive and requires a triggering environmental event. Several underlying mechanisms may lead to *hypercoagulable states* in the newborn. *Polycythemia* has been reported in association with neonatal stroke (27). Neonatal *prothrombotic risk factors* reported in the literature in patients with perinatal stroke are mutations of Factor V (G1691A) (30), Factor V Leiden (R506Q) (22, 36, 63, 64), Factor II (G20210A) (30), methylene tetrahydrofolate reductase mutations (T667T) (30), hyperhomocysteinemia (30), elevated Factor VIIIc (30), lipoprotein (a) (30, 36), deficiencies of antithtrombin III, protein C (28) or protein S (30), and anticardiolipin antibodies (30). A multicenter case control study found that term neonates with a symptomatic ischemic stroke were 6.7 times more likely to have at least one prothrombotic disorder when compared to age and sex matched controls (8). In contrast, the mechanism for arterial thromboembolic disease is most likely multifactorial (8, 30). Kurnik et al. (30) reported a triggering condition in 71% of patients with a prothrombotic condition and a recurrent thrombotic event, suggesting that both the genome and the environment contribute to this complex disorder.

PATHOGENESIS

Stroke in the fetus or newborn is most likely a complex disorder and therefore most certainly multifactorial in nature (2). The most prominent pathogenetic mechanisms are trauma, hypoxia (or impairment of energy metabolism), coagulopathies/hypercoagulable states, and endothelial damage. Genetic susceptibilities are directly responsible for some cases of fetal and neonatal strokes and most likely create a tendency to stroke in others. This is well exemplified by familial porencephaly, for which an autosomal dominant mode of inheritance has also been reported. The defect in this entity was mapped to collagen IV-a1 gene on chromosome 13 (65, 66). Subsequently it was shown in an animal model that mice carrying mutations in

Table 7-4   Reported Pathologies Associated with Fetal and Neonatal Stroke

	Fetal stroke	Neonatal stroke
Maternal conditions	*Trauma* (6) *History of infertility* (7) *Hematological disorders* - Immune thrombocytopenic purpura (9) *Metabolic disease* - Diabetes (5, 11) *Pharmacological* - Salicilate ingestion (12) - Warfarin use (13) - Antiepileptic medication (14) - Cocaine exposure (15) *Maternal epilepsy* (14) *Other unclassified* - Pancreatitis (16) - Fever with gastroenteritis (17)	*History of infertility* (7) *Metabolic disease* - Diabetes (8) *Immunological disorders* - Systemic lupus erytematosus (10) - Anticardiolipin antibodies (10)

Pregnancy or labor related disorders	*Placental/cord abnormalities*
	- Placental hemorrhage (18)
	- Placental thromboses (18)
	- Abruptio placenta (18)
	- Complicated multiple gestations (11)
	- Preeclampsia/gestational
	  hypertension (20)
	Infection
	- Chorioamnionitis (7)
	Oligohydramnios (7)
	Polyhydramnios (21)
	IUGR and fetal distress (22)
		Placental/cord abnormalities
		- Preeclampsia (7)
		- Cord abnormalities (7)
		- Fetomaternal hemorrhage (19)
		Infection
		- Chorioamnionitis (7)
		Labor related
		- Prolonged rupture of membranes (7)
		- Prolonged second stage of labor (7)
		- Vacuum assistance (7)
		- Emergency cesarean delivery (7)
		- Hypoxic ischemic encephalopathy
		  (7, 8, 22)
		- Birth trauma (22, 23)

Fetal/neonatal conditions	*Hematological disorders*
	- Alloimmune thrombocytopenia (24–26)
	- Von Willebrand's disease (29)
	- Factor V Leiden mutation (31)
	- Protein C deficiency (32)
	- Fetal anemia (22)
	Inborn errors of metabolism
	- Pyruvate decarboxylase deficiency (35)
	- Carnitine palmitoyl transferase
	  deficiency (38, 39)
	Infection
	- CMV infection (41)
	- Non-A non-B hepatitis (42)
		Hematologic disorders
		- Polycythemia (27)
		- Protein C deficiency (28)
		- Protein S deficiency (30)
		- Antithrombin III deficiency (30)
		- Factor V Leiden mutation (22)
		- MTFHR mutation (8, 33, 34)
		- Hyperhomocisteinemia (30)
		- Lipoprotein (a)(59, 108)
		- Vitamin K deficiency (37)
		Infection
		- Septicemia (8, 22)
		- Bacterial meningitis (40)
		Inborn errors of metabolism
		- Alpha-1-antitrypsin deficiency (43–46)
		*Cardiac disorders and surgical
		  complications*
		- Congenital heart disease (47, 48)
		- Extracorporeal membrane
		  oxygenation (49, 50)
		- Vascular catheterization (51, 52)
		Dehydration (53)
		Trauma (53)

the COL4A1 gene experience intracerebral hemorrhage in the perinatal period resulting from alterations in the structural integrity of vessels (67). Environmental factors play an important role as exemplified by trauma, drug-related causes, or infection.

PATHOLOGY

Pathology of Fetal Stroke

Classification of intracranial hemorrhage includes five groups: intraventricular, intra-parenchymal, infratentorial (cerebellar), subdural, and subarachnoid hemorrhages.

Tissue reaction to a hemorrhagic or ischemic insult is dependent on fetal brain maturity. In the second trimester the damaged tissue undergoes pure liquefaction necrosis with subsequent resorption without scar formation, resulting in cavities. Porencephaly, multicystic encephalomalacia, and hydranencephaly are terms used for different patterns of cavities (56). More mature fetal brain reacts to injury with gliosis (56).

The majority (83%) of the cases in our series were hemorrhagic. There was no significant difference in timing of diagnosis between hemorrhagic or nonhemorrhagic cases ($p = 0.46$), cases with or without porencephaly ($p = 0.46$), cases with or without intraparenchymal hemorrhage ($p = 0.17$). Associated ventriculomegaly was found in 64% of fetal cases, as shown in Table 7-2.

Pathology of Neonatal Stroke

In the term neonate arterial ischemic stroke is most likely related to a focal ischemic lesion in the distribution of a specific cerebral artery. Miller (68) reported that 83% of the arterial ischemic strokes occurred in the MCA territory. Lee et al. (7) reported a similar incidence (70%). Lesions of the anterior or posterior cerebral artery territories are much less commonly reported (68, 69). Lesions are left sided in almost 53–75% of perinatal stroke cases (7, 68–70). Infarcts are hemorrhagic in 20% of these cases (71).

INCIDENCE

The true incidence and prevalence of stroke in the fetal and neonatal period remains poorly defined. There is no unbiased, evidence-based study on the incidence of fetal or neonatal stroke. There are few studies on the incidence of antenatal cases and thus the true incidence of fetal stroke is unknown (53, 72). This is due to both deficiencies in diagnosis and a lack of understanding of the etiologies of this injury (5). A recent report from a tertiary referral center indicated an incidence of antenatal hemorrhagic or ischemic events of 0.46 per 1000 deliveries (38). It should be kept in mind, however, that a considerable fraction of fetal stroke cases result in intrauterine death or stillbirth, while another group does only present late in the infancy and that these factors may be hiding a likely higher true incidence.

An analysis of several studies reveals a very broad range numbers for the incidence of neonatal stroke, ranging from 17 to 93 per 10 000 live births and as high as 5.4% in neonatal autopsies (Table 7-5). The incidence varies according to the methods used, which include national registries, autopsy studies, and studies analyzing neonatal seizures. Fullerton et al. (74) noted that this incidence is 17 times higher than the incidence of childhood ischemic stroke and as high as the incidence of large-vessel ischemic stroke in patients older than 18 years. According to the results of the Canadian Childhood Stroke Registry the incidence of perinatal stroke is $93/10^5$ (75). In this registry the neonates accounted for 25% of acute ischemic

Table 7-5   Studies on Incidence of Fetal and Neonatal Stroke

Study	Incidence/ prevalence	Inclusion criteria	Comments
Elchalal et al., 2005 (38)	Incidence 4.6 per 10^5 deliveries	Antenatal hemorrhagic and ischemic insults detected at two tertiary obstetric centers	Antenatal hemorrhage and ischemia
Lee et al., 2005 (7)	Prevalence 20 per 10^5 live births	Strokes occurring in utero or until 28 days after birth diagnosed by MRI/CT	
Kylan-Lynch and Nelson, 2001 (53)	Prevalence 26.4 per 10^5 live births per year	Stroke incidence for neonates	- National Hospital Discharge Survey - 6.7 per 10^5 hemorrhagic and 17.8 per 10^5 ischemic cases
deVeber, 2000 (55)	93 per 10^5 live births	Perinatal ischemic events	Canadian Pediatric Stroke Registry
Govaert et al., 2000 (22)	35 per 10^5 live births	Arterial stroke on routine US	- Retrospective analysis - Prevalence: $12/10^3$ for neonates admitted to the NICU - 45% of the affected were premature (mostly with deep lesions)
Günther et al., 2000 (8)	1.35 per 10^5 live births	Full-term neonates with symptomatic ischemic stroke	Results of the German Childhood Stroke Study Group
Estan and Hope, 1997 (69)	26.95 per 10^5 newborns >31 wks	Arterial stroke on US performed for neonatal seizures	- Retrospective analysis - Strokes identified only in term neonates
Perlman et al., 1994 (70)	20 per 10^5 deliveries	Arterial stroke on US performed for symptomatic neonate	- Retrospective analysis - Strokes identified only in term neonates
Barmada et al., 1979 (73)	5.4% in neonatal autopsies	Arterial stroke on neonatal autopsies	- Strokes more common in term neonates - Multiple small strokes in prematures - Most commonly embolic

strokes in childhood. In the National Hospital Discharge Survey the rate of stroke was $26.4/10^5$ live births per year in infants younger than 30 days of age (53). Barmada et al. (73) reported a 5.4% incidence of arterial stroke in neonatal autopsies. Most of these were term neonates and presented with embolic lesions.

After perinatal asphyxia, stroke is the most common cause of seizures in the term infant (69, 76, 77). Statistics obtained from studies on neonatal seizures therefore have been one of the early resources on incidence of fetal/neonatal stroke. In these studies the incidence has been estimated at between $24.7/10^5$ and $35/10^5$. Govaert et al. (22) in their retrospective study of routinely performed ultrasounds in the neonatal intensive care unit (NICU) over a 10-year period found the incidence to be 0.35 per 10^3 live births. Estan and Hope (69) found a slightly lower incidence in newborns with seizures (11/44.518). It should be kept in mind, however, that information derived from these studies likely underestimates the incidence. An unknown proportion of fetal and neonatal stokes remain undiagnosed in the fetal and neonatal period and some are completely silent. Seizures are not the only mode of presentation and incidence of seizures varies considerably among studies, which may add another level of bias. Additionally a significant proportion of stroke cases may be missed by routine ultrasound studies which complicates the matter even further (69, 78, 79).

Gender Effect in the Incidence of Stroke

Among the fetal cases that we have analyzed gender information was available in 46 cases. No gender predilection could be found when all cases or cases less than 28 weeks were taken into consideration. In contrast, in their study of 66 term children with neonatal arterial stroke and 32 term children with neonatal cerebral sinovenous thrombosis, all confirmed by MRI or CT, Golomb et al. (80) have reported that both entities were more commonly diagnosed in boys (62.1 and 78.1%, respectively). Thus the true effect of gender in the incidence of stroke needs further study.

CLINICAL MANIFESTATIONS

The clinical picture in both the fetal and neonatal period is very subtle (2, 5). Focal signs are uncommon in the early neonatal period (69, 81). Perinatal arterial ischemic stroke most commonly occurs in term neonates (53, 69, 70, 72). Almost 60% become manifest in the acute neonatal period (7).

Neonatal Encephalopathy

Patients with fetal or perinatal stroke may present with nonspecific clinical signs, such as hypotonia, which will require differential diagnosis from hypoxic, metabolic, or infectious disorders. In one study of stroke, 25% of patients presented with apnea and hypotonia (70). Similarly, Kurnik et al. (30) reported that 13% of their patients presented with apneas and 10% presented with hypotonia.

Spastic Hemiplegic Cerebral Palsy

It is estimated that 20–30% of cases of hemiplegic cerebral palsy (CP) are related to fetal or neonatal stroke. For those who are born at term, it is reported to be responsible for 50–70% of the spastic hemiplegic CP (82). Similarly, data from Sweden also suggest that congenital hemiplegia due to prenatal or perinatal brain damage is the most common form of CP among children born at term and the second most common form of CP among prematures (83). Two-thirds of these are of normal intelligence (83).

The spasticity is more marked in the upper extremities and transitory hemiparesis or generalized tone anomalies may be seen in the neonatal period for a course of days (81, 84, 85). In some cases this spastic paresis is preceded by a transient hypotonia contralateral to the affected side (85).

Seizures

Govaert et al. (22) reported that cortical lesions are over 5 times more commonly associated with neonatal seizures than deep-seated infarcts classically found in fetal or preterm stroke. Infants with cortical lesions were more likely to be term, present with neonatal seizures, and survive (22). In contrast, deep gray and periventricular white matter infarctions were less likely to result in neonatal seizures and/or hemiparesis than a complete infarction of the MCA (22).

Arterial ischemic stroke is the second most common identifiable cause of focal neonatal seizures (76). In an otherwise healthy neonate presenting with seizures the reported probability of a cerebral infarct ranges from 12 to 30% (22, 69, 77). Conversely, the incidence reported for a seizure presentation ranges from 85 to 92% for infants with stroke (69, 86).

Lee et al. (7) in their analysis of 40 cases of neonatal/fetal stroke concluded that 70% presented with neonatal seizures. Similarly, in the cohort reported by Perlman et al. (70), 75% presented with seizures. Of these, 50% were focal motor, 33% were generalized motor, and 17% were subtle seizures. Of 12 cases (who presented with seizures) reported by Estan and Hope (69), 67% were focal motor, there was generalized motor in 25% and subtle seizures in the remaining 8%. In these infants, seizures usually occurred within the first 72 hours after birth (69, 87).

DIAGNOSIS

The mean gestational age at diagnosis of fetal stroke in our review of 128 cases was 29 ± 5.3 weeks and the median age was 30 weeks (range 22–37 weeks), with 34% of the fetuses diagnosed between 14 and 28 weeks and 66% diagnosed after 29 weeks.

A number of patients remain undiagnosed during the fetal and neonatal periods and only become manifest in late infancy; these children are commonly diagnosed as "delayed presentation" in the current literature (18, 34, 85, 87). This presumptive fetal or neonatal event usually manifests as an asymmetry of reach and grasp at a median of 6 months (34, 87). Seizures and language delay were also seen (87). An interesting observation is that internal capsule damage is significantly more common among those cases who presented later in childhood, suggesting that this injury may be relatively silent in the fetal and neonatal time periods (87).

Role of Ultrasound

The diagnosis of fetal intraventricular hemorrhage (IVH) and stroke first became possible with the use of fetal cranial ultrasonography (US) (16, 88). Considering that a significant percentage of fetal stroke cases remain asymptomatic, in utero ultrasound with its wide availability and low cost is a practical screening tool. Screening fetal US is usually performed during the early portion of the second trimester, a time before stroke typically occurs (89, 90). When late second or third trimester US is performed, however, it is an effective screening tool since both cerebral cavitary lesions and hemorrhage are easily diagnosed by this modality. Although being practical, the ultrasound imaging lacks the sensitivity of CT and MRI for the detection of either acute or small ischemic lesions (58, 91–97). In a recent study of fetal strokes, in 21% of the cases MRI enabled a more accurate diagnosis of injury than either other modality (38). Estan and Hope (69) reported that US scans failed to demonstrate lesions that were present on CT in 9 out of 12 (75%) of their cohort.

Role of CT

Because of its superior tissue resolution CT was used primarily or as an adjunct to ultrasound in the imaging of fetal or perinatal stroke (98). Sreenan et al. (81) concluded that the extent of stroke on CT did not correlate with long-term outcome. Although CT provides much morphological information it has been largely replaced by MRI (11, 78, 94, 99, 100, 101).

Role of Fetal MRI

As a recently introduced imaging modality, fetal MRI now permits better definition of anatomical and functional injury to the fetal cerebrum and the extent of ongoing plasticity. Signal characteristics of infarct and hemorrhage are well established in the adult and pediatric population. However, at present, no such information is present for fetuses (102). Prior to 2000, 11% of fetal stroke cases had MRI studies and this increased to 48% in the period between 2000 and 2006. MRI technology is an ever changing one and new technologies improve its applicability.

The use of diffusion-weighted imaging for diagnosis of cerebral infarction in the neonate was first reported in 1994 (103). Further reports established this modality as the most sensitive imaging modality for the detection of acute stroke in the fetus or the newborn (101). Another technique, functional MRI, presents an appealing strategy to study functional consequences of the insult.

Treatment

Today there is no definitive treatment for fetal or neonatal stroke (104). Late diagnosis of the entity further limits potential therapies, and current efforts are directed at understanding the underlying pathology. Maternal thrombocyte infusion via cordocentesis is used in fetal alloimmune thrombocytopenia (25, 105). Pooled immunoglobulins may be administered to the mother with maternal ITP (9). The only potential therapy to treat maternal warfarin use is fresh frozen plasma transfusion through cordocentesis as fetal bioavailability of maternal vitamin K administration is only 1/20 of the maternal levels (13).

PROGNOSIS

Prognosis of Fetal Stroke

Mortality

Outcome data were available for 118 of 128 cases of fetal stroke (92%). Fifty-eight pregnancies resulted in fetal death, stillbirth, or were terminated (49% of fetal stroke cases with a known outcome). Of 60 cases which were born alive, 12 died in the neonatal period and 2 cases were deceased in early childhood.

Recurrence

There have been at least two reports of neonatal ischemic stroke cases who had a US-confirmed in utero stroke (18, 106). Similarly we have found 8 cases (6%) of acute fetal stroke incidents associated with a porencephalic cyst, which most likely indicates a secondary insult before 20–22 weeks.

Long-term Outcome

There is very limited information on the outcome of fetal cases. In our earlier publication of 54 cases of fetal stroke cases, we found 46 cases with a reported outcome; over half (51%) resulted in fetal or neonatal death and 55% of the survivors were handicapped at follow-up ages of 3 months to 6 years (5). Ghi et al. (54) published the findings of 109 cases of fetal intracranial hemorrhages, which included 16 of their cases and 93 cases from the literature. They reported that 40% of their cases died in utero or within the first month after birth. Only 53% of the reported newborns who survived were normal at a median follow-up of 11.6 months (54).

Indicators of Long-term Prognosis

Several studies have shown that fetal stroke with ventriculomegaly is associated with a poor outcome. In our analysis ventriculomegaly was present in 79 (62%) of the cases. Only eight of these were alive and normal at the last follow-up (10%).

Two studies commenting on the association of the ultrasound findings with postnatal outcome stated that in lower grade hemorrhages the complete disappearance of the hemorrhage on follow-up imaging was associated with a better postnatal neurologic outcome while progression to a higher grade indicated a worse prognosis (38, 54).

Prognosis of Neonatal Stroke

Mortality

In the USA the infant mortality rate related to stroke during 1995–1998 was 5.33/100 000. The rates were 2.21/100 000 for the perinatal period and 3.49/100 000 in the neonatal period. According to the National Hospital Discharge Survey from 1980 through 1998 the neonatal in-hospital mortality related to stroke was 10.1%. Similarly the Canadian Pediatric Stroke Registry reported mortality less than 10% following neonatal stroke. When comparing term and premature cases with cerebral arterial infarction, Govaert et al. (22) found an over 6 times higher likelihood of neonatal death in the premature group.

Recurrence

There are no conclusive studies on the risk of recurrence of neonatal stroke. However, reported risk is well below that of childhood or adult stroke. Lee et al. reported no recurrence in the follow-up of 176 patients for a median of 41 months. In a recent prospective follow-up study, Kurnik et al. (30) found a 1.86% risk of recurrent cerebral arterial stroke and a total of 3.3% risk of arterial or venous thrombosis with a median follow-up of 3.5 years. The highest incidence of recurrence was reported by the Canadian Pediatric Stroke Registry and ranged from 3 to 5% (55). A higher incidence of prothrombotic disorders in this cohort may be responsible for this higher incidence, which at the same time supports the notion that the risk of recurrence is determined by the underlying pathology (30, 55).

Long-term Prognosis

Much of the information on long-term prognosis following neonatal stroke is based on retrospective analysis. This is further complicated by the variance in stroke types, follow-up duration, methods of assessment, and the populations studied (1). Major studies reporting outcome of fetal and neonatal stroke are

Table 7-6   Major Studies on Outcome of Fetal and Neonatal Stroke

Study	N[a]	Inclusion criteria	Follow-up (months)	Recurrence rate	Late assessment	Neurodevelopmental outcome
Ment et al., 1984 (106)	11	Infants admitted to intensive care unit with a CT diagnosis of cerebral infarction	Mean 6.5 ± 2.1	N/A	No strict criteria	Dead 18% Normal in infancy 27% Hemi-/quadriplegic 36%
Sran and Baumann, 1988	17	Roentgenographically imaged brain infarct within 30 days after birth (clinical evidence of neonatal onset)	Mean 38 (range 12–132)	None	No strict criteria	1 dead The longer the follow-up, the worse the outcome
Trauner et al., 1993 (107)	29	Single unilateral cerebral infarction of fetal or neonatal onset. Multiple lesions, structural abnormalities (tumor, CVM), cases with global insults excluded	Mean 44 ± 5.4	None	Neurologic exam and intelligence tests	Hemiparesis in 72% Sensory deficit 35% Visual field cut 24%
Estan and Hope, 1997 (69)	12	Infants with gestational age ≥32 weeks with unilateral cerebral infarction	Median 33 (range 11–60)	None	No strict criteria	No motor, cognitive or seizure disorders 92% Hemiplegia in 8%
Sreenan et al., 2000 (81)	47	Term neonates with cerebral infarction as diagnosed on CT	Mean 42.1 (range 18–164)	None	No strict criteria	No sequelae 33% CP 48% Visual impairment 15% Epilepsy 46% Cognitive impairment 40%
Golomb et al., 2001 (34)	22	Hemiparesis with onset after 2 months of age, normal neonatal neurologic exam, remote cortical infarct on MRI	Median 48 (range 8–198)	None	No strict criteria	Persistent hemiparesis in all Speech, behavior, or learning problems in 55% Epilepsy in 23%
Mercuri et al., 1998 and 2004 (108)	22	Full-term infants with infarction on neonatal MRI done for work-up of neonatal seizures	Until school age	None	Structured neurologic exam and movement assessment battery for children	No motor sequelae 40% Hemiplegia 30% Other motor deficit 30%
Lee et al., 2005 (87)	176	Strokes occurring in utero or until 28 days after birth diagnosed by MRI/CT	Median 41 (range 1–89)	None	Chart review	No sequelae 19% CP 58% Epilepsy 39% Language delay 25% Behavioral abnormalities 22%
de Vries et al., 2005 (109)	15	Infants with gestational age ≥35 weeks with an arterial ischemic stroke or borderzone infarction found on MRI made for neonatal encephalopathy or seizures	12 of 14 survivors followed >18 months	None	MRI, neurologic exam	1 dead Hemiplegia in 36% Hemiparesis in 1 Epilepsy in 1

[a]Only term neonates included in the table.

listed in Table 7-6. Several authors indicate a relatively poor outcome (81, 106, 107, 110, 111). Lynch et al. (53) in their literature review of 415 cases over a 30-year period reported that only 40% of the patients had a normal development and that 3% had died. In the Canadian Pediatric Stroke Registry, outcome was normal in a third (55). Sreenan et al. (81) reported that two-thirds of their cases were affected by some mental-motor deficit. Lee et al. (87) found that only 19% had a normal outcome. Estan and Hope (69), on the contrary, reported a better outcome, indicating that 11 of 12 cases with unilateral cortical infarction had a normal neuromotor development at a median of 33 months. In their analysis, de Vries and Levene (112) concluded that over 50% of infants with neonatal cerebral infarction were entirely normal at the age of 12–18 months. In a more recent study by de Vries et al. (71) the authors found that when the neonatal thromboembolic event involved the main branch of the MCA the patients had significant morbidity, while the involvement of other branches had a more favorable outcome.

For all strokes, motor deficits are generally diagnosed during infancy or early childhood, but cognitive and behavioral deficits usually become manifest at later ages. As discussed previously, spastic hemiplegia in the most common sequel of neonatal stroke.

Indicators of Long-term Prognosis

Certain symptomatology, EEG, and imaging findings may be indicative of late outcome (1). Although abnormal neurologic exam at discharge from the NICU has been associated with long-term disability by Sreenan et al. (81), this finding has not been supported by other studies (113). Several authors have also suggested that cases presenting beyond the neonatal period had a higher incidence of permanent neurologic problems (34) and CP (87).

Diffuse or multifocal injury as demonstrated by diffuse background abnormality in the neonatal EEG is suggestive of increased risk for epilepsy (85). In a study by Mercuri et al. (113) an abnormal background in an EEG study within the first week after stroke correlated with future hemiplegia in 83% of cases. Sreenan et al. (81) in their study of 47 term neonates with cerebral infarction as diagnosed on CT interestingly reported that the absence of seizures in the neonatal period was associated with no long-term disability.

Localization or the extent of findings on CT were not correlated with long-term outcome (81). MRI may be of practical importance in predicting long-term outcome. Hemiplegia was reported in only a small proportion of cases with cerebral infarction on neonatal MRI and was present only in children who had concomitant involvement of hemisphere, internal capsule, and basal ganglia (108). The same study concluded that involvement of the internal capsule is always associated with motor disturbance to some degree when assessed at school age (108). De Vries et al. (109) confirmed that the involvement of cortex, basal ganglia, and the internal capsule invariably resulted in hemiplegia. Another study looking at the visual function of patients with perinatal stroke concluded that the presence or severity of visual abnormalities could not always be predicted by the site and extent of the lesion seen on imaging (114). Similarly, Mercuri (84) reported that in full-term infants with neonatal arterial ischemic stroke the presence of large porencephalies on MRI was associated with a high rate of epilepsy and cognitive deficits. In that series, 9 of 14 (64%) surviving infants with adverse long-term outcome were noted to have either parenchymal hemorrhage or focal hemispheric porencephaly, in contrast to 2 of 8 (25%) infants with normal neurodevelopmental outcome (84). It is not known, however, what proportion of this cohort can be attributed to antenatal events.

Several studies have indicated a normal intelligence in children with neonatal stroke (107, 115–117). However, lower IQs have been documented in children with

Table 7-7   Comparison of Fetal and Neonatal Stroke

	Fetal stroke	Neonatal stroke
Time of diagnosis	14 GA to onset of labor resulting in delivery	Labor resulting in delivery through 28 PND
Incidence	4.6 per 10 000 deliveries (excludes intrauterine death and delayed presentation)	17 to 93 per 10 000 live births
Gender predilection	None reported	Male predominance reported in one study
Hemorrhage	>80%	20%
Most common etiologies	- Complicated twin gestation - Alloimmune thrombocytopenia - Maternal trauma - No evident cause in roughly half of the cases	- Most likely multifactorial - Prothromotic disorders - Polycythemia - Cardiac disorders - Preeclampsia - Labor-related insults - Chorioamnionitis
Presentation	- Neonatal seizures - Neonatal encephalopathy - Cerebral palsy - Delayed onset motor symptoms - May be clinically silent	- Seizures - Cerebral palsy - Neonatal encephalopathy - May be clinically silent
Outcome	Fetal or neonatal death in over half Severe disability in over half of survivors	Normal neurological development in 19–40%
Recurrence	Only few cases reported	Up to 5% reported

epilepsy and children with more widespread infarcts (117). A study of fetal and neonatal stoke cases with unilateral brain damage found no evidence of clinically significant behavioral or emotional problems between affected individuals and control individuals, even when the frontal lobe was involved (107).

CONCLUSIONS

For the developing brain, stroke is most certainly a complex disorder. While the true incidence of fetal stroke remains largely unexplored, stroke occurs in 2–9 per 1000 live term births. Stroke in the fetus is almost always hemorrhagic, while stroke in the term neonate is more commonly caused by embolic or thromboembolic events. Similarly, the most common causes of stroke in the fetus are twin gestation, alloimmune thrombocytopenia, and maternal trauma while prothrombotic disorders, cardiac disorders, polycythemia, preeclampsia, prolonged rupture of membranes, and chorioamnionitis are most commonly diagnosed in series of neonatal stroke. A quick comparison is provided in Table 7-7. Table 7-8 presents all reported cases of fetal stroke in the current literature.

Finally, stroke – whether fetal or neonatal – appears to result in significant disability in childhood and beyond. For this reason, better definitions of injury and targeted population, genetic, and environmental risk factor studies are needed to prevent this injury to the developing brain.

Table 7-8 Fetal Stroke Cases in Present Literature

Reference (year)	Patient	Gest age at Dx	Sex	Mode of prenatal diagnosis	Prenatal radiological findings	Postnatal radiological or postmortem findings	Pregnancy complications	Birth history	Outcome
Kim et al. (16) (1982)	1	28 wks	M	US	IPH, IVH, VM	Prenatal findings confirmed by autopsy	Maternal fever with pancreatitis 26–28 wks, placental thromboses	IUFD	Death
Lustig-Gillman et al. (88) (1983)	2	31 wks	M	US	IVH, VM	Massive IVH with parenchyma hemorrhage	–	Died at birth	Death
McGahan et al. (118) (1984)	3	34 wks	M	US, CT	IVH, VM	Ventriculomegaly, IVH	–	Preterm delivery	Shunted hydrocephalus, hemiparetic at 3 months
Donn et al. (119) (1984)	4	32 wks	M	US	Supratentorial and posterior fossa hemorrhage, IVH, VM	–	–	Stillbirth	Death
Bondurant et al. (120) (1984)	5	26 wks	M	US	IPH	Prenatal findings confirmed by autopsy	Preeclampsia, placental abruption	Stillbirth	Death
Minkoff et al. (14) (1985)	6	32 wks	M	US	IVH, VM	Prenatal findings confirmed by autopsy	Maternal epilepsy; seizures during 2nd and 3rd trimesters	IUFD	Death
Mintz et al. (21) (1985)	7	29 wks	M	US	IVH, VM	Massive intraparenchymal hemorrhage confirmed by autopsy	Polyhydramnios	Stillbirth	Death
Pretorius et al. (121) (1986)	8	33 wks	F	US	IPH	Ventriculomegaly, intraparenchymal hemorrhage	-	Preterm delivery	NL at 16 months
DeVries et al. (25) (1988)	9	35 wks	M	US	IPH	Ventriculomegaly, subcortical hemorrhage, cystic encephalomalacia	Fetal alloimmune thrombo-cytopenia	Neonatal seizures	N/A

Reference (year)	Case	GA	Sex	Modality	Dx	Imaging findings	Maternal/pregnancy factors	Clinical course / delivery	Outcome
Leidig et al. (42) (1988)	10	29 wks	F	US	IVH, VM	Ventriculomegaly, IVH	Complicated twin pregnancy	Preterm delivery	Shunted hydrocephalus; Long-term follow-up N/A
	11	37 wks	M	US	IPH, VM	Subependymal hemorrhage confirmed by US and at autopsy	Oligohydramnios, IUGR	Hepatic insufficiency, thrombocytopenia, pulmonary hypoplasia, congenital hepatitis	Neonatal death
Zorzi et al. (122) (1988)	12	36 wks	M	US	IVH, VM	Porencephaly, subependymal cyst, IVH	—	Preterm delivery	Shunted hydrocephalus, long-term follow-up N/A
Stoddard et al. (123) (1988)	13	34 wks	F	US	PVH, IVH	Ventriculomegaly, cavitation, parenchymal hypodensity	Oligohydramnios, IUGR	Preterm delivery	Microcephaly, developmental delay at 8 months
Gunn et al. (124) (1988)	14	26 wks	N/A	US	IPH, IVH	Prenatal findings confirmed by autopsy	Complicated twin pregnancy	Stillbirth	Death
Sims et al. (125) (1988)	15	34 wks	N/A	US	IVH	—	Trauma	Term	Hemiplegia, shunted hydrocephalus
Burrows et al. (126) (1988)	16	34 wks	N/A	US	Porencephaly	—	Fetal alloimmune thrombocytopenia	—	Normal
Chambers et al. (20) (1988)	17	36 wks	N/A	US	IVH	—	Hypertensive mother	—	Shunted hydrocephalus
Fogarty et al. (17) (1989)	18	25 wks	M	US	PVH, IVH	Periventricular hemorrhage, IVH	Maternal fever and diarrhea 1 wk prior to dx, placental thromboses	Preterm delivery	N/A
Stirling et al. (127) (1989)	19	35 wks	N/A	US	IVH, VM	Intraparenchymal hemorrhage	Maternal gastroenteritis and hypertension at 35 wks	Preterm delivery	Long term follow-up N/A, patient shunted but later became shunt independent

(continued)

Table 7-8 Fetal Stroke Cases in Present Literature—cont'd

Reference (year)	Patient	Gest age at Dx	Sex	Mode of prenatal diagnosis	Prenatal radiological findings	Postnatal radiological or postmortem findings	Pregnancy complications	Birth history	Outcome
Jennett et al. (128) (1990)	20	35 wks	M	US	PVH, posterior fossa hemorrhage	–	–	–	Neonatal death
Giovangrandi et al. (129) (1990)	21	20 wks	N/A	US	IVH, VM	–	Fetal alloimmune thrombocytopenia	–	Neonatal death
Mullaart et al. (29) (1991)	22	32 wks	F	US	IPH, VM	Ventriculomegaly, intraparenchymal hemorrhage	Fetal von Willebrand disease	Term, abnormal EEG	Hemiparesis at 6 months
Scher et al. (18) (1991)	23	32 wks	M	US	Porencephaly	Porencephaly	Placental hemorrhage	Term	Spastic hemiparesis
	24	32 wks	M	US	Porencephaly, IVH	Porencephaly, IVH and ventriculomegaly on MRI	Hx maternal thrombophebitis and prophylactic heparin throughout pregnancy	Term	Hemiparesis, dystonia, shunted hydrocephalus
Edmondson et al. (130) (1992)	25	30 wks	M	US	IPH	Hydranencephaly confirmed by CT and at autopsy	None	Preterm delivery	Neonatal death
Achiron et al. (131) (1993)	26	27 wks	N/A	US	Massive IPH	N/A	Complicated twin pregnancy Preeclampsia	Preterm delivery Stillbirth	Neonatal death
	27	26 wks	N/A	US	IVH, VM	N/A	N/A	Preterm delivery	Death
	28	29 wks	N/A	US	PVH	Germinal matrix hemorrhage on US			Normal at 12 months
	29	30 wks	N/A	US	PVH, VM	Ventriculomegaly, PVL	N/A	Term	Normal at 18 months
	30	36 wks	N/A	US	Massive IVH, VM	Ventriculomegaly, intraparencyhmal hemorrhage, IVH	N/A	Term	Severe developmental retardation, death at 7 months
Ville et al. (13) (1993)	31	33 wks	N/A	US	Massive IPH, posterior fossa cyst with cerebellar hypoplasia	Prenatal findings confirmed by autopsy	Maternal pulmonary embolism at 26 wks, warfarin use with a surge	IUFD	Death

32		29 wks	N/A	US	Massive IVH	Prenatal findings confirmed by autopsy	Maternal warfarin use for congenital cardiac disease throughout pregnancy up to INR of 8.6 at 28 wks	IUFD	Death
33	Sibony et al. (132) (1993)	26 wks	N/A	US	IPH	–	Preeclampsia	Pregnancy terminated	Death
34	Anderson et al. (41) (1994)	20 wks	N/A	US	IPH, VM	Polymicrogyria and intraparenchymal hematoma	CMV-related changes in fetus	Pregnancy terminated	Death
35	Hadi et al. (133) (1994)	36 wks	N/A	US	Posterior fossa hemorrhage	–	–	–	Neonatal death
36	Dean et al. (134) (1995)	34 wks	M	US	IPH, IVH, VM	–	Fetal alloimmune thrombocytopenia	Premature delivery	Shunted hydrocephalus
37	Tampakoudis et al. (9) (1995)	32 wks	N/A	US	IPH, VM	Ventriculomegaly, porencephaly	Maternal idiopathic thrombocytopenic purpura	Preterm delivery	Neonatal death secondary to untreated hydrocephalus
38	Reiss et al. (135) (1996)	22 wks	M	US/MRI	IPH	Porencephaly	–	Term	Normal at 18 months
39	Vergani et al. (136) (1996)	23 wks	N/A	US	IVH, VM	–	–	–	Normal at 30 months
40		34 wks	N/A	US	IVH, VM	–	–	–	Normal at 30 months
41		31 wks	N/A	US	Posterior fossa hemorrhage, IVH, VM	–	–	–	Developmental delay
42		33 wks	N/A	US/MRI	Cortical infarct, IVH, VM	–	–	–	Developmental delay, shunted hydrocephalus
43	Pilu et al. (137) (1997)	29 wks	N/A	US	Porencephaly, VM	N/A	–	Term	Severe retardation, shunted hydrocephalus
44		36 wks	N/A	US	Porencephaly, VM	N/A	–	Term	Severe retardation, shunted hydrocephalus
45		33 wks	N/A	US	Porencephaly, VM	N/A	–	Term	

(continued)

Table 7-8 Fetal Stroke Cases in Present Literature—cont'd

Reference (year)	Patient	Gest age at Dx	Sex	Mode of prenatal diagnosis	Prenatal radiological findings	Postnatal radiological or postmortem findings	Pregnancy complications	Birth history	Outcome
	46	32 wks	N/A	US	IVH, porencephaly, VM	N/A	Fetal alloimmune thrombocyto-penia	Term	Severe retardation, shunted hydrocephalus Death
	47	35 wks	N/A	US	IVH, porencephaly, VM	N/A	–	Term	Severe retardation, shunted hydrocephalus Death
	48	25 wks	N/A	US	Porencephaly, VM	–	Complicated twin pregnancy	Preterm delivery	Death
	49	24 wks	N/A	US	Porencephaly, VM	–	Complicated twin pregnancy	Pregnancy terminated	Death
	50	22 wks	N/A	US	Porencephaly	–	–	Pregnancy terminated	Death
	51	32 wks	N/A	US	Porencephaly	Schizencephaly	–	Term	Death
	52	34 wks	N/A	US	Porencephaly	–	–	Term	Severe retardation
Kirkinen et al. (138) (1997)	53	36 wks	N/A	US/MRI	VM, choroidal hemorrhage	Ventriculomegaly, IVH	N/A	–	Shunted hydrocephalus Long-term follow-up N/A
	54	32 wks	N/A	US/MRI	IPH, VM	Prenatal findings confirmed by autopsy	N/A	Stillbirth	Death
	55	33 wks	N/A	US/MRI	VM	–	N/A	N/A	Shunted hydrocephalus Long-term follow-up N/A
Guerriero et al. (139) (1997)	56	25 wks	N/A	US	IVH	–	Preeclampsia	Preterm delivery	Neonatal death
Sherer et al. (15) (1998)	57	23 wks	N/A	US	IVH	–	Complicated twin pregnancy	N/A	N/A

Reference	Case	GA	Sex	Modality	Findings	Additional findings	Risk factor/cause	Delivery	Outcome
Ohba et al. (140) (1998)	58	32 wks	M	US/MRI	PVH, IVH, VM, aqueductal obstruction	N/A	Epileptic mother, seizures 3–4/month, on multiple medications	IUFD	Death
Canapicchi et al. (141) (1998)	59	34 wks	M	US/MRI	PVH, VM	Ventriculomegaly, subependymal chronic hemorrhage, IVH	N/A	Term, NL	Shunted hydrocephalus, otherwise NL at 12 months
Brun et al. (35) (1999)	60	29 wks	F	US	PVH, VM, intraventricular synechiae	Same findings with progressive PVL	Pyruvate carboxylase deficiency	Preterm delivery, severe metabolic disturbance	Neonatal death
Hashimoto et al. (142) (1999)	61	37 wks	N/A	US/MRI	IVH, VM	–	N/A	N/A	N/A
Kirkinen et al. (32) (2000)	62	33 wks	F	US/MRI	IPH, VM, intraorbital mass	Ventriculomegaly, subependymal hemorrhage	Protein C deficiency	Preterm delivery	Shunted hydrocephalus, blindness secondary to vitrous hemorrhage
Groothuis et al. (90) (2000)	63	26 wks	F	US	IVH, VM	Grade 4 IVH	Partial placental abruption at 25 wks	Preterm delivery	N/A
Strigini et al. (6) (2001)	64	28 wks	F	US/MRI	IPH	Intraparenchymal hemorrhage Ventriculomegaly	Car accident within 24h of US	IUFD	Death
(2001)	65	34 wks	F	US/MRI	PVH, IVH, VM	Ventriculomegaly	Car accident within 72 h of US	Term	Shunted hydrocephalus Hemiparesis at 12 months
	66	38 wks	M	US	IVH, VM	N/A	Fall while gardening within 24 h of US	Term	Shunted hydrocephalus Spasticity, motor impairment at 6 months
Bassez et al. (24) (2001)	67	28 wks	F	US	IPH	Prenatal findings confirmed by autopsy	Fetal alloimmune thrombocytopenia	IUFD	Death
Fukui et al. (143) (2001)	68	32 wks	F	US/MRI	IVH, VM	Ventriculomegaly, subependymal hemorrhage, IVH	None	Term	Shunted hydrocephalus, otherwise NL at 15 months

(continued)

Table 7-8 Fetal Stroke Cases in Present Literature—cont'd

Reference (year)	Patient	Gest age at Dx	Sex	Mode of prenatal diagnosis	Prenatal radiological findings	Postnatal radiological or postmortem findings	Pregnancy complications	Birth history	Outcome
	69	36wks	M	US/MRI	IVH, VM	Ventriculomegaly, IVH, aqueductal obstruction by hematoma	None	Term, NL	Shunted hydrocephalus, otherwise NL at 12 months
Laveaucoupet et al. (11) (2001)	70	29 wks	F	US/MRI	Multicystic encephalomalacia, IVH	IVH, PVL, ventriculomegaly	Maternal diabetes, severe ketoacidosis	Pregnancy terminated	Death
	71	32 wks	F	US/MRI	Porencephaly	Cerebral necrosis at autopsy	N/A	Pregnancy terminated	Death
	72	35 wks	M	US/MRI	Periventricular ischemia	Cerebral necrosis at autopsy	N/A	Pregnancy terminated	Death
	73	34 wks	M	US/MRI	Porencephaly, IVH	Porencephaly	N/A	N/A	N/A
	74	32 wks	F	US/MRI	Cystic infarct in the internal capsule	Same	Complicated twin pregnancy	Term	Normal at 20 months
Elpeleg et al. (39) (2001)	75	22 wks	N/A	US	IPH, calcifications, VM	–	Carnitine palmitoijyl trsf deficiency	Pregnancy terminated	Death
Dale et al., (60) (2002)	76	20wks	F	US/MRI	Porencephaly, VM	–	Fetal alloimmune thrombocytopenia	Premature delivery	Microcephaly, epilepsy
Hildebrandt et al. (26) (2002)	77	34 wks	N/A	US/MRI	Schizencephaly, IPH, cerebellar hypoplasia,	Same	Fetal alloimmune thrombocytopenia	N/A	N/A
Ghi et al. (54) (2003)	78	32 wks	N/A	US	IVH	–	None	Live birth	Mild ventriculomegaly at birth Long-term follow-up N/A
	79	22 wks	N/A	US	IVH	–	None	Live birth	Normal neonatal US Long-term follow-up N/A
	80	21 wks	N/A	US	IVH	–	None	Live birth	Normal neonatal US Long-term follow-up N/A

81	24 wks	N/A	US	IVH	—	Hydrops fetalis	Live birth	Shunted hydrocephalus
82	29 wks	N/A	US	IVH, VM	—	—	Pregnancy terminated	Death
83	28 wks	N/A	US	IVH, VM	—	—	IUFD	Death
84	29 wks	N/A	US	IVH, VM	—	Trauma	Live birth	Mental retardation, shunted hydrocephalus
85	33 wks	N/A	US	IVH, VM	—	None	Live birth	Shunted hydrocephalus
86	24 wks	N/A	US	IPH, VM	—	Complicated twin pregnancy	Live birth	Normal
87	22 wks	N/A	US	IPH	Prenatal findings confirmed by autopsy	—	Pregnancy terminated	Death
88	22 wks	N/A	US	Posterior fossa hemorrhage	Prenatal findings confirmed by autopsy	Rh isoimmunization with hydrops	Pregnancy terminated	Death
89	22 wks	N/A	US	Posterior fossa hemorrhage	Cerebellar hypoplasia	Rh isoimmunization with hydrops	Live birth	Normal at 12 months
Current Yale cohort 90	31 wks	M	US/MRI	Porencephaly, IVH, VM	Progressive hydrocephalus	Complicated twin pregnancy Maternal heparin use	Term	Hemiparesis, delay, shunted hydrocephalus
91	34 wks	F	US/MRI	Cortical ischemia, IPH, IVH, VM	Ventriculomegaly, colpocephaly	Gestational diabetes	Term, hypotonic, neonatal seizures	Tetraparesis, delay, epilepsy, hydrocephalus
92	32 wks	F	US/MRI	Porencephaly, IPH, IVH, VM	Progressive hydrocephalus	None	Term	Hemiparesis, epilepsy, delay, shunted hydrocephalus
93	22 wks	F	US/MRI	Porencephaly, VM	Porencephaly, ventriculomegaly	Oligohydramnios	Term	Normal
94	34 wks	F	US	IVH, VM	Ventriculomegaly, lenticular hemorrhage, IVH	None	Term	Normal
95	22 wks	F	US	PVH	Subependymal ischemic changes	Pyruvate carboxylase deficiency, gestational diabetes	Term, severe metabolic disturbance, neonatal seizures	Death

(continued)

Table 7-8 Fetal Stroke Cases in Present Literature—cont'd

Reference (year)	Patient	Gest age at Dx	Sex	Mode of prenatal diagnosis	Prenatal radiological findings	Postnatal radiological or postmortem findings	Pregnancy complications	Birth history	Outcome
	96	35 wks	M	US/MRI	IPH, IVH, VM	Same	Fetal alloimmune thrombocytopenia	Preterm delivery	Spasticity
	97	24 wks	F	US/MRI	Porencephaly	Same	Maternal JRA	Term	Shunted hydrocephalus, developmental delay
	98	31 wks	F	US/MRI	IPH	Same	Fetal alloimmune thrombocytopenia, maternal diabetes	Preterm delivery	Normal cognitive testing
	99	18 wks	M	US	PVH, IVH	–	Possible genetic defect Mother positive for MTHFR mutatins, treated	Pregnancy terminated	Death
	100	19 wks	M	US/MRI	PVH, IVH	–	Possible genetic defect Mother positive for MTHFR mutatins, treated	Pregnancy terminated	Death
Elchalal et al. (38) (2006)	101	22 wks	N/A	US	PVH,VM	Prenatal findings confirmed by autopsy	–	Pregnancy terminated	Death
	102	22 wks	N/A	US/MRI	IVH, VM	Prenatal findings confirmed by autopsy	–	Pregnancy terminated	Death
	103	28 wks	N/A	US/MRI	IVH, VM	Prenatal findings confirmed by autopsy	Complicated twin pregnancy	Pregnancy terminated	Death

104	22 wks	N/A	US	IVH, VM	Prenatal findings confirmed by autopsy	–	IUFD	Death
105	23 wks	N/A	US/MRI	IVH, VM, calcifications	Same on neonatal US	–	Term	Normal at 48 months
106	28 wks	N/A	US/MRI	IVH, VM	Spontaneous regression	Complicated twin pregnancy	Preterm delivery	Normal at 30 months
107	24 wks	N/A	US	IVH, VM	Neonatal US confirmation of VM	Rh isoimmunization with hydrops	Preterm delivery	Normal 48 months
108	33 wks	N/A	US/MRI	IVH, VM	–	–	IUFD	Death
109	40 wks	N/A	US	IVH, VM	Confirmed at postmortem CT	–	IUFD	Death
110	30 wks	N/A	US/MRI	IVH, VM	Confirmed at neonatal CT	–	IUFD	Death
111	34 wks	N/A	US/MRI	IVH, VM	Aquaductal stenosis on neonatal MRI, IVH	–	Preterm delivery	Shunted hydrocephalus, developmental delay
112	26 wks	N/A	US/MRI	IPH, VM	–	–	IUFD	Death
113	29 wks	N/A	US	IPH,VM	Prenatal findings confirmed by autopsy	–	IUFD	Death
114	24 wks	N/A	US	IPH, porencephaly	Confirmed at postmortem CT	–	IUFD	Death
115	34 wks	N/A	US	IPH, VM, calcifications	Prenatal findings confirmed by autopsy, dystrophic calcifications, CMV negative	–	IUFD	Death
116	24 wks	N/A	US	IPH, VM, calcifications	Prenatal findings confirmed by autopsy and postmortem CT	–	IUFD	Death
117	21 wks	N/A	US	IPH, porencephaly, VM	Prenatal findings confirmed by autopsy and postmortem CT	–	IUFD	Death
118	19 wks	N/A	US	IPH, VM, calcifications	–	Carnitine palmitoyl-transferase deficiency	IUFD	Death
119	22 wks	N/A	US	IPH,VM	–	–	IUFD	Death

(continued)

Table 7-8 **Fetal Stroke Cases in Present Literature—cont'd**

Reference (year) Patient	Gest age at Dx	Sex	Mode of prenatal diagnosis	Prenatal radiological findings	Postnatal radiological or postmortem findings	Pregnancy complications	Birth history	Outcome
120	23 wks	N/A	US/MRI	IPH, VM	Prenatal findings confirmed by autopsy	IUGR	IUFD	Death
121	32 wks	N/A	US/MRI	IPH	Same on neonatal US	IUGR	Premature delivery	Moderate psychomotor retardation
122	31 wks	N/A	US	Porencephaly, VM	Confirmed at neonatal CT	–	Term	Mental retardation, shunted hydrocephalus
123	22 wks	N/A	US	Porencephaly, VM	Confirmed at neonatal CT	Polyhydramnios	Term	Mental retardation, hemiplegia, blindness, shunted hydrocephalus
124	34 wks	N/A	US	Porencephaly	Confirmed at neonatal CT	Polyhydramnios	Premature delivery	Severe neurodevelopmental retardation
125	30 wks	N/A	US/MRI	Posterior fossa hemorrhage	Neonatal MRI revealed absence of left cerebellar lobe	–	Term	Severe neurological impairment
126	14 wks	N/A	US	Porencephaly, VM	Confirmed at neonatal CT	Complicated twin pregnancy	Premature delivery	Neonatal death
127	32 wks	N/A	US/MRI	IPH	Confirmed at neonatal CT	–	Premature delivery	Severe neuromotor impairment
128	23 wks	N/A	US/MRI	IPH	–	Complicated twin pregnancy	Term	Hemiparesis

Acknowledgments

The authors wish to thank Drs. Gabrielle deVeber and Donna Ferreiro for scientific advice. K.O. was supported by Anna Fuller Fund. L.R.M. was supported by NS 27116 and NS 35476.

REFERENCES

1. Lynch JK, Hirtz DG, DeVeber G, et al. Report of the National Institute of Neurological Disorders and Stroke workshop on perinatal and childhood stroke. Pediatrics 109:116–23, 2002.
2. Chalmers EA. Perinatal stroke: risk factors and management. Br J Haematol 130:333–43, 2005.
3. Bissonnette JM, Hohimer AR, Richardson BS, et al. Regulation of cerebral blood flow in the fetus. J Dev Physiol 6:275–80, 1984.
4. El-Khoury N, Braun A, Hu F, et al. Astrocyte end-feet in germinal matrix, cerebral cortex, and white matter in developing infants. Pediatr Res 59:673–9, 2006.
5. Ozduman K, Pober BR, Barnes P, et al. Fetal stroke. Pediatr Neurol 30:151–62, 2004.
6. Strigini FA, Cioni G, Canapicchi R, et al. Fetal intracranial hemorrhage: is minor maternal trauma a possible pathogenetic factor? Ultrasound Obstet Gynecol 18:335–42, 2001.
7. Lee J, Croen LA, Backstrand KH, et al. Maternal and infant characteristics associated with perinatal arterial stroke in the infant. JAMA 293:723–9, 2005.
8. Günther G, Junker R, Strater R, et al. Symptomatic ischemic stroke in full-term neonates: role of acquired and genetic prothrombotic risk factors. Stroke 31:2437–41, 2000.
9. Tampakoudis P, Bili H, Lazaridis E, et al. Prenatal diagnosis of intracranial hemorrhage secondary to maternal idiopathic thrombocytopenic purpura: a case report. Am J Perinatol 12:268–70, 1995.
10. Cervera R, Piette JC, Font J, et al. Antiphospholipid syndrome: clinical and immunologic manifestations and patterns of disease expression in a cohort of 1,000 patients. Arthritis Rheum 46:1019–27, 2002.
11. de Laveaucoupet J, Audibert F, Guis F, et al. Fetal magnetic resonance imaging (MRI) of ischemic brain injury. Prenat Diagn 21:729–36, 2001.
12. Govaert P, Staelens V, Vanhaesebrouch P. Perinatal intracranial hemorrhage due to maternal salicylate ingestion. Clin Pediatr (Phila) 34:174–5, 1995.
13. Ville Y, Jenkins E, Shearer MJ, et al. Fetal intraventricular haemorrhage and maternal warfarin. Lancet 341:1211, 1993.
14. Minkoff H, Schaffer RM, Delke I, et al. Diagnosis of intracranial hemorrhage in utero after a maternal seizure. Obstet Gynecol 65:22S–24S, 1985.
15. Sherer DM, Anyaegbunam A, Onyeije C. Antepartum fetal intracranial hemorrhage, predisposing factors and prenatal sonography: a review. Am J Perinatol 15:431–41, 1998.
16. Kim MS, Elyaderani MK. Sonographic diagnosis of cerebroventricular hemorrhage in utero. Radiology 142:479–80, 1982.
17. Fogarty K, Cohen HL, Haller JO. Sonography of fetal intracranial hemorrhage: unusual causes and a review of the literature. J Clin Ultrasound 17:366–70, 1989.
18. Scher MS, Belfar H, Martin J, et al. Destructive brain lesions of presumed fetal onset: antepartum causes of cerebral palsy. Pediatrics 88:898–906, 1991.
19. Boyce LH, Khandji AG, DeKlerk AM, et al. Fetomaternal hemorrhage as an etiology of neonatal stroke. Pediatr Neurol 11:255–7, 1994.
20. Chambers SE, Johnstone FD, Laing IA. Ultrasound in-utero diagnosis of choroid plexus haemorrhage. Br J Obstet Gynaecol 95:1317–20, 1988.
21. Mintz MC, Arger PH, Coleman BG. In utero sonographic diagnosis of intracerebral hemorrhage. J Ultrasound Med 4:375–6, 1985.
22. Govaert P, Matthys E, Zecic A, et al. Perinatal cortical infarction within middle cerebral artery trunks. Arch Dis Child Fetal Neonatal Ed 82:F59–63, 2000.
23. Roessmann U, Miller RT. Thrombosis of the middle cerebral artery associated with birth trauma. Neurology 30:889–92, 1980.
24. Bassez G, Kaplan C, Vauthier-Brouzes D, et al. A case of antenatal cerebral haemorrhage resulting from maternal alloimmunisation against fetal platelets. Childs Nerv Syst 17:302–4, 2001.
25. de Vries LS, Connell J, Bydder GM, et al. Recurrent intracranial haemorrhages in utero in an infant with alloimmune thrombocytopenia. Case report. Br J Obstet Gynaecol 95:299–302, 1988.
26. Hildebrandt T, Powell T. Repeated antenatal intracranial haemorrhage: magnetic resonance imaging in a fetus with alloimmune thrombocytopenia. Arch Dis Child Fetal Neonatal Ed 87:F222–3, 2002.
27. Amit M, Camfield PR. Neonatal polycythemia causing multiple cerebral infarcts. Arch Neurol 37:109–10, 1980.
28. van Kuijck MA, Rotteveel JJ, van Oostrom CG, et al. Neurological complications in children with protein C deficiency. Neuropediatrics 25:16–19, 1994.
29. Mullaart RA, Van Dongen P, Gabreels FJ, et al. Fetal periventricular hemorrhage in von Willebrand's disease: short review and first case presentation. Am J Perinatol 8:190–2, 1991.
30. Kurnik K, Kosch A, Strater R, et al. Recurrent thromboembolism in infants and children suffering from symptomatic neonatal arterial stroke: a prospective follow-up study. Stroke 34:2887–92, 2003.
31. Varelas PN, Sleight BJ, Rinder HM, et al. Stroke in a neonate heterozygous for factor V Leiden. Pediatr Neurol 18:262–4, 1998.

32. Kirkinen P, Salonvaara M, Nikolajev K, et al. Antepartum findings in fetal protein C deficiency. Prenat Diagn 20:746–9, 2000.

33. Ganesan V, Prengler M, McShane MA, et al. Investigation of risk factors in children with arterial ischemic stroke. Ann Neurol 53:167–73, 2003.

34. Golomb MR, MacGregor DL, Domi T, et al. Presumed pre- or perinatal arterial ischemic stroke: risk factors and outcomes. Ann Neurol 50:163–8, 2001.

35. Brun N, Robitaille Y, Grignon A, et al. Pyruvate carboxylase deficiency: prenatal onset of ischemia-like brain lesions in two sibs with the acute neonatal form. Am J Med Genet 84:94–101, 1999.

36. Nowak-Gottl U, Günther G, Kurnik K, et al. Arterial ischemic stroke in neonates, infants, and children: an overview of underlying conditions, imaging methods, and treatment modalities. Semin Thromb Hemost 29:405–14, 2003.

37. Aydinli N, Citak A, Caliskan M, et al. Vitamin K deficiency: late onset intracranial haemorrhage. Eur J Paediatr Neurol 2:199–203, 1998.

38. Elchalal U, Yagel S, Gomori JM, et al. Fetal intracranial hemorrhage (fetal stroke): does grade matter? Ultrasound Obstet Gynecol 26:233–43, 2005.

39. Elpeleg ON, Hammerman C, Saada A, et al. Antenatal presentation of carnitine palmitoyltransferase II deficiency. Am J Med Genet 102:183–7, 2001.

40. Ment LR, Ehrenkranz RA, Duncan CC. Bacterial meningitis as an etiology of perinatal cerebral infarction. Pediatr Neurol 2:276–9, 1986.

41. Anderson MW, McGahan JP. Sonographic detection of an in utero intracranial hemorrhage in the second trimester. J Ultrasound Med 13:315–18, 1994.

42. Leidig E, Dannecker G, Pfeiffer KH, et al. Intrauterine development of posthaemorrhagic hydro-cephalus. Eur J Pediatr 147:26–9, 1988.

43. Bussel JB, Zabusky MR, Berkowitz RL, et al. Fetal alloimmune thrombocytopenia. N Engl J Med 337:22–6, 1997.

44. Hope PL, Hall MA, Millward-Sadler GH, et al. Alpha-1-antitrypsin deficiency presenting as a bleeding diathesis in the newborn. Arch Dis Child 57:68–70, 1982.

45. Jenkins HR, Leonard JV, Kay JD, et al. Alpha-1-antitrypsin deficiency, bleeding diathesis, and intracranial haemorrhage. Arch Dis Child 57:722–3, 1982.

46. Payne NR, Hasegawa DK. Vitamin K deficiency in newborns: a case report in alpha-1-antitrypsin deficiency and a review of factors predisposing to hemorrhage. Pediatrics 73:712–16, 1984.

47. Kumar K. Neurological complications of congenital heart disease. Indian J Pediatr 67:S15–19, 2000.

48. Miller G, Mamourian AC, Tesman JR, et al. Long-term MRI changes in brain after pediatric open heart surgery. J Child Neurol 9:390–7, 1994.

49. Cilley RE, Zwischenberger JB, Andrews AF, et al. Intracranial hemorrhage during extracorporeal membrane oxygenation in neonates. Pediatrics 78:699–704, 1986.

50. Watson JW, Brown DM, Lally KP, et al. Complications of extracorporeal membrane oxygenation in neonates. South Med J 83:1262–5, 1990.

51. Bull MJ, Schreiner RL, Garg BP, et al. Neurologic complications following temporal artery catheterization. J Pediatr 96:1071–3, 1980.

52. Ruff RL, Shaw CM, Beckwith JB, et al. Cerebral infarction complicating umbilical vein catheterization. Ann Neurol 6:85, 1979.

53. Lynch JK, Nelson KB. Epidemiology of perinatal stroke. Curr Opin Pediatr 13:499–505, 2001.

54. Ghi T, Simonazzi G, Perolo A, et al. Outcome of antenatally diagnosed intracranial hemorrhage: case series and review of the literature. Ultrasound Obstet Gynecol 22:121–30, 2003.

55. DeVeber G. Canadian pediatric ischemic stroke registry. Pediatr Child Health A17:5–14, 2000.

56. Barkovich AJ. Brain and spine injuries in infancy and childhood. In (Pediatric Neuroimaging. Philadelphia, PA. Lippincott, Williams and Wilkins, 2000, pp. 157–240.

57. Levine D. Case 46: encephalomalacia in surviving twin after death of monochorionic co-twin. Radiology 223:392–5, 2002.

58. Levine D. MR imaging of fetal central nervous system abnormalities. Brain Cogn 50:432–48, 2002.

59. Johnson JA, Ryan G, al-Musa A, et al. Prenatal diagnosis and management of neonatal alloimmune thrombocytopenia. Semin Perinatol 21:45–52, 1997.

60. Dale ST, Coleman LT. Neonatal alloimmune thrombocytopenia: antenatal and postnatal imaging findings in the pediatric brain. Am J Neuroradiol 23:1457–65, 2002.

61. Pineda M, Campistol J, Vilaseca MA, et al. An atypical French form of pyruvate carboxylase deficiency. Brain Dev 17:276–9, 1995.

62. Wong LT, Davidson AG, Applegarth DA, et al. Biochemical and histologic pathology in an infant with cross-reacting material (negative) pyruvate carboxylase deficiency. Pediatr Res 20:274–9, 1986.

63. Gurgey A, Mesci L, Renda Y, et al. Factor V Q 506 mutation in children with thrombosis. Am J Hematol 53:37–9, 1996.

64. Pipe SW, Schmaier AH, Nichols WC, et al. Neonatal purpura fulminans in association with factor V R506Q mutation. J Pediatr 128:706–9, 1996.

65. Breedveld G, de Coo RF, Lequin MH, et al. Novel mutations in three families confirm a major role of COL4A1 in hereditary porencephaly. J Med Genet 43:490–5, 2006.

66. van der Knaap MS, Smit LM, Barkhof F, et al. Neonatal porencephaly and adult stroke related to mutations in collagen IV A1. Ann Neurol 59:504–11, 2006.

67. Gould DB, Phalan FC, Breedveld GJ, et al. Mutations in Col4a1 cause perinatal cerebral hemorrhage and porencephaly. Science 308:1167–71, 2005.

68. Miller V. Neonatal cerebral infarction. Semin Pediatr Neurol 7:278–88, 2000.

69. Estan J, Hope P. Unilateral neonatal cerebral infarction in full term infants. Arch Dis Child Fetal Neonatal Ed 76:F88–93, 1997.

70. Perlman JM, Rollins NK, Evans D. Neonatal stroke: clinical characteristics and cerebral blood flow velocity measurements. Pediatr Neurol 11:281–4, 1994.

71. de Vries LS, Groenendaal F, Eken P, et al. Infarcts in the vascular distribution of the middle cerebral artery in preterm and fullterm infants. Neuropediatrics 28:88–96, 1997.

72. deVeber G. Stroke and the child's brain: an overview of epidemiology, syndromes and risk factors. Curr Opin Neurol 15:133–8, 2002.

73. Barmada MA, Moossy J, Shuman RM. Cerebral infarcts with arterial occlusion in neonates. Ann Neurol 6:495–502, 1979.

74. Fullerton HJ, Wu YW, Zhao S, et al. Risk of stroke in children: ethnic and gender disparities. Neurology 61:189–94, 2003.

75. deVeber G. Canadian paediatric ischaemic stroke registry: Analysis of children with arterial ischaemic stroke. Canadian Pediatric Stroke Study Group. Ann Neurol 48:526, 2000.

76. Levy SR, Abroms IF, Marshall PC, et al. Seizures and cerebral infarction in the full-term newborn. Ann Neurol 17:366–70, 1985.

77. Lien JM, Towers CV, Quilligan EJ, et al. Term early-onset neonatal seizures: obstetric characteristics, etiologic classifications, and perinatal care. Obstet Gynecol 85:163–9, 1995.

78. Krishnamoorthy KS, Soman TB, Takeoka M, et al. Diffusion-weighted imaging in neonatal cerebral infarction: clinical utility and follow-up. J Child Neurol 15:592–602, 2000.

79. Mercuri E, Cowan F, Rutherford M, et al. Ischaemic and haemorrhagic brain lesions in newborns with seizures and normal Apgar scores. Arch Dis Child Fetal Neonatal Ed 73:F67–74, 1995.

80. Golomb MR, Dick PT, MacGregor DL, et al. Neonatal arterial ischemic stroke and cerebral sinovenous thrombosis are more commonly diagnosed in boys. J Child Neurol 19:493–7, 2004.

81. Sreenan C, Bhargava R, Robertson CM. Cerebral infarction in the term newborn: clinical presentation and long-term outcome. J Pediatr 137:351–5, 2000.

82. Uvebrant P. Hemiplegic cerebral palsy. Aetiology and outcome. Acta Paediatr Scand Suppl 345:1–100, 1988.

83. Hagberg B, Hagberg G, Beckung E, et al. Changing panorama of cerebral palsy in Sweden. VIII. Prevalence and origin in the birth year period 1991–94. Acta Paediatr 90:271–7, 2001.

84. Mercuri E. Early diagnostic and prognostic indicators in full term infants with neonatal cerebral infarction: an integrated clinical, neuroradiological and EEG approach. Minerva Pediatr 53:305–11, 2001.

85. Scher MS, Wiznitzer M, Bangert BA. Cerebral infarctions in the fetus and neonate: maternal-placental-fetal considerations. Clin Perinatol 29:693-724, vi–vii, 2002.

86. deVeber G, Monagle P, Chan A, et al. Prothrombotic disorders in infants and children with cerebral thromboembolism. Arch Neurol 55:1539–43, 1998.

87. Lee J, Croen LA, Lindan C, et al. Predictors of outcome in perinatal arterial stroke: a population-based study. Ann Neurol 58:303–8, 2005.

88. Lustig-Gillman I, Young BK, Silverman F, et al. Fetal intraventricular hemorrhage: sonographic diagnosis and clinical implications. J Clin Ultrasound 11:277–80, 1983.

89. Catanzarite VA, Schrimmer DB, Maida C, et al. Prenatal sonographic diagnosis of intracranial haemorrhage: report of a case with a sinusoidal fetal heart rate tracing, and review of the literature. Prenat Diagn 15:229–35, 1995.

90. Groothuis AM, de Kleine MJ, Oei SG. Intraventricular haemorrhage in utero. A case-report and review of the literature. Eur J Obstet Gynecol Reprod Biol 89:207–11, 2000.

91. Kostovic I, Judas M, Rados M, et al. Laminar organization of the human fetal cerebrum revealed by histochemical markers and magnetic resonance imaging. Cereb Cortex 12:536–44, 2002.

92. Levine D. Fetal magnetic resonance imaging. Top Magn Reson Imaging 12:1–2, 2001.

93. Levine D. Magnetic resonance imaging in prenatal diagnosis. Curr Opin Pediatr 13:572–8, 2001.

94. Levine D. Ultrasound versus magnetic resonance imaging in fetal evaluation. Top Magn Reson Imaging 12:25–38, 2001.

95. Levine D, Edelman RR. Fast MRI and its application in obstetrics. Abdom Imaging 22:589–96, 1997.

96. Levine D, Hatabu H, Gaa J, et al. Fetal anatomy revealed with fast MR sequences. AJR Am J Roentgenol 167:905–8, 1996.

97. Trop I, Levine D. Hemorrhage during pregnancy: sonography and MR imaging. AJR Am J Roentgenol 176:607–15, 2001.

98. Ment LR, Freedman RM, Ehrenkranz RA. Neonates with seizures attributable to perinatal complications: computed tomographic evaluation. Am J Dis Child 136:548–50, 1982.

99. Annick Sevely CM. Magnetic resonance imaging of the fetal brain. In Rutherford MA (ed). MRI of the Neonatal Brain. London: Harcourt/WB Saunders, 2002, pp. 287–94.

100. Kirkinen P, Partanen K, Ryynanen M, et al. Fetal intracranial hemorrhage. Imaging by ultrasound and magnetic resonance imaging. J Reprod Med 42:467–72, 1997.

101. Venkataraman A, Kingsley PB, Kalina P, et al. Newborn brain infarction: clinical aspects and magnetic resonance imaging. CNS Spectr 9:436–44, 2004.

102. Garel C. MRI of the Fetal Brain: Normal Development and Cerebral Pathologies. Berlin: Springer Verlag, 2004.

103. Cowan FM, Pennock JM, Hanrahan JD, et al. Early detection of cerebral infarction and hypoxic ischemic encephalopathy in neonates using diffusion-weighted magnetic resonance imaging. Neuropediatrics 25:172–5, 1994.

104. Adams DF, Ment LR, Vohr B. Antenatal therapies and the developing brain. Semin Neonatol 6:173–83, 2001.
105. Dickinson JE, Marshall LR, Phillips JM, et al. Antenatal diagnosis and management of fetomaternal alloimmune thrombocytopenia. Am J Perinatol 12:333–5, 1995.
106. Ment LR, Duncan CC, Ehrenkranz RA. Perinatal cerebral infarction. Ann Neurol 16:559–68, 1984.
107. Trauner DA, Nass R, Ballantyne A. Behavioural profiles of children and adolescents after pre- or perinatal unilateral brain damage. Brain 124:995–1002, 2001.
108. Mercuri E, Barnett A, Rutherford M, et al. Neonatal cerebral infarction and neuromotor outcome at school age. Pediatrics 113:95–100, 2004.
109. de Vries LS, Van der Grond J, Van Haastert IC, et al. Prediction of outcome in new-born infants with arterial ischaemic stroke using diffusion-weighted magnetic resonance imaging. Neuropediatrics 36:12–20, 2005.
110. Koelfen W, Freund M, Varnholt V. Neonatal stroke involving the middle cerebral artery in term infants: clinical presentation, EEG and imaging studies, and outcome. Dev Med Child Neurol 37:204–12, 1995.
111. Mantovani JF, Gerber GJ. "Idiopathic" neonatal cerebral infarction. Am J Dis Child 138:359–62, 1984.
112. de Vries LS, Levene MI. Cerebral Ischaemic Lesions. Edinburgh: Churchill Livingstone, 1995.
113. Mercuri E, Rutherford M, Cowan F, et al. Early prognostic indicators of outcome in infants with neonatal cerebral infarction: a clinical, electroencephalogram, and magnetic resonance imaging study. Pediatrics 103:39–46, 1999.
114. Mercuri E, Atkinson J, Braddick O, et al. Visual function and perinatal focal cerebral infarction. Arch Dis Child Fetal Neonatal Ed 75:F76–81, 1996.
115. Goodman R, Yude C. IQ and its predictors in childhood hemiplegia. Dev Med Child Neurol 38:881–90, 1996.
116. Vargha-Khadem F, Isaacs E, Muter V. A review of cognitive outcome after unilateral lesions sustained during childhood. J Child Neurol 9(Suppl 2):67–73, 1994.
117. Vargha-Khadem F, Isaacs E, van der Werf S, et al. Development of intelligence and memory in children with hemiplegic cerebral palsy. The deleterious consequences of early seizures. Brain 115:315–29, 1992.
118. McGahan JP, Haesslein HC, Meyers M, et al. Sonographic recognition of in utero intraventricular hemorrhage. AJR Am J Roentgenol 142:171–3, 1984.
119. Donn SM, Barr M Jr, McLeary RD. Massive intracerebral hemorrhage in utero: sonographic appearance and pathologic correlation. Obstet Gynecol 63:28S–30S, 1984.
120. Bondurant S, Boehm FH, Fleischer AC, et al. Antepartum diagnosis of fetal intracranial hemorrhage by ultrasound. Obstet Gynecol 63:25S–27S, 1984.
121. Pretorius DH, Singh S, Manco-Johnson ML, et al. In utero diagnosis of intracranial hemorrhage resulting in fetal hydrocephalus. A case report. J Reprod Med 31:136–8, 1986.
122. Zorzi C, Angonese I, Nardelli GB, et al. Spontaneous intraventricular haemorrhage in utero. Eur J Pediatr 148:83–5, 1988.
123. Stoddard RA, Clark SL, Minton SD. In utero ischemic injury: sonographic diagnosis and medicolegal implications. Am J Obstet Gynecol 159:23–5, 1988.
124. Gunn TR, Mora JD, Becroft DM. Congenital hydrocephalus secondary to prenatal intracranial haemorrhage. Aust N Z J Obstet Gynaecol 28:197–200, 1988.
125. Sims ME, Mann E. Communicating hydrocephalus secondary to fetal intracranial hemorrhage. J Perinatol 8:371–3, 1988.
126. Burrows RF, Caco CC, Kelton JG. Neonatal alloimmune thrombocytopenia: spontaneous in utero intracranial hemorrhage. Am J Hematol 28:98–102, 1988.
127. Stirling HF, Hendry M, Brown JK. Prenatal intracranial haemorrhage. Dev Med Child Neurol 31:807–11, 1989.
128. Jennett RJ, Daily WJ, Tarby TJ, et al. Prenatal diagnosis of intracerebellar hemorrhage: case report. Am J Obstet Gynecol 162:1472–4; discussion 1474–5, 1990.
129. Giovangrandi Y, Daffos F, Kaplan C, et al. Very early intracranial haemorrhage in alloimmune fetal thrombocytopenia. Lancet 336:310, 1990.
130. Edmondson SR, Hallak M, Carpenter RJ Jr, et al. Evolution of hydranencephaly following intracerebral hemorrhage. Obstet Gynecol 79:870–1, 1992.
131. Achiron R, Pinchas O, Reichman B, et al. Fetal intracranial haemorrhage: clinical significance of in utero ultrasonographic diagnosis. Br J Obstet Gynaecol 100:995–9, 1993.
132. Sibony O, Fondacci C, Oury JF, et al. In utero fetal cerebral intraparenchymal hemorrhage associated with an abnormal cerebral Doppler. Fetal Diagn Ther 8:126–8, 1993.
133. Hadi HA, Finley J, Mallette JQ, et al. Prenatal diagnosis of cerebellar hemorrhage: medicolegal implications. Am J Obstet Gynecol 170:1392–5, 1994.
134. Dean LM, McLeary M, Taylor GA. Cerebral hemorrhage in alloimmune thrombocytopenia. Pediatr Radiol 25:444–5, 1995.
135. Reiss I, Gortner L, Moller J, et al. Fetal intracerebral hemorrhage in the second trimester: diagnosis by sonography and magnetic resonance imaging. Ultrasound Obstet Gynecol 7:49–51, 1996.
136. Vergani P, Strobelt N, Locatelli A, et al. Clinical significance of fetal intracranial hemorrhage. Am J Obstet Gynecol 175:536–43, 1996.
137. Pilu G, Falco P, Perolo A, et al. Differential diagnosis and outcome of fetal intracranial hypoechoic lesions: report of 21 cases. Ultrasound Obstet Gynecol 9:229–36, 1997.

138. Kirkinen P, Orden MR, Partanen K. Cerebral blood flow changes associated with fetal intracranial hemorrhages. Acta Obstet Gynecol Scand 76:308–12, 1997.

139. Guerriero S, Ajossa S, Mais V, et al. Color Doppler energy imaging in the diagnosis of fetal intracranial hemorrhage in the second trimester. Ultrasound Obstet Gynecol 10:205–8, 1997.

140. Ohba T, Yoshimura T, Ohyama K, et al. A case of fetal intracranial bleeding complicated by hydrocephalus in a woman with frequent epileptic seizures. J Maternal-Fetal Invest 8:98–100, 1998.

141. Canapicchi R, Cioni G, Strigini FA, et al. Prenatal diagnosis of periventricular hemorrhage by fetal brain magnetic resonance imaging. Childs Nerv Syst 14:689–92, 1998.

142. Hashimoto I, Tada K, Nakatsuka M, et al. Fetal hydrocephalus secondary to intraventricular hemorrhage diagnosed by ultrasonography and in utero fast magnetic resonance imaging. A case report. Fetal Diagn Ther 14:248–53, 1999.

143. Fukui K, Morioka T, Nishio S, et al. Fetal germinal matrix and intraventricular haemorrhage diagnosed by MRI. Neuroradiology 43:68–72, 2001.

Chapter 8

Diagnosis and Treatment of Neonatal Seizures

Mark S. Scher, MD

Introduction
Recognition of Neonatal Seizures
Clinical Seizure Criteria
Nonepileptic Behaviors of Neonates
Electrographic Seizure Criteria
Subcortical Seizures versus Nonictal Functional Decortication
Seizures in the Clinical Context of Maternal–Fetal–Placental Diseases:
  Following a Diagnostic Algorithm
Principles of Therapy
Summary

Unresolved issues remain with respect to the recognition and treatment of newborns exhibiting seizures. Current controversies bring into sharp focus clinical and translational research findings concerning epidemiologic factors, neurobiologic and pathophysiologic mechanisms which can improve our understanding of seizure generation and consequences for the immature brain. Diagnostic and therapeutic algorithms must be based on prenatal, peripartum, and postnatal contributions to neonatal seizures in the neonate, with or without the expression of neonatal encephalopathy. Novel neonatal seizure classifications must consider specific etiologies and the continuum of anatomically specific brain injury when designing therapeutic protocols for rescue/repair as well as antiepileptogenesis.

INTRODUCTION

Basic issues still remain regarding the recognition and treatment of neonatal seizures (Table 8-1). Who and how to treat newborns with seizures continue to occupy much discussion and controversy in written and oral presentations. While clinical seizures remain a common occurrence in neonatal intensive care settings, with an incidence as high as 2.6 per thousand live births for term infants and 30–130 per thousand live preterm births, increasing use of bedside electrophysiologic monitoring has resulted in the growing recognition that the incidence of seizures may be even higher. Yet the "who" question in the algorithm to diagnose and treat neonatal seizures includes a heterogeneous cohort of newborns who may present throughout the neonatal period (i.e., 30 days post-term). The manner of clinical presentation will reflect alternative diagnostic explanations for seizure recurrence based on timing, etiology, or brain region of injury (1). Presentation may imply part of a longer-standing encephalopathic process prior to and/or during parturition in

Table 8-1   Questions and Controversies Concerning Neonatal Seizures

Questions	Controversies
Who should be treated?	Timing of brain insult, age at presentation, presence or absence of an encephalopathy, underlying etiology
What constitutes a seizure?	Clinical versus electrical criteria for seizures, what constitutes status epilepticus
What is appropriate treatment?	Specific therapeutic choices
	Define the endpoints of treatment to assess efficacy based on etiology, timing, and location
How long to treat?	Ability to predict risk for sequelae (e.g., epilepsy, neurodevelopmental disorders)
Why to treat?	To distinguish seizures as an epiphenomena versus a neuronal process that contributes to epileptic-induced brain damage

some newborns. Other infants present with isolated seizures or ictal events that herald the onset of new postnatal disease or an otherwise silent antepartum process.

Seizure occurrence must be based on a reliance of both clinical sign recognition and coincident electrographic expression to define the exact onset and offset of seizure duration. This is also essential to more accurately define status epilepticus. The issue of seizure recognition highlights the controversy regarding the assessment of treatment efficacy, linking to etiologic process, as well as location and timing of injury. Unresolved questions also include the unknown duration of treatment for a neonate who experienced seizures after emergent treatment in the neonatal intensive care unit. Long-term treatment may be required for the child at an increased risk for childhood seizures and neurocognitive/neurobehavioral sequelae at older ages.

Finally, there remains a controversy as to whether electrical versus clinical seizures are more detrimental to normal brain structure and function. Based on current epilepsy models in the immature and older populations, epileptic-induced brain damage can occur either as a direct result of the metabolic consequences of the seizures themselves, and/or the underlying etiologies in which seizures are imbedded. Therefore the final section of this chapter will discuss the current innovations which augment our understanding of seizures in the immature brain. Proposed and current research may lead to novel therapeutic approaches that are relevant to the pathophysiologic mechanisms responsible for both seizures and nonepileptic paroxysmal movement disorders, in the context of the associated etiologies, location, and timing of injury in the immature brain.

RECOGNITION OF NEONATAL SEIZURES

There remains a fundamental controversy regarding seizure recognition (2). Many intensivists continue to rely on primarily clinical criteria for the diagnosis of neonatal seizures, while acknowledging that electrographic confirmation of seizures may also be necessary. This controversy has been fueled by the technological advances at the bedside using synchronized video-electroencephalographic monitoring. Simultaneous documentation of suspicious clinical behaviors with electrographic seizures is considered the neurophysiologic gold standard. With this technology, new classifications of neonatal seizures can draw a clearer distinction between "epileptic" versus "nonepileptic" events. Failure to document electrographic seizures by scalp recordings suggests the possibility that clinical events may be either nonepileptic paroxysmal behaviors or subcortical seizure events. While commonly diagnosed in older childhood and adult populations, such explanations for neonates are less actively described. However, several authors argue that traditionally described "subtle seizures" have no coincidental electrographic seizure occurrence on scalp recordings, underscoring the controversy. EEG recordings are therefore helpful to avoid treatment choices with traditional antiepileptic medications for paroxysmal nonepileptic events.

The advocacy for electrographic confirmation should include the use of automated screening devices in concert with traditional EEG studies. First designed in the late 1960s using only one channel of EEG, these devices usually rely on a single computerized algorithm to detect a "pattern" for neonatal seizures. A limited number of channels are inadequate to document the electrographic expression of seizures that may originate distant from the electrode site or to be of such low amplitude and/or duration to avoid definitive conclusions regarding the presence or duration of seizures (3). There is as yet no consensus regarding the comparison of screening recordings with traditional EEG studies with respect to the detection of seizures with acceptable false negative and false positive results. Two-tiered recording paradigms need to be incorporated in future studies to combine the results from screening devices with more traditional comprehensive neurophysiologic protocols.

CLINICAL SEIZURE CRITERIA

Neonatal seizures are presently listed separately from the traditional classification of seizures and epilepsy during childhood. The International League Against Epilepsy's classification adopted by the World Health Organization still considers neonatal seizures within an unclassified category (4). A recent classification scheme now suggests a more strict distinction of clinical seizure (nonepileptic) events from electrographically confirmed (epileptic) seizures, with respect to possible treatment interventions (5). Continued refinement of such novel classifications is needed to reconcile the variable agreement between clinical and EEG criteria for establishing a seizure diagnosis (6, 7) in the context of nonepileptic movement disorders caused by acquired diseases, malformations and/or medications.

Several caveats (Table 8-2) may be useful in the identification of suspected neonatal seizures and raise questions regarding our diagnostic acumen using only clinical criteria.

The clinical criteria for neonatal seizure diagnosis were historically subdivided into five clinical categories: focal clonic, multifocal or migratory clonic, tonic, myoclonic, and subtle seizures (8). A more recent classification expands the clinical subtypes, adopting a strict temporal occurrence of specific clinical events with coincident electrographic seizures, to distinguish neonatal clinical "nonepileptic" seizures from "epileptic" seizures (Tables 8-3 and 8-4) (5).

Table 8-2	Caveats Concerning Recognition of Neonatal Seizures
1	Specific stereotypic behaviors occur in association with normal neonatal sleep or waking states, medication effects, and gestational maturity
2	Consider that any abnormal repetitive activity may be a clinical seizure if out of context for expected neonatal behavior
3	Attempt to document coincident electrographic seizures with the suspected clinical event
4	Abnormal behavioral phenomena may have inconsistent relationships with coincident EEG seizures, suggesting a subcortical seizure focus
5	Nonepileptic pathologic movement disorders are events that are independent of the seizure state, and may also be expressed by neonates

Table 8-3   Clinical Characteristics, Classification, and Presumed Pathophysiology of Neonatal Seizures

Classification	Characterization
Focal clonic	Repetitive, rhythmic contractions of muscle groups of the limbs, face, or trunk May be unifocal or multifocal May occur synchronously or asynchronously in muscle groups on one side of the body May occur simultaneously but asynchronously on both sides Cannot be suppressed by restraint Pathophysiology: epileptic
Focal tonic	Sustained posturing of single limbs Sustained asymmetrical posturing of the trunk Sustained eye deviation Cannot be provoked by stimulation or suppressed by restraint Pathophysiology: epileptic
Generalized tonic	Sustained symmetrical posturing of limbs, trunk, and neck May be flexor, extensor, or mixed extensor/flexor May be provoked or intensified by stimulation May be suppressed by restraint or repositioning Presumed pathophysiology: nonepileptic
Myoclonic	Random, single, rapid contractions of muscle groups of the limbs, face, or trunk Typically not repetitive or may recur at a slow rate May be generalized, focal, or fragmentary May be provoked by stimulation Presumed pathophysiology: may be epileptic or nonepileptic
Spasms	May be flexor, extensor, or mixed extensor/flexor May occur in clusters Cannot be provoked by stimulation or suppressed by restraint Pathophysiology: epileptic
Motor automatisms	
Ocular signs	Random and roving eye movements or nystagmus (distinct from tonic eye deviation) May be provoked or intensified by tactile stimulation Presumed pathophysiology: nonepileptic
Oral-buccal-lingual movements	Sucking, chewing, tongue protrusions May be provoked or intensified by stimulation Presumed pathophysiology: nonepileptic
Progression movements	Rowing or swimming movements Pedaling or bicycling movements of the legs May be provoked or intensified by stimulation May be suppressed by restraint or repositioning Presumed pathophysiology: nonepileptic
Complex purposeless movements	Sudden arousal with transient increased random activity of limbs May be provoked or intensified by stimulation Presumed pathophysiology: nonepileptic

From Mizrahi EM, Kellaway P. Diagnosis and Management of Neonatal Seizures. Philadelphia, PA: Lippincott-Raven, 1998.

Subtle Seizure Activity

This is the most frequently observed category of neonatal seizures and includes repetitive buccolingual movements, orbital–ocular movements, unusual bicycling or peddling, and autonomic findings (Fig. 8-1A). Subtle paroxysmal events which interrupt the expected behavioral repertoire of neonatal state and which appear stereotypic or repetitive should heighten the clinician's level of suspicion for seizures. However, alterations in cardiorespiratory regularity, body movements,

Table 8-4 Classification of Neonatal Seizures Based on Electroclinical Findings

Clinical seizures with a consistent electrocortical signature (pathophysiology: epileptic)

Focal clonic	Unifocal
	Multifocal
	Hemiconvulsive
	Axial
Focal tonic	Asymmetrical truncal posturing
	Limb posturing
	Sustained eye deviation
Myoclonic	Generalized
	Focal
Spasms	Flexor
	Extensor
	Mixed extensor/flexor

Clinical seizures without a consistent electrocortical signature (pathophysiology: presumed nonepileptic)

Myoclonic	Generalized
	Focal
	Fragmentary
Generalized tonic	Flexor
	Extensor
	Mixed extensor/flexor
Motor automatisms	Oral-buccal-lingual movements
	Ocular signs
	Progression movements
	Complex purposeless movements

Electrical seizures without clinical seizure activity

From Mizrahi EM, Kellaway P. Diagnosis and Management of Neonatal Seizures. Philadelphia, PA: Lippincott-Raven, 1998.

and other behaviors during active (REM) and quiet (NREM) sleep or waking segments also must be recognized before proceeding to a seizure evaluation (9, 10). Within the subtle category of neonatal seizures are stereotypic changes in heart rate, blood pressure, oxygenation, or other autonomic signs, particularly during pharmacologic paralysis for ventilatory care. Other autonomic events include penile erections, skin changes, salivation, and tearing. Autonomic expressions may be intermixed with motoric findings. Isolated autonomic signs such as apnea, unless accompanied by other clinical findings, are rarely associated with coincident electrographic seizures (Fig. 8-1B) (11, 12). Since subtle seizures are both clinically difficult to detect and only variably coincident with EEG seizures, synchronized video/EEG/polygraphic recordings are recommended to document temporal relationships between clinical behaviors and coincident electrographic events (5, 13–15). Despite the "subtle" expression of this seizure category, these children may still have suffered significant brain injury.

Clonic Seizures

Rhythmic movements of muscle groups in a focal distribution which consist of a rapid phase followed by a slow return movement are clonic seizures, to be distinguished from the symmetric "to-and-fro" movements of tremulousness or jitteriness (1). Gentle flexion of the affected body part easily suppresses the tremor, while clonic seizures persist. Clonic movements can involve any body part such as the face, arm, leg, and even diaphragmatic or pharyngeal muscles. Generalized clonic activities can occur in the newborn but rarely consist of a classical tonic followed by

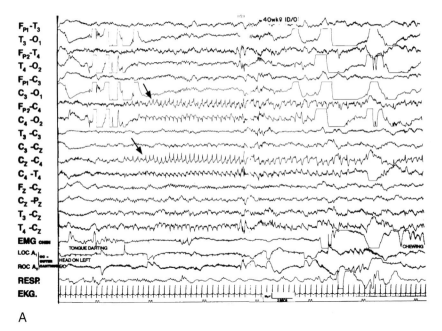

A

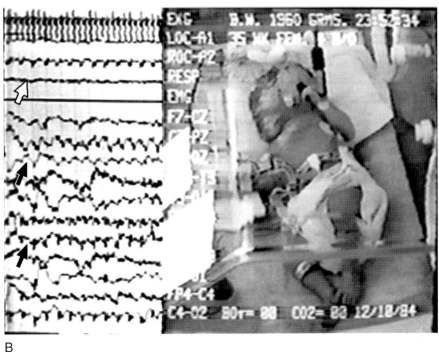

B

Figure 8-1 (A) EEG segment of a 40-week gestation, 1-day-old female following severe asphyxia resulting from rupture of velamentous insertion of the umbilical cord during delivery. An electrical seizure in the right central/midline region is recorded, (arrows) coincident with buccolingual and eye movements (see comments and eye channels on record). (From Scher MS, Painter MJ. Electrographic diagnosis of neonatal seizures. Issues of diagnostic accuracy, clinical correlation and survival. In Wasterlain CG, Vert P (eds). Neonatal Seizures. New York: Raven Press, 1990, p. 17, with permission.) (B) Synchronized video-EEG record of a 35-week gestation, 1-day-old female with *E. coli* meningitis and cerebral abscesses. The open arrow notes apnea coincident with prominent right hemispheric and midline electrographic seizures (closed arrows). In addition to apnea, other motoric signs coincident to EEG seizures were noted at other times during the record. (From Scher MS, Painter MJ. Controversies concerning neonatal seizures. Pediatr Clin North Am 36:288, 1989, with permission.)

127

clonic phase, characteristic of the generalized motor seizure noted in older children and adults. Focal clonic and hemiclonic seizures have been described with localized brain injury usually from cerebrovascular lesions (13, 16–18) (Fig. 8-2A) but can also be seen with generalized brain abnormalities. As with older patients, focal seizures in the neonate may be followed by transient motor weakness, historically referred to as a transient Todd's paresis or paralysis (19), to be distinguished by a more persistent hemiparesis over multiple days to weeks. Clonic movements without EEG-confirmed seizures have been described in neonates with normal EEG backgrounds and their neurodevelopment outcome will more likely be normal (14). The less experienced clinician may misclassify myoclonic as clonic movements. Recent computational studies suggest strategies to extract quantitative information from video recordings of neonatal seizures as a method by which clinicians can differentiate myoclonic from focal clonic seizures, as well as distinguish normal infant behaviors (20).

Multifocal (Fragmentary) Clonic Seizures

Multifocal or migratory clonic activities spread over body parts in either a random or an anatomically appropriate fashion. Such seizure movements may alternate from side to side and appear asynchronously between the two halves of the child's body. The word fragmentary was historically applied to distinguish this event from the more classical generalized tonic–clonic seizure seen in the older child. Multifocal clonic seizures may also resemble myoclonic seizures which alternatively consist of brief shock-like muscle twitching of the midline and/or extremity musculature. Neonates with this seizure description often suffer death or significant neurological morbidity (21).

Tonic Seizures

Tonic seizure refers to a sustained flexion or extension of axial or appendicular muscle groups. Tonic movements of a limb or sustained head or eye turning may also be noted. Tonic activity with coincident EEG needs to be carefully documented, since 30% of such movements lack a temporal correlation with electrographic seizures (22) (Figs. 8-3A–C). "Brainstem release" resulting from functional decortication after severe neocortical dysfunction or damage is one physiologic explanation for this nonepileptic activity, to be discussed below. Extensive neocortical damage or dysfunction permits the emergence of uninhibited subcortical expressions of extensor movements (23) (see Fig. 8-6). Tonic seizures may also be misidentified, when the nonepileptic movement disorder of dystonia is the more appropriate behavioral description (Figs. 8-2C and 8-3A). Both tonic movements and dystonic posturing may also simultaneously occur.

Myoclonic Seizures

Myoclonic movements are rapid, isolated jerks which can be generalized, multifocal, or focal in an axial or appendicular distribution. Myoclonus lacks the slow return phase of the clonic movement complex described above. Healthy preterm infants commonly exhibit myoclonic movements without seizures or a brain disorder. EEG, therefore, is recommended to confirm the coincident appearance of electrographic discharges with these movements (Fig. 8-4A). Pathologic myoclonus in the absence of EEG seizures also can occur in severely ill preterm or full-term infants after suffering severe brain dysfunction or damage (24). As with older children and adults, myoclonus may reflect injury

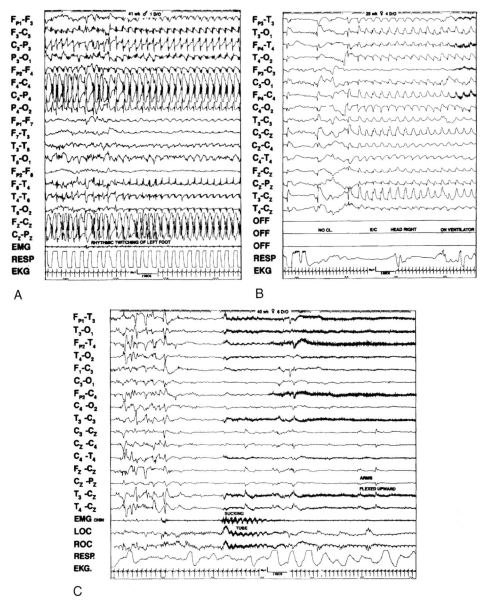

A

B

C

Figure 8-2 (A) Segment of EEG of a 41-week gestation, 1-day-old male with an electroclinical seizure characterized by rhythmic clonic movements of the left foot coincident with bihemispheric electrographic discharges of higher amplitude in the right hemisphere. This seizure was documented prior to antiepileptic medication. (B) Segment of EEG of a 25-week gestation, 4-day-old female with an electrographic seizure without clinical accompaniments. (C) Segment of an EEG of a 40-week gestation, 6-day-old infant with stereotypic flexion posturing in the absence of electrographic seizures (note muscle artifact). (From Scher MS. Pediatric electroencephalography and evoked potentials. In Swaiman KS (ed). Pediatric Neurology: Principles and Practice. St. Louis, MO: CV Mosby, 1999, p. 164, with permission.)

at multiple levels of the neuraxis from the spine, brainstem to cortical regions. Stimulus-evoked myoclonus with either coincident single coincident spike discharges or sustained electrographic seizures have been reported (24) (Figs. 8-4A and 8-4B). An extensive evaluation must be initiated to exclude metabolic, structural, and genetic causes. Rarely, healthy sleeping neonates exhibit abundant myoclonus which subsides with arousal to the waking state (25, 26), termed benign sleep myoclonus of the newborn.

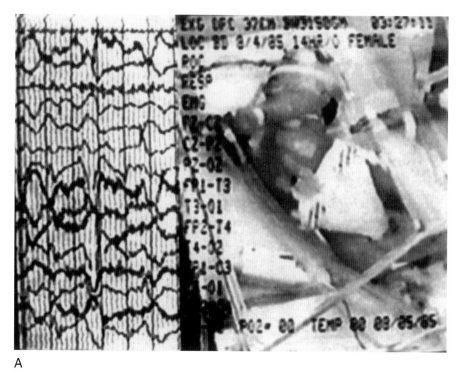

A

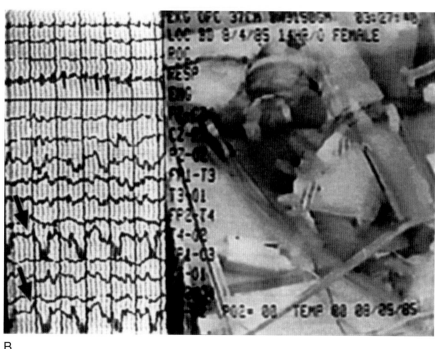

B

Figure 8-3 (A) Segment of a synchronized video-EEG record of a 37-week gestation, 1-day-old female who suffered asphyxia, demonstrating prominent opisthotonos with left arm extension in the absence of coincident electrographic seizure activity. (From Scher MS. Neonatal seizures: an expression of fetal or neonatal brain disorders. In Stevenson DK (ed). Fetal and Neonatal Brain Injury: Mechanisms, Management and the Risks of Practice, 3rd edition. West Nyack, NY: Cambridge University Press, 2003, p.735.) (B) Synchronized video-EEG record of the same patient as in (A), documenting electrographic seizure in the right posterior quadrant (arrows), following cessation of left arm tonic movements and persistent opisthotonos. (From Scher MS, Painter MJ. Controversies concerning neonatal seizures. In Pellock JM (ed). Seizure Disorders. Pediatr Clin North Am. Philadelphia, PA: WB Saunders, 36:292, 1989, with permission.)

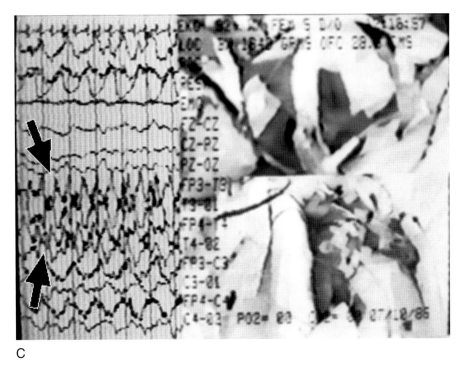

C

Figure 8-3. cont'd, (C) Segment of a video-EEG recording documenting a fixed tonic neck reflex with coincident electrographic seizures in the temporal regions (arrows), described as a tonic seizure. (From Scher MS, Painter MJ. Controversies concerning neonatal seizures. In Pellock JM (ed). Seizure Disorders. Pediatr Clin North Am. Philadelphia, PA: WB Saunders, 36:292, 1989, with permission.)

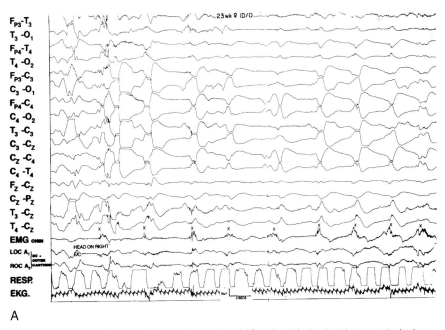

A

Figure 8-4 (A) EEG segment of a 23-week gestation, 1-day-old female with Grade III intraventricular hemorrhage and progressive ventriculomegaly. An electroclinical seizure is noted with coincident myoclonic movements of the diaphragm (× marks). (From Scher MS. Pathological myoclonus of the newborn: electrographic and clinical correlations. Pediatr Neurol 1:342–8, 1985, with permission.)

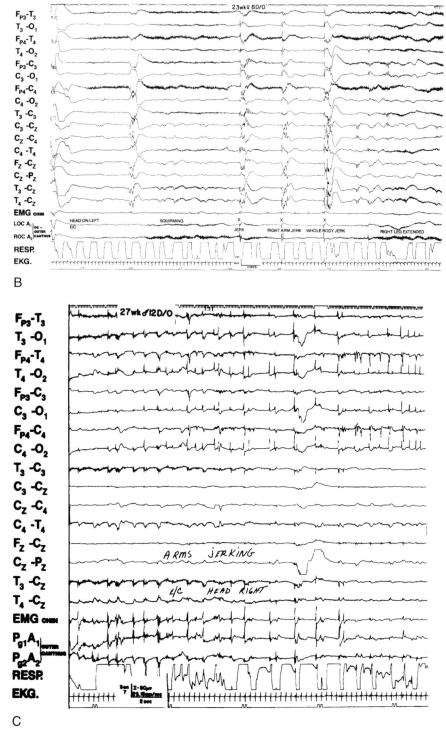

Figure 8-4. cont'd, (B) Segment of an EEG recording of an asymptomatic 23-week, 8-day-old female with sponta- neous generalized focal myoclonus without electrographic discharges other than myogenic spike potentials. (From Scher MS. Pathological myoclonus of the newborn: electrographic and clinical correlations. Pediatr Neurol 1:342–8, 1985, with permission.) (C) Segment of an EEG recording of an encephalopathic 27-week, 12-day-old male with herpes encephalitis who exhibits nonepileptic multifocal myoclonus (myogenic potentials as EEG artifacts).

Specific nonepileptic neonatal movement repertoires continually challenge the physician's attempt to reach an accurate diagnosis of seizures and avoid the unnecessary use of antiepileptic medications. Coincident synchronized video/EEG/polygraphic recordings is now the suggested diagnostic tool to confirm the temporal relationship between the suspicious clinical phenomena and electrographic expression of seizures (27). The following three examples of nonepileptic movement disorders incorporate a new classification scheme (5), based on the absence of coincident EEG seizures.

Tremulousness or Jitteriness with EEG Correlates

Tremors are frequently misidentified as clonic activity. Unlike the unequal phases of clonic movements described above, the flexion and extension phases of tremor are equal in amplitude. Children are generally alert or hyperalert but may also appear somnolent. Passive flexion and repositioning of the affected tremulous body part diminishes or eliminates the movement. Such movements are usually spontaneous but can be provoked by tactile stimulation. Metabolic or toxin-induced encephalopathies including mild asphyxia, drug withdrawal, hypoglycemia-hypocalcemia, intracranial hemorrhage, hypothermia, and growth restriction are common clinical scenarios when such movements occur. Neonatal tremors generally decrease with age. For example, 38 full-term infants with excessive tremulousness resolved spontaneously over a six-week period, with 92% neurologically normal at three years of age (28). Medications are rarely considered to treat this particular movement disorder (29).

Neonatal Myoclonus without EEG Seizures

Myoclonic movements are bilateral and synchronous, or asymmetric and asynchronous in appearance. Clusters of myoclonic activity occur more predominantly during active (REM) sleep, and are more predominant in the preterm infant (9, 30) (Fig. 8-4B), although can occur in healthy full-term infants. Benign movements are not stimulus-sensitive, have no coincident electrographic seizure correlates, or are associated with EEG background abnormalities. When these movements occur in the healthy full-term neonate, the activity is suppressed during wakefulness. The clinical description of benign neonatal sleep myoclonus must be a diagnosis of exclusion, after a careful consideration of pathologic diagnoses (25).

Infants with severe central nervous system dysfunction also may present with nonepileptic spontaneous or stimulus-evoked myoclonus. Different forms of metabolic encephalopathies (such as glycine encephalopathy), cerebrovascular lesions, brain infections, or congenital malformations may present with nonepileptic pathologic myoclonus (Fig. 8-4C) (24). Encephalopathic neonates may respond to tactile or painful stimulation by either isolated focal, segmental, or generalized myoclonic movements. Rarely, cortically generated spike or sharp wave discharges as well as seizures may also be noted on the EEG recordings which are coincident with these myoclonic movements (Figs. 8-5A and 8-5B) (31). Medication-induced myoclonus as well as other stereotypic movements have also been described (32), which resolve when the responsible drug is withdrawn.

A rare familial disorder has been described in the neonatal and early infancy periods, specifically termed hyperekplexia. These movements usually are misinterpreted as a hyperactive startle reflex. Infants are stiff, with severe hypertonia which may lead to apnea and bradycardia. Forced flexion of the neck or hips sometimes alleviates these events. EEG background rhythms are generally age-appropriate.

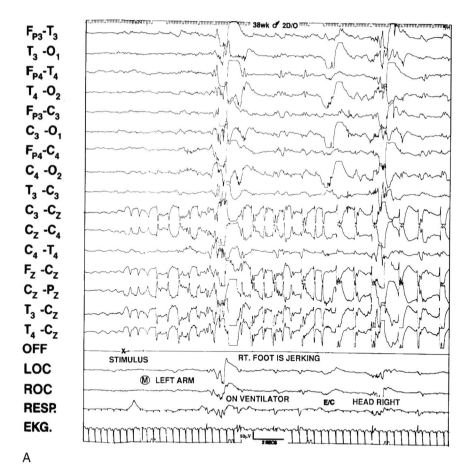

A

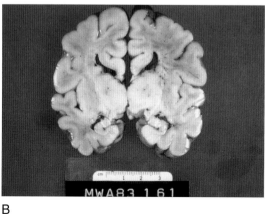

B

Figure 8-5 (A) Segment of an EEG recording of a 38-week, 2-day-old male with glycine encephalopathy who has stimulus-sensitive generalized and multifocal myoclonus. Note the onset of a midline (C_z onset) electrographic seizure with a painful stimulus, followed by right foot myoclonus. (From Scher MS. Neonatal seizures: an expression of fetal or neonatal brain disorders. In Stevenson DK (ed). Fetal and Neonatal Brain Injury: Mechanisms, Management and the Risks of Practice, 3rd edition. West Nyack, NY: Cambridge University Press, 2003, p.745.) (B) Coronal section of the brain for the patient described in (A), with agenesis of the corpus callosum, bat-winged shape of lateral ventricles. Spongy myelinosis was noted on microscopic examination. (From Scher MS. Pathological myoclonus of the newborn: electrographic and clinical correlations. Pediatr Neurol 1:342–8, 1985.)

The postulated defect for these individuals involve regulation of brainstem centers which facilitate myoclonic movements (33). Occasionally benzodiazepines or valproic acid lessen the startling, stiffening, or falling events (34). Neurologic prognosis is reported to be variable.

Neonatal Dystonia without EEG Seizures

Dystonia is a third commonly misdiagnosed movement disorder that is often misrepresented as tonic seizures. Dystonia can be associated with either acute or chronic disease states involving basal ganglia structures or the extrapyramidal pathways which innervate these regions. Antepartum or intrapartum adverse events such as commonly severe asphyxia (i.e., termed status mamoratus) (8) or rarely such as specific inherited metabolic diseases (35, 36) result in injury to these structures. Alternatively, posturing may reflect subcortical motor pathways that are functionally unopposed because of a diseased or malformed neocortex (23) (Figs. 8-2C, 8-3A, and 8-6). Documentation of EEG seizures with coincident video/EEG/polygraphic recordings help avoid misdiagnosis as seizures and inappropriate treatment.

ELECTROGRAPHIC SEIZURE CRITERIA

Over the last few decades electrographic/polysomnographic studies have become invaluable tools for the assessment of suspected seizures (5, 13, 22, 27, 37–39). Technical and interpretative skills of normal and abnormal neonatal EEG sleep patterns must be mastered before one can develop a confident visual analysis style for seizure recognition (9, 10, 40–42).

Corroboration with the EEG technologist is always an essential part of the diagnostic process, since physiologic and nonphysiologic artifacts can masquerade as EEG seizures. The physician must also anticipate expected behaviors for the child for a specific gestational maturity, medication use, and state of arousal, in the context of potential artifacts. Synchronized video-EEG documentation permits careful off-line analysis for more accurate documentation.

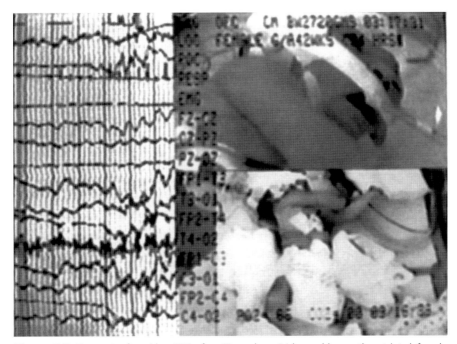

Figure 8-6 Segment of a video-EEG of a 42-week, < 24-hour-old growth-restricted female demonstrating stereotypic posturing and eye opening with no coincident electrographic seizure. The child presented with nonimmune hydrops fetalis with significant neocortical injury from a fetal time period. The EEG background is markedly slow and suppressed, representing a severe interictal electrographic abnormality. (From Scher MS. Neonatal siezures: an expression of fetal or neonatal brain disorders. In Stevenson DK (ed). Fetal and Neonatal Brain Injury: Mechanisms, Management and the Risks of Practice, 3rd edition. West Nyack, NY: Cambridge University Press, 2003, p.749.)

As with the epileptic older child and adult, it is generally accepted that the epileptic seizure is a clinical paroxysm of altered brain function with the simultaneous presence of an electrographic event on an EEG recording. Therefore, when assessing the suspected clinical event in the neonate, synchronized video/EEG/polygraphic monitoring is a useful tool to distinguish an epileptic from a nonepileptic event. Some advocate the use of single- or dual-channel computerized devices for continuous prolonged monitoring (43) given the multiple logistical challenges with the use of conventional multichannel recording devices at the cribside of a critically ill newborn. This specific device may consequentially fail to detect focal or regional seizures if the single-channel recording is not near the brain region involved with seizure expression, is sufficiently short in duration, or low in amplitude (3). For example, a recent study reported that fewer than 3 out of 10 neonates with suspected seizures on a single-channel device could be verified by conventional EEG (44). Others have suggested that modified four-, five-, or nine-channel EEG can efficiently detect seizures when verified by continuous video-EEG telemetry (3, 45).

Epilepsy monitoring services for older children and adults readily utilize intracerebral or surface electrocorticography to detect seizures. Such recording strategies, however, are not ethically appropriate or practical for the neonatal patient. Subcortical foci are consequentially difficult to definitively eliminate from consideration, as will be discussed below.

Ictal EEG Patterns: A More Reliable Marker for Seizure Onset, Duration, and Severity

Neonatal EEG seizure patterns commonly consist of a repetitive sequence of waveforms which evolve in frequency, amplitude, electrical field, and/or morphology. Four types of ictal patterns have been described: focal ictal patterns with normal background, focal patterns with abnormal background, multifocal ictal patterns (42), and focal monorhythmic periodic patterns of various frequencies. It is generally suggested that a minimal duration of 10 seconds for the evolution of discharges is required to distinguish electrographic seizures from repetitive but nonictal epileptiform discharges (13, 46, 47) (Figs. 8-1A, 8-2A, and 8-2B). Clinical neurophysiologists separately classify brief or prolonged repetitive discharges which lack an electrographic evolution as nonictal abnormal epileptiform patterns but not confirmatory of seizures (48). The unique features of neonatal electrographic seizure duration and topography are discussed below.

Seizure Duration and Topography

Few studies have quantified minimal or maximal seizure durations in neonates (5, 13, 46). Most notably, the definition of the most severe expression of seizures, status epilepticus, which potentially promotes brain injury can be problematic. For the older patient, status epilepticus is defined as at least 30 minutes of continuous seizures or two consecutive seizures with an interictal period during which the patient fails to return to full consciousness. This definition is not easily applied to the neonate for whom the level of arousal may be difficult to assess, particularly if sedative medications are given. One study arbitrarily defined neonatal status epilepticus as continuous seizure activity for at least 30 minutes, or 50% of the recording time (46); 33% or 11 of 34 full-term infants had status epilepticus with a mean duration of 29.6 minutes prior to antiepileptic drug use, with another 9% or 3 out of the 34 preterm infants who also had status epilepticus with an average duration of 5.2 minutes per seizure (i.e., 50% of the recording time).

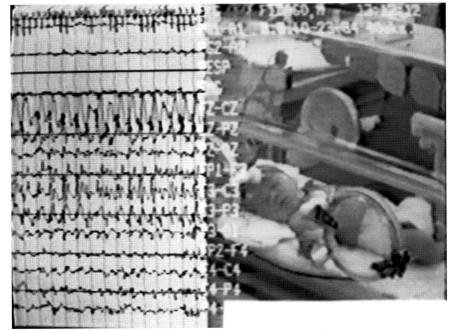

Figure 8-7 (A) Segment of a synchronized video-EEG of a 40-week, 1-day-old male with electrographic status epilepticus noted in the left central/midline regions, after antiepileptic medication administration. Focal right shoulder clonic activity was only intermittently noted, while continuous electrographic seizures were documented mostly without clinical expression. This phenomenon of uncoupling of electrical and clinical seizure activities is associated with antiepileptic drug administration use (see text). (From Scher MS, Painter MJ. Controversies concerning neonatal seizures. In Pellock JM (ed). Seizure Disorders. Pediatr Clin North Am. Philadelphia, PA: WB Saunders, 36:290, 1989, with permission.)

The mean seizure duration was longer in the full-term infant (i.e., 5 minutes) compared to the preterm infant (i.e., 2.7 minutes). Given that more than 20% of this study group fit the criteria for status epilepticus based on EEG documentation, concerns must be raised regarding the underdiagnosis of the more severe form of seizures that potentially contribute to brain injury, if only clinical criteria is applied.

Uncoupling of the clinical and electrographic expressions of neonatal seizures after antiepileptic medication administration also contributes to an underestimation of the true seizure duration, including status epilepticus (Fig. 8-7). One study estimated that 25% of neonates expressed persistent electrographic seizures despite resolution of their clinical seizure behaviors after receiving antiepileptic medications (49), termed electroclinical uncoupling. Other pathophysiological mechanisms besides medication effect also might explain uncoupling (7).

Most neonatal electrographic seizures arise focally from one brain region. Generalized synchronous and symmetrical repetitive discharges can also occur. In one study, 56% of seizures were seen in a single location at onset; specific sites included temporal-occipital (15%), temporal-central (15%), central (10%), frontotemporal central (6%), frontotemporal (5%), and vertex (5%). Multiple locations at the onset of the electrographic seizures were noted in 44% (13). Electrographic discharges may be expressed as specific EEG frequency ranges from fast to slow, including beta, alpha, theta, or delta activities. Multiple electrographic seizures can also be expressed independently in anatomically unrelated brain regions.

NEUROLOGY

SUBCORTICAL SEIZURES VERSUS NONICTAL FUNCTIONAL DECORTICATION

Experimental animal models offer conflicting neuronal mechanisms to explain clinical events which do not have coincident EEG confirmation. Most clinical neurophysiologists require documentation of an ictal pattern by surface EEG electrodes. However, subcortical seizures with only intermittent propagation to the surface may occur. At the other end of the spectrum, nonictal "brainstem release" phenomena must be considered, particularly if EEG seizures are never expressed (22). A more integrated electroclinical approach has been suggested to classify clinical events as seizures versus nonepileptic movement disorders, based on documentation by synchronized video-EEG monitoring (5).

Brainstem Release Phenomena

Synchronized video/EEG/polygraphic monitoring provides the physician with documentation of a suspicious event with a concurrent electrographic pattern on surface recordings (15). The temporal relationship between clinical and electrographic phenomena has been described, based on the synchronized video/EEG/polygraphic monitoring. Based on 415 clinical seizures in 71 babies, clonic seizure activity had the best correlation with coincident electrographic seizures. "Subtle" clinical events, on the other hand, had a more inconsistent relationship with coincident EEG seizure activity suggesting a nonepileptic brainstem release phenomena for at least a proportion of such events. Functional decortication resulting from neocortical damage without coincident EEG seizures (22) has therefore been suggested, such as with tonic posturing, as illustrated in Figure 8-3A. Newborns with nonseizure brainstem release activity may express a different functional pattern of metabolic dysfunction, detected as altered glucose uptake on single photon emission tomography studies than neonates with seizures (50). A recent suggestion to document increased prolactin levels with clinical seizures has also been reported (51), but such levels have not yet been correlated with electrographic seizures.

Electroclinical Dissociation Suggesting Subcortical Seizures

Experimental studies of immature animals also support the possibility that subcortical structures may initiate seizures, which subsequently, although intermittently, propagate to the cortical surface (52–54). While EEG depth recordings in adults and adolescents help document subcortical seizures both with and without clinical expression, this technology is not applicable or appropriate to the neonate. Only one anecdotal report of a human infant documented seizures possibly emanated from deep gray matter structures (55).

Electroclinical dissociation (ECD) is one proposed mechanism by which subcortical seizures may only intermittently appear on surface-recorded EEG studies (6). ECD has been defined as a reproducible clinical event that occurs both with and without coincidental electrographic seizures. In one group of 51 infants with electroclinical seizures, 33 infants simultaneously expressed both electrical and clinical seizure phenomena. Extremity movements were more significantly associated with synchronized electroclinical seizures. However, a subset of 18 of 51 neonates (34%) also expressed ECD on EEG recordings. For neonates who expressed ECD, the clinical seizure component always preceded the electrographic seizure expression, suggesting that a subcortical focus may have initiated the seizure state. Some of these children also expressed synchronized electroclinical seizures, even on the same EEG record. It may be useful to classify clinical events without either simultaneous or disassociated electrographic patterns as nonepileptic movement disorders, requiring alternative treatment pathways.

Controversy remains whether subcortical seizures versus nonictal functional decortication best categorize suspicious clinical behaviors without coincident EEG seizure documentation. This dilemma should encourage the clinician to use the EEG as a neurophysiologic yardstick by which more exact seizure start and end-points can be assigned, before offering pharmacologic treatment with antiepileptic drugs (AEDs) (27). Neonates certainly exhibit electrographic seizures that go undetected unless EEG is utilized (56–61). Two examples are neonates who are pharmacologically paralyzed for ventilatory assistance (Fig. 8-8A), or clinical seizures which are suppressed by the use of AEDs (Fig. 8-8B) (13 ,49, 56, 59–61). In one cohort of 92 infants, 60% of whom were pretreated with antiepileptic medications, 50% of neonates had electrographic seizures with no clinical accompaniment (49). Both clinical and electrographic seizure criteria were noted for 45% of 62 preterms and 53% of 33 full-term infants. Seventeen infants were pharmacologically paralyzed when the EEG seizure was first documented. A later cohort of 60 infants, none of whom were pretreated with antiepileptic medications, included 7% of infants with only electrographic seizures prior to AED administration (49), and 25% who expressed electroclinical uncoupling after AED use.

The underestimation of seizures in the newborn period may also result from inadequate monitoring for specific neurologic signs. Autonomic changes in respirations, blood pressure, oxygenation, heart rate, pupillary size, skin color, and salivation are examples of subtle ictal signs (Figs. 8-9A and 8-9B). In one study, autonomic seizures accompanied electrographic seizures in 37% of 19 preterm neonates (56). Newer classifications of neonatal seizures emphasize documentation of autonomic findings on EEG recordings (5).

Variation in the Incidence of Neonatal Seizures Based on Clinical versus EEG Criteria

Overestimation and underestimation of neonatal seizures are consequentially reported whether clinical or electrical criteria are used. Using clinical criteria, seizure incidences ranged from 0.5% in term infants to 22.2% in preterm neonates (62–65). Discrepancies in incidence reflect not only varying postconceptional ages of the study populations chosen, but also poor interobserver reliability (66) and the hospital setting in which the diagnosis was made. Hospital-based studies (56) which include high-risk deliveries generally report a higher seizure incidence. Population studies (67) which include less medically ill infants from general nurseries report lower percentages. Incidence figures based only on clinical criteria without EEG confirmation include "false positives," consisting of the neonates with either normal or nonepileptic pathologic neonatal behaviors. Conversely, the absence of scalp-generated EEG seizures may include a subset of "false negatives" who express seizures only from subcortical brain regions without expression on the cortical surface. Closer consensus between clinical and EEG criteria is still needed.

SEIZURES IN THE CLINICAL CONTEXT OF MATERNAL–FETAL–PLACENTAL DISEASES: FOLLOWING A DIAGNOSTIC ALGORITHM

Once seizures are confirmed by EEG, the neurologist must place these events into the context of clinical, historical, and laboratory findings to determine the pathogenesis and timing of an encephalopathic process in the symptomatic neonate.

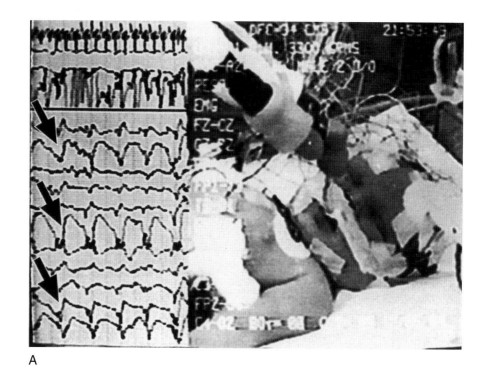

A

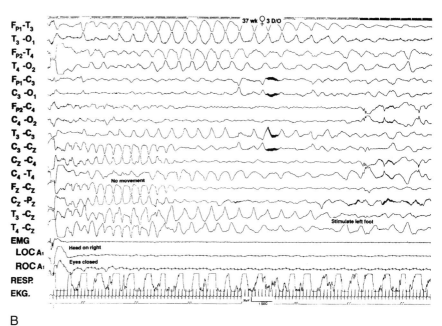

B

Figure 8-8 (A) Segment of a synchronized video-EEG record of a 38-week gestation, 2-day-old male who is pharmacologically paralyzed for ventilatory care. A seizure is noted in the right posterior quadrant and midline (arrows). (From Scher MS, Painter MJ. Controversies concerning neonatal seizures. In Pellock JM (ed). Seizure Disorders. Pediatr Clin North Am. Philadelphia, PA: WB Saunders, 36:287, 1989, with permission.) (B) EEG segment for a 37-week, 3-day-old female after antiepileptic drug use with multifocal electrical seizures in the delta frequency range in the temporal and midline regions. Note the marked suppression of normal EEG background. (From Scher MS. Neonatal seizures. Seizures in special clinical settings. In Wyllie E (ed). The Treatment of Epilepsy. Principles and Practice, 2nd edition. Baltimore, MD: Williams & Wilkins, 1997, p. 608, with permission.)

Seizures associated with neonates after asphyxia support either acute intrapartum events and/or antepartum disease processes. Does the child with seizures also express clinical and laboratory signs of evolving cerebral edema? The presence of a bulging fontanel with neuroimaging evidence of increased intracranial pressure and cerebral edema (i.e., obliterated ventricular outline and abnormal diffusion-weighted magnetic resonance images) strongly suggest a more recent asphyxial disease process, in or around the intrapartum period. Hyponatremia and increased urine osmolality suggest the syndrome of inappropriate secretion of antidiuretic hormone accompanying acute or subacute cerebral edema.

Alternatively, failure to document evolving cerebral edema during the first 3 days after asphyxia, or documentation of encephalomalacia or cystic brain lesions on neuroimaging shortly after birth (i.e., even in the encephalopathic newborn) suggests a more chronic disease process and remote antepartum brain injury. Liquefaction necrosis requires longer than 2 weeks after the presumed in utero asphyxial event to produce a cystic cavity (68), which is then visible on neuroimaging.

Isolated seizures in an otherwise asymptomatic neonate also suggest a disease process that occurs either during the postnatal or antepartum period. Neonates present with seizures as a result of postnatal illnesses from intracranial infection, cardiovascular lesions, drug toxicity, or inherited metabolic diseases. Children with

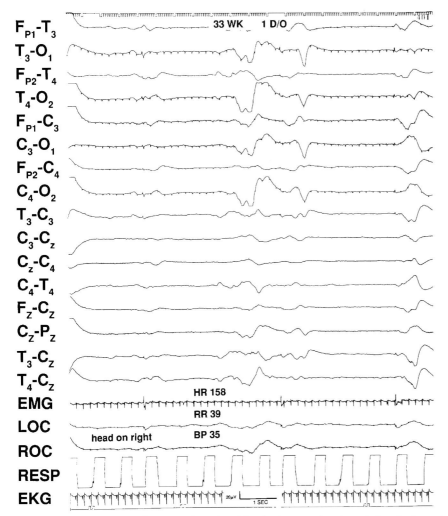

Figure 8-9 EEG segments of a 33-week, 1-day-old male documenting drops in heart rate and blood pressure measurements after the onset of an electrographic seizure.

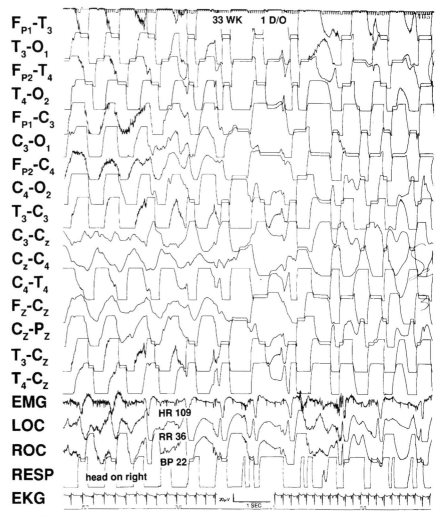

Figure 8-9, cont'd.

antepartum injury may express isolated seizures after in utero cerebrovascular injury on the basis of thrombolytic and/or embolic disease of the mother, placenta, or fetus. Fetal injury alternatively may occur after ischemic-hypoperfusion events from circulatory disturbances, such as maternal shock, chorioamnionitis, or placental fetal vasculopathy (69). Other antepartum congenital or acquired factors may include familial epilepsy or preeclampsia.

Only a percentage of neonates with remote in utero cerebrovascular disease before labor and delivery present with neonatal seizures (70). Many remain asymptomatic until later during infancy or childhood. Neonatal expression of seizures may reflect acute or subacute physiologic stress during or in proximity to parturition which lowers seizure threshold in vulnerable brain regions that have been previously damaged.

Following a careful review of the medical histories of the mother, fetus, and newborn, determination of serum glucose, electrolytes, ammonia, lactate, pyruvate, magnesium, calcium, and phosphorus levels may diagnose correctable metabolic conditions in newborns with seizures who will not require antiepileptic medications. Spinal fluid analyses include cell count, protein, glucose, lactate, pyruvate, amino acids, and culture studies to consider central nervous system infection, intracranial hemorrhage, and metabolic disease. Metabolic acidosis on serial arterial blood gas determinations may alternatively suggest an inherited metabolic disease, particularly if intrapartum asphyxia was not judged to be severe. Absence of multi-organ dysfunction may alert the clinician to other etiologies for seizures besides intrapartum asphyxia. Signs of chronic in utero stress such as growth restriction, early hypertonicity after neonatal depression, joint contractures, or elevated nucleated red blood cell values all suggest longer-standing antepartum stress to the fetus. Careful review of placental and cord specimens can also be extremely useful. Neuroimaging, preferably using magnetic resonance imaging, can help localize and grade the severity and possibly time an insult (71). Identification of genetic or syndromic conditions can contribute to the expression neonatal encephalopathies independent to asphyxial injury (72). Ancillary studies may also include long-chain fatty acids and chromosomal/DNA analyses, as deemed necessary by family and clinical histories. Finally, serum and urine organic acid and amino acid determinations may be needed to delineate a specific biochemical disorder for the child with a persistent metabolic acidosis. Lysosomal enzyme studies are also occasionally considered to diagnose specific enzymatic deficiencies in children with neonatal seizures.

PRINCIPLES OF THERAPY

The goal for treating neonatal seizures remains the prevention of long-term brain damage in the context of the medical management of the underlying etiology for a brain disorder. The two-tiered objective of medical management for neonatal seizures is the initial treatment of etiologic factors that may be responsible for seizure generation followed by the cessation of seizures of epileptic origin with either traditional antiepileptic medications or etiology-specific therapeutic agents. These goals may not be achievable since many etiologic factors are not determined for all neonates, and the potential causes for seizures are as yet unknown. As discussed in previous sections, certain clinical seizures with no electrographic expression on surface recordings may in fact be nonepileptic in physiologic origin and therefore may not respond to traditional antiepileptic medications. Alternative treatment choices that stop or lessen nonepileptic movement disorders may be required. Alternatively, antiepileptic medications may be ineffective in children with clinical and/or electrographic expression of presumed cortically propagated seizures, despite high doses of one or multiple antiepileptic medications. Finally, there is a "double-edged blade" to therapeutic interventions to prevent seizures. Antiepileptic medications used to control seizures may have short-term negative consequences by causing cerebral perfusion secondary to systemic hypotension, contributing to adverse consequences on brain growth and development.

There are three stages in the current acute management of neonates with seizures: (i) initial medical management; (ii) etiology-specific therapy; and (iii) antiepileptic medication treatment. These stages should be patient-specific for the clinical profile for the individual neonate. A hypothesized fourth level of treatment will be discussed which refers to the current level of understanding regarding seizure generation in the immature brain related to specific etiologies, brain region, and timing of injury.

General principles of medical management should always include maintaining the newborn's airway, providing adequate ventilation, and preserving cardiovascular circulation. In neonates with seizures, particularly those with recurrent or prolonged seizures, elevations in respiration, heart rate, and blood pressure may occur. Measures must therefore be taken to ensure adequate ventilatory support, and circulatory perfusion of neonates with seizures during the initial stage of evaluation and therapy. This approach will potentially avoid the autonomic side effects that may occur as a result of recurrent seizures that can compromise multiorgan system function, leading to secondary brain damage.

If a specific reason for seizures has been identified as potentially treatable, etiology-specific therapy needs to be initiated. These treatable causes are critical to seizure management, and will not respond to traditional antiepileptic medications. Examples of common treatable metabolic etiologies include hypoglycemia, hypocalcemia, and hypomagnesemia. The neonatal intensivist must consider the associated brain disorders that may accompany such treatable metabolic derangements, such as asphyxia, intracranial infection, or craniocerebral trauma. Therapeutic protocols associated with these common etiologies are listed in Table 8-5.

Although uncommon, there are other inherited metabolic conditions that may respond to specific nutritional supplementation. This form of treatment is exemplified by the therapy for pyridoxine deficiency, requiring 50 to 500 mg of pyridoxine with coincident EEG monitoring. This is a "potentially treatable" cause of medically refractory seizures. It is an exceedingly rare condition but should always be considered in an attempt to control seizures that do not respond to more conventional medical management. Other epileptic encephalopathies associated with metabolic disturbances include folinic acid deficiency and sulfite oxide/molybdenum deficiencies. Some of these metabolic disorders of metabolism can mimic traditional signs of postasphyxial encephalopathy (72).

Emergent Antiepileptic Drug Treatment

It remains controversial which first-line AED agents should be used for neonatal seizure management. There have traditionally been three drug categories: barbiturates, phenytoin, and benzodiazepines. As listed in Table 8-5 regarding loading doses, subsequent doses may then be required for persistent seizure activity that did not respond to the initial loading doses. Adverse events must be anticipated with the administration of these antiepileptic medications, including alteration in levels of arousal, systemic hypotension, bradycardia, respiratory depression, and cardiac arrhythmias.

While the initial loading doses are approximated by the use of the neonate's body weight, certain researchers advocate the use of protein characteristics for antiepileptic medications in assigning the initial dosing. The unbound or free fraction of each of these drugs is pharmacologically active in the protein-binding characteristics of neonates which vary to the extent that uniform dosing scheduled by weight does not provide the same efficacy and safety for the individual child. Preemptive binding profiles calculated for the individual neonate *at risk* for seizures may allow more accurate establishment of a customized loading dose of each drug for that child, thus avoiding toxicity for that individual neonate. This procedure is not universally available. However, these pharmacologic findings underscore the potential pharmacokinetic and pharmacodynamic variability among neonates regarding the utilizations of these drugs.

A "relative consensus" still exists regarding the choice of a specific antiepileptic medication as either a first- or second-line AED, while phenytoin remains the secondary choice (73). Additional AEDs in the benzodiazepine family of drugs continue to be suggested. Controversy remains regarding these choices, given the evidence-based medicine which questions the efficacy to control seizures with specific AEDs (74).

If the decision to treat neonates with antiepileptic medications is reached, important questions must be addressed with respect to who should be treated, when to begin treatment, which drug to use, and for how long neonates should be treated. Some authors suggest that only neonates with clinical seizures should

Table 8-5   Anticonvulsant Drugs for Neonatal Seizures

Drug	Loading dose	Maintenance dose	Withdrawal	Side effects	Monitoring
Phenobarbital	20 mg/kg i.v. max. 40 mg/kg	3–5 mg/kg per 24 h i.v. or p.o.	Irritability, altered sleep, tremors	Drowsiness	Blood pressure
Midazolam	>35 wks 0.05 mg/kg i.v. (in 10 min)	0.15 mg/kg/h	If seizure free for 24 h	Temporary reduction of blood pressure and cerebral blood flow	Blood pressure
Lidocaine	2 mg/kg i.v.	6 mg/kg/h i.v.	After 24 h of treatment: 4 mg/kg/h After 36 h: 2 mg/kg/h After 48 h: stop If seizure free for 24 h	Arrhythmia, seizures, hypotension	ECG, EEG, blood pressure
Clonazepam	0.15 mg/kg i.v. repeat 1× or 2×	0.1 mg/kg per 24 h			
Phenytoin	20 mg/kg i.v. (infusion rate 1 mg/kg/min)	3–4 mg/kg per 24 h i.v.	At removal of i.v. lines	Dysrhythmia	EEG
Pyridoxine	50–100 mg	50–100 mg	If no effect: stop		EEG
Thiopental	10 mg/kg i.v.	Increase dose until EEG shows burst suppression	After 24 h	Hypotension	EEG, blood pressure

From van de Bor M. The recognition and management of neonatal seizures. Curr Paediatr 12:382–7, 2002.

receive medications; brief electrographic seizures need not be treated. Others suggest more aggressive treatment of EEG seizures, since uncontrolled seizures potentially have an adverse effect on immature brain development. An alternative observation suggests that early administration of an AED, such as Phenobarbital, may have adverse effects on outcome in term infants.

Phenobarbital and phenytoin, nonetheless, remain the most widely used antiepileptic medications; benzodiazepines, primidone, and valproic acid have been anecdotally reported. The half-life of Phenobarbital ranges from 45 to 173 hours in the neonate (75–77); the initial loading dose is recommended at 20 mg/kg, with a maintenance dose of 3–4 mg/kg/day. Therapeutic levels are generally suggested to be between 16 and 40 μg/mL; however, there is no consensus with the respect to drug maintenance.

The preferred loading dose of phenytoin is 15–20 mg/kg (75, 76). Serum levels of phenytoin are difficult to maintain because this drug is rapidly redistributed to body tissues. Blood levels cannot be well maintained using an oral preparation.

Benzodiazepines may also be used to control neonatal seizures. The drug most widely used is diazepam. One study suggests a half-life of 54 hours in preterm infants to 18 hours in full-term infants (78). Intravenous administration is recommended since it is slowly absorbed after an intramuscular injection. Diazepam is highly protein bound; alteration of bilirubin binding is low. Recommended intravenous doses for acute management should begin at 0.5 mg/kg. Deposition into muscle precludes its use as a maintenance antiepileptic medication, since profound hypotonia and respiratory depression may result, particularly if barbiturates have also been administered. Lidocaine rather than diazepam infusion has more recently been suggested (79).

Efficacy of Treatment

Conflicting studies report varying efficacy with Phenobarbital or phenytoin. Most studies only apply a clinical endpoint to seizure cessation. One study (76) found that only 36% of neonates with clinical seizures responded to Phenobarbital, while another study noted cessation of clinical seizures with Phenobarbital in only 32% of neonates (75). With doses as high as 40 mg/kg (80), seizure control was reported to be 85%. A more recent study reported that the earlier administration of high-dose Phenobarbital in a group of asphyxiated infants was associated with a 27% reduction in clinical seizures and better outcome than a group who did not receive high dosages (81). However, coincident EEG studies are now suggested to verify the resolution of electrographic seizures. A recent report suggests that 30% of neonates have persistent electrographic seizures after suppression of clinical seizure behaviors following drug administration (49). With EEG as an endpoint to judge cessation of seizures, neither Phenobarbital nor phenytoin was effective to control seizure activity (82).

The use of free or drug-bound fractions of AEDs has been suggested to better assess both efficacy and potential toxicity of AEDs in pediatric populations (83). Drug binding in neonates with seizures has only recently been reported, and can be altered in a sick neonate with organ dysfunction. Toxic side effects may result from elevated free fractions of a drug which adversely affect cardiovascular and respiratory function. To guard against untoward effects, evaluation of treatment and efficacy must take into account both total and free AED fractions, in the context of the newborn's progression or resolution of systemic illness.

Once an antiepileptic drug is chosen, the clinician must closely monitor that seizures are not worsened by the administration of such a drug choice. AEDs may cause worsening of seizures by either aggravating previous seizures or triggering new seizure types as described in four neonates after midazolam was administered (84).

Discontinuation of Drug Use

The clinician's decision to maintain or discontinue antiepileptic drug use is also uncertain (85, 86). Discontinuation of drugs before discharge from the neonatal unit is generally recommended, since clinical assessments of arousal, tone, and behavior will not be hampered by medication effect. However, newborns with congenital or destructive brain lesions on neuroimaging, or those with persistently abnormal neurologic examinations at the time of discharge may suggest to the clinician that a slower taper-off medication is required over several weeks or months. Most children with neonatal seizures rarely reoccur during the first 2 years of life, and prophylactic AED administration need not be maintained past 3 months of age, even in the child at risk. This is supported by a recent study suggesting a low risk of seizure reoccurrence after early withdrawal of AED therapy in the neonatal period (87). Also, older infants who present with specific epileptic syndromes, such as infantile spasms, will not respond to the conventional AEDs that were initially begun during the neonatal period. This honeymoon period without seizures commonly persists for many years in most children before isolated or recurrent seizures appear.

The potential damage of the developing central nervous system by AEDs also emphasizes the need to consider early discontinuation of these agents in the newborn period. Adverse effects on the morphology and metabolism of neuronal cells have been extensively reported from collective research performed over the last few decades (88).

Novel Antiepileptic Drug Approaches

Mechanisms of seizure generation, propagation, and termination are different during early brain development as compared with more mature ages. These age-related mechanisms have partially been elucidated (89). Given that traditional antiepileptic medications have unacceptable efficacy to stop neonatal seizures for specific subsets of newborns, alternative medication options must be developed.

New antiepileptic alternatives to treat neonatal seizures are now being studied. One class of medications are the N-methyl-D-aspartate antagonists, such as topiramate (90). Experimental models of asphyxia-induced seizure activity in immature brain animals have indicated a certain degree of efficacy.

Such models provide data regarding pharmacologic and physiologic characteristics of neuronal responses after an asphyxial stress which causes excessive release of excitotoxic neurotransmitters (91), such as glutamate. Specific cell membrane receptors termed metabotropic glutamate receptors (MGluRs) are sensitive to extracellular glutamate release and may play a role in epileptogenesis and seizure-induced brain damage (92). One class of membrane receptor, for example, has been studied in rat pups after hypoxia-induced seizures, suggesting that MGluRs' downregulation can be associated with epileptogenesis in the absence of cell loss (89). Subclasses of MGluRs will lead to investigations of novel drugs which block these membrane receptors as the mode of treatment for neonatal seizures (93).

Another therapeutic approach is suggested by experimental studies that demonstrate enhanced seizure susceptibility in the developing brain because gamma-aminobutyric acid (GABA) exerts a depolarizing excitatory rather than repolarizing inhibitory action in immature subjects (94). This paradoxical action of GABA early in development may be due in part to age-related differences in chloride homeostasis (95). Chloride transport is a function of two membrane pumps with different time courses of expression. Early in development (i.e., in the rat, P3–P15 after birth), the Na^+–K^+–$2Cl^-$ cotransporter (NKCC1) imports large amounts of chloride into the neuron (along with sodium and potassium to maintain electroneutrality). This pump sets the chloride equilibrium potential positive to the resting potential so that when the GABA$_A$ receptor is activated, chloride flows out of the neuron, depolarizing it. Over time, NKCC1 expression diminishes, and another chloride transporter, KCC2, is expressed. KCC2 has the opposite effect; it extrudes chloride out of the neuron, placing the equilibrium potential more negative than the resting potential so that GABA$_A$ receptor activation allows extracellular chloride to flow into the neuron, hyperpolarizing it and endowing GABA with inhibitory action.

Researchers have termed this the developmental "switch" in chloride homeostasis. This maturational aspect to the chloride ion may influence seizure susceptibility in the neonatal brain. The additional depolarization that is due to GABA$_A$ receptor activation augments excitation that may be initiated by the glutamate neurotransmission. As a result there is a shift in the excitation–inhibition balance towards excessive excitation, and thus towards seizure activity. These conclusions have been suggested by Dzhala et al. (96), who described the developmental profile of NKCC1 in the human neonate. In the early postnatal period, NKCC1 rises to a peak and then declines to adult levels. This rearrangement of membrane receptors occurs over the first few months of life. In the same time period, KCC2 expression gradually rises to adult levels. By blocking NKCC1 function with a commonly used diuretic known as bumetanide there is a prevention of the accumulation of intercellular chloride which therefore counteracts the depolarizing action of GABA$_A$ receptor activation. Bumetanide reduces kainic-induced seizures in neonatal, but not adult, rats, and bursts firing in hippocampus slices. As further evidence, for genetically engineered mice who lack NKCC1, bumetanide is not effective in ameliorating seizures, supporting its role as a specific inhibitor of NKCC1. Therefore, bumetanide is now considered a promising AED with a developmental target, namely the immature chloride cotransporter NKCC1. Some claim that this particular diuretic can be safely used for the neonate, although its long-term safety profile needs to be better studied. It has also been recently suggested that pharmacologic agents that can diminish bursting behavior in neonatal neurons can add an additional level to the control of seizures. Dzhala et al. (96) demonstrated that bumetanide rapidly suppresses synchronous bursts of network activity in P4–P8 hippocampus slices in the rat model. This supports the use of this agent as a potential antiepileptic medication in this age group. Clinical trials need to demonstrate that bumetanide or other similar diuretics can inhibit seizure activity (97). One needs to establish that these agents can reach the brain in appropriate concentrations and lack short- as well as long-term effects.

There are still crucial issues regarding the theory that GABA-mediated excitation may have an important aspect human neonatal seizures, amenable to the treatment as discussed above. It is yet unknown why some GABAergic agents such as Phenobarbital and benzodiazepine fail to have adequate efficacy for human neonatal seizure control. Though seizures can be halted in a percentage of newborns, additional understanding of epileptogenesis in the immature brain must consider the etiology-specific aspects of GABA-mediated mechanisms of seizures as it relates to asphyxia, infection, or trauma. A specific etiology may alter seizure threshold by epigenetic modification, changing the specific genetic variability within individuals. Based on up- or downregulation of genetic expression, individuals who suffer asphyxia, infection, or trauma may have variable vulnerability or resistance to GABA-mediated mechanisms for seizures. This generalization is further complicated by the timing and the specific brain region of damage which may have occurred remotely during the antepartum as opposed to the intrapartum or neonatal periods, and selectively affected deep gray matter as well as neocortical structures. Therefore one must consider the question of whether neonatal seizures represent novel brain injury or are surrogates of injury resulting from etiologies either varied in brain location or during time periods beginning during fetal life (98). The neurologist must place events leading to seizures in the context of clinical, historical and laboratory findings to determine both the pathogenesis and timing of an encephalopathic process in a neonate who is symptomatic with seizures. A new classification of neonatal seizures which integrates electrographic expression, brain region, etiology, and timing may then have more relevance to the choice of anti-epileptic medication both during the neonatal period, as well as later during child-hood (99).

SUMMARY

Recognition and classification of seizures remain problematic. The clinician should rely on synchronized video/EEG/polygraphic recordings to correlate suspicious behaviors with electrographic seizures. This monitoring technique will limit mis-diagnosis and overtreatment of nonepileptic abnormal behaviors, and define an exact endpoint for cortically propagated seizures. This practice must be integrated with an appreciation of pathophysiologic mechanisms responsible for brain injury in a variety of anatomical sites during antepartum time periods from maternal–fetal–placental diseases as well as during the intrapartum or neonatal periods (99).

REFERENCES

1. Scher MS. Seizures in the neonate: diagnostic and therapeutic considerations. In Spitzer AR (ed). Intensive Care of the Fetus and Neonate, 2nd edition. Philadelphia, PA: Elsevier-Mosby, 2005.
2. Scher MS. Neonatal seizures: an expression of fetal or neonatal brain disorders. In Stevenson DK, Sunshine P (eds). Fetal and Neonatal Brain Injury. Cambridge: Cambridge University Press, 2002, pp. 735–84.
3. Clancy RR. Prolonged electroencephalogram monitoring for seizures and their treatment. Clin Perinatol 33:649–665, vi, 2006.
4. Commission on Classification and Terminology of the International League Against Epilepsy. Proposal for revised clinical and electroencephalographic classification of epileptic seizures. Epilepsia 22:489–501, 1981.
5. Mizrahi EM, Kellaway P. Diagnosis and Management of Neonatal Seizures. Philadelphia, PA: Lippincott-Raven, 1998.
6. Weiner SP, Painter MJ, Geva D, et al. Neonatal seizures: electroclinical dissociation. Pediatr Neurol 7:363–8, 1991.
7. Biagioni E, Ferrari F, Boldrini A, et al. Electroclinical correlation in neonatal seizures. Eur J Paediatr Neurol 2:117–25, 1998.
8. Volpe JJ. Neonatal seizures. In Neurology of the Newborn, 4th edition. Philadelphia, PA: WB Saunders, 2001, pp. 178–214.
9. Scher MS. Electroencephalography of the newborn: normal and abnormal features. In Niedermeyer E, Lopes da Silva F (eds). Electroencephalography: Basic Principles, Clinical Applications, and Related Fields, 5th edition. Philadelphia, PA: Lippincott Williams and Wilkins, 2005, pp. 937–89.
10. Scher MS. Normal electrographic-polysomnographic patterns in preterm and fullterm infants. Semin Pediatr Neurol 3:2–12, 1996.
11. DaSilva O, Guzman GMC, Young GB. The value of standard electroencephalograms in the evaluation of the newborn with recurrent apneas. J Perinatol 18:377–80, 1998.
12. Fenichel GM, Olson BJ, Fitzpatrick JE. Heart rate changes in convulsive and nonconvulsive neonatal apnea. Ann Neurol 7:577–82, 1980.
13. Bye AM, Flanagan D. Spatial and temporal characteristics of neonatal seizures. Epilepsia 36:1009–16, 1995.
14. Boylan GB, Pressler RM, Rennie JM, et al. Outcome of electroclinical, electrographic, and clinical seizures in the newborn infant. Dev Med Child Neurol 41:819–25, 1999.
15. Mizrahi EM, Kellaway P. Characterization and classification of neonatal seizures. Neurology 37:1837–44, 1987.
16. Scher MS, Klesh KW, Murphy TF, et al. Seizures and infarction in neonates with persistent pulmonary hypertension. Pediatr Neurol 2:332–9, 1986.
17. Clancy R, Malin S, Laraque D, et al. Focal motor seizures heralding stroke in full-term neonates. Am J Dis Child 139:601–6, 1985.
18. Levy SR, Abroms IF, Marshall PC, et al. Seizures and cerebral infarction in the full-term newborn. Ann Neurol 17:366–70, 1985.
19. Holmes G. Diagnosis and management of seizures in childhood. In Markowitz M (ed). Major Problems in Clinical Pediatrics. Philadelphia, PA: WB Saunders, 1987, pp. 237–61.

20. Karayiannis NB, Srinivasan S, Bhattacharya R, et al. Extraction of motion strength and motor activity signals from video recordings of neonatal seizures. IEEE Trans Med Imaging 20:965–80, 2001.

21. Rose AL, Lombroso CT. A study of clinical, pathological, and electroencephalographic features in 137 full-term babies with a long-term follow-up. Pediatrics 45:404–25, 1970.

22. Kellaway P, Hrachovy RA. Status epilepticus in newborns: a perspective on neonatal seizures. In Delgado-Escueta AV, Wasterlain CG, Treiman DM, et al. (eds). Status Epilepticus: Mechanisms of Brain Damage and Treatment. New York: Raven Press, 1983, Vol. 34, pp. 93–9.

23. Sarnat HB. Anatomic and physiologic correlates of neurologic development in prematurity. In Sarnat HB (ed). Topics in Neonatal Neurology. Orlando, FL: Grune and Stratton, 1984, pp. 1–25.

24. Scher MS. Pathologic myoclonus of the newborn: electrographic and clinical correlations. Pediatr Neurol 1:342–8, 1985.

25. Coulter DL, Allen RJ. Benign neonatal sleep myoclonus. Arch Neurol 39:191–2, 1982.

26. Resnick TJ, Moshe SL, Perotta L, et al. Benign neonatal sleep myoclonus. Relationship to sleep states. Arch Neurol 43:266–8, 1986.

27. Clancy RR. The contribution of EEG to the understanding of neonatal seizures. Epilepsia 37(Suppl 1):S52–9, 1996.

28. Shuper A, Zalzberg J, Weitz R, et al. Jitteriness beyond the neonatal period: a benign pattern of movement in infancy. J Child Neurol 6:243–5, 1991.

29. Parker S, Zuckerman B, Bauchner H, et al. Jitteriness in full-term neonates: prevalence and correlates. Pediatrics 85:17–23, 1990.

30. Hakamada S, Watanabe K, Hara K, et al. Development of the motor behavior during sleep in newborn infants. Brain Dev 3:345–50, 1981.

31. Sexson WR, Thigpen J, Stajich GV. Stereotypic movements after lorazepam administration in premature neonates: a series and review of the literature. J Perinatol 15:146–49; quiz 150–1, 1995.

32. Scher MS, Belfar H, Martin J, et al. Destructive brain lesions of presumed fetal onset: antepartum causes of cerebral palsy. Pediatrics 88:898–906, 1991.

33. Brown P, Rothwell JC, Thompson PD, et al. The hyperekplexias and their relationship to the normal startle reflex. Brain 114:1903–28, 1991.

34. Andermann F, Andermann E. Startle disorders of man: hyperekplexia, jumping and startle epilepsy. Brain Dev 10:213–22, 1988.

35. Barth PJ. Inherited progressive disorders of the fetal brain: a field in need of recognition. In Fukuyama Y, Suzuki Y, Kamoshia S, et al. (eds). Fetal and Perinatal Neurology: Basel: Karger, 1992, pp. 299–313.

36. Lyon G, Adams RD, Kolodny EH. Hypoglycemia. In Neurology of Hereditary Metabolic Diseases of Children, 2nd edition. New York: McGraw-Hill, 1996, pp. 6–44.

37. Scher MS. Seizures in the newborn infant. Diagnosis, treatment, and outcome. Clin Perinatol 24:735–72, 1997.

38. Oliveira AJ, Nunes ML, da Costa JC: Polysomnography in neonatal seizures. Clin Neurophysiol 111(Suppl 2):S74–80, 2000.

39. Watanabe K, Kuroyanagi M, Hara K, et al. Neonatal seizures and subsequent epilepsy. Brain Dev 4:341–6, 1982.

40. Hrachovy R, Mizrahi E, Kellaway P. Electroencephalography of the newborn. In Daly D, Pedley T (eds). Current Practice of Clinical Electroencephalography, 2nd edition. New York: Raven Press, 1990, pp. 201–42.

41. Stockard-Pope JE, Werner SS, Bickford RG. Atlas of Neonatal Electroencephalography, 2nd edition. New York: Raven Press, 1992.

42. Lombroso CT. Neonatal polygraphy in full-term and premature infants: a review of normal and abnormal findings. J Clin Neurophysiol 2:105–55, 1985.

43. Hellstrom-Westas L. Comparison between tape-recorded and amplitude-integrated EEG monitoring in sick newborn infants. Acta Paediatr 81:812–19, 1992.

44. Klebermass K, Kuhle S, Kohlhauser-Vollmuth C, et al. Evaluation of the Cerebral Function Monitor as a tool for neurophysiological surveillance in neonatal intensive care patients. Childs Nerv Syst 17:544–50, 2001.

45. Alfonso I, Jayakar P, Yelin K, et al. Continuous-display four-channel electroencephalographic monitoring in the evaluation of neonates with paroxysmal motor events. J Child Neurol 16:625–8, 2001.

46. Scher MS, Hamid MY, Steppe DA, et al. Ictal and interictal electrographic seizure durations in preterm and term neonates. Epilepsia 34:284–8, 1993.

47. Clancy RR, Legido A. The exact ictal and interictal duration of electroencephalographic neonatal seizures. Epilepsia 28:537–41, 1987.

48. Sheth RD. Electroencephalogram confirmatory rate in neonatal seizures. Pediatr Neurol 20:27–30, 1999.

49. Scher MS, Alvin J, Gaus L, et al. Uncoupling of EEG–clinical neonatal seizures after antiepileptic drug use. Pediatr Neurol 28:277–80, 2003.

50. Alfonso I, Papazian O, Litt R, et al. Single photon emission computed tomographic evaluation of brainstem release phenomenon and seizure in neonates. J Child Neurol 15:56–8, 2000.

51. Kilic S, Tarim O, Eralp O. Serum prolactin in neonatal seizures. Pediatr Int 41:61–4, 1999.

52. Browning RA. Role of the brain-stem reticular formation in tonic–clonic seizures: lesion and pharmacological studies. Fed Proc 44:2425–31, 1985.

53. Caveness WF, Kato M, Malamut BL, et al. Propagation of focal motor seizures in the pubescent monkey. Ann Neurol 7:213–21, 232–5, 1980.

54. Hosokawa S, Iguchi T, Caveness WF, et al. Effects of manipulation of the sensorimotor system on focal motor seizures in the monkey. Ann Neurol 7:222–9, 236–7, 1980.

55. Danner R, Shewmon DA, Sherman MP. Seizures in an atelencephalic infant. Is the cortex essential for neonatal seizures? Arch Neurol 42:1014–16, 1985.

56. Scher MS, Aso K, Beggarly ME, et al. Electrographic seizures in preterm and full-term neonates: clinical correlates, associated brain lesions, and risk for neurologic sequelae. Pediatrics 91:128–34, 1993.

57. Coen RW, McCutchen CB, Wermer D, et al. Continuous monitoring of the electroencephalogram following perinatal asphyxia. J Pediatr 100:628–30, 1982.

58. O'Meara MW, Bye AM, Flanagan D. Clinical features of neonatal seizures. J Paediatr Child Health 31:237–40, 1995.

59. Staudt F, Roth JG, Engel RC. The usefulness of electroencephalography in curarized newborns. Electroencephalogr Clin Neurophysiol 51:205–8, 1981.

60. Eyre JA, Oozeer RC, Wilkinson AR. Continuous electroencephalographic recording to detect seizures in paralysed newborn babies. Br Med J (Clin Res Ed) 286:1017–18, 1983.

61. Goldberg RN, Goldman SL, Ramsay RE, et al. Detection of seizure activity in the paralyzed neonate using continuous monitoring. Pediatrics 69:583–6, 1982.

62. Ronen GM, Penney S, Andrews W. The epidemiology of clinical neonatal seizures in Newfoundland: a population-based study. J Pediatr 134:71–5, 1999.

63. Eriksson M, Zetterstrom R. Neonatal convulsions. Incidence and causes in the Stockholm area. Acta Paediatr Scand 68:807–11, 1979.

64. Seay AR, Bray PF. Significance of seizures in infants weighing less than 2500 grams. Arch Neurol 34:381–2, 1977.

65. Saliba RM, Annegers FJ, Waller DK, et al. Risk factors for neonatal seizures: a population-based study, Harris County, Texas, 1992–1994. Am J Epidemiol 154:14–20, 2001.

66. Lanska MJ, Lanska DJ, Baumann RJ, et al. Interobserver variability in the classification of neonatal seizures based on medical record data. Pediatr Neurol 15:120–3, 1996.

67. Lanska MJ, Lanska DJ, Baumann RJ, et al. A population-based study of neonatal seizures in Fayette County, Kentucky. Neurology 45:724–32, 1995.

68. Friede RL. Porencephaly, hydranencephaly, multilocular cystic encephalopathy. In Developmental Neuropathology. New York: Springer-Verlag, 1975, pp. 102–13.

69. Miller V. Neonatal cerebral infarction. Semin Pediatr Neurol 7:278–88, 2000.

70. de Vries LS, Groenendaal F, Eken P, et al. Infarcts in the vascular distribution of the middle cerebral artery in preterm and fullterm infants. Neuropediatrics 28:88–96, 1997.

71. Leth H, Toft PB, Herning M, et al. Neonatal seizures associated with cerebral lesions shown by magnetic resonance imaging. Arch Dis Child Fetal Neonatal Ed 77:F105–10, 1997.

72. Enns GM. Inborn errors of metabolism masquerading as hypoxic-ischemic encephalopathy. NeoReviews 6:e549–58, 2005.

73. Carmo KB, Barr P. Drug treatment of neonatal seizures by neonatologists and paediatric neurologists. J Paediatr Child Health 41:313–16, 2005.

74. Sankar R, Painter MJ. Neonatal seizures: after all these years we still love what doesn't work. Neurology 64:776–7, 2005.

75. Lockman LA, Kriel R, Zaske D, et al. Phenobarbital dosage for control of neonatal seizures. Neurology 29:1445–9, 1979.

76. Painter MJ, Pippenger C, MacDonald H, et al. Phenobarbital and diphenylhydantoin levels in neonates with seizures. J Pediatr 92:315–19, 1978.

77. Painter MJ, Pippenger C, Wasterlain C, et al. Phenobarbital and phenytoin in neonatal seizures: metabolism and tissue distribution. Neurology 31:1107–12, 1981.

78. Smith BT, Masotti RE. Intravenous diazepam in the treatment of prolonged seizure activity in neonates and infants. Dev Med Child Neurol 13:630–4, 1971.

79. Malingre MM, Van Rooij LG, Rademaker CM, et al. Development of an optimal lidocaine infusion strategy for neonatal seizures. Eur J Pediatr 165:598–604, 2006.

80. Gal P, Toback J, Boer HR, et al. Efficacy of phenobarbital monotherapy in treatment of neonatal seizures: relationship to blood levels. Neurology 32:1401–4, 1982.

81. Hall RT, Hall FK, Daily DK. High-dose phenobarbital therapy in term newborn infants with severe perinatal asphyxia: a randomized, prospective study with three-year follow-up. J Pediatr 132:345–8, 1998.

82. Painter MJ, Scher MS, Stein AD, et al. Phenobarbital compared with phenytoin for the treatment of neonatal seizures. N Engl J Med 341:485–9, 1999.

83. Painter MJ, Minnigh B, Mollica L, et al. Binding profiles of anticonvulsants in neonates with seizures. Ann Neurol 22:413, 1987.

84. Montenegro MA, Guerreiro MM, Caldas JP, et al. Epileptic manifestations induced by midazolam in the neonatal period. Arq Neuropsiquiatr 59:242–3, 2001.

85. Scher MS, Painter MJ. Controversies concerning neonatal seizures. Pediatr Clin North Am 36:281–310, 1989.

86. Camfield PR, Camfield CS. Neonatal seizures: a commentary on selected aspects. J Child Neurol 2:244–51, 1987.

87. Hellstrom-Westas L, Blennow G, Lindroth M, et al. Low risk of seizure recurrence after early withdrawal of antiepileptic treatment in the neonatal period. Arch Dis Child Fetal Neonatal Ed 72:F97–101, 1995.

88. Mizrahi EM. Acute and chronic effects of seizures in the developing brain: lessons from clinical experience. Epilepsia 40(Suppl 1):S42–50; discussion S64–6, 1999.

89. Sanchez RM, Jensen FE. Maturational aspects of epilepsy mechanisms and consequences for the immature brain. Epilepsia 42:577–85, 2001.

90. Koh S, Jensen FE. Topiramate blocks perinatal hypoxia-induced seizures in rat pups. Ann Neurol 50:366–72, 2001.

91. Jensen FE, Wang C. Hypoxia-induced hyperexcitability in vivo and in vitro in the immature hippocampus. Epilepsy Res 26:131–40, 1996.

92. Aronica EM, Gorter JA, Paupard MC, et al. Status epilepticus-induced alterations in metabotropic glutamate receptor expression in young and adult rats. J Neurosci 17:8588–95, 1997.

93. Lie AA, Becker A, Behle K, et al. Up-regulation of the metabotropic glutamate receptor mGluR4 in hippocampal neurons with reduced seizure vulnerability. Ann Neurol 47:26–35, 2000.

94. Brooks-Kayal AR. Rearranging receptors. Epilepsia 46(Suppl 7):29–38, 2005.

95. Staley KJ. Wrong-way chloride transport: is it a treatable cause of some intractable seizures? Epilepsy Currents 6:124–7, 2006.

96. Dzhala VI, Talos DM, Sdrulla DA, et al. NKCC1 transporter facilitates seizures in the developing brain. Nat Med 11:1205–13, 2005.

97. Haglund MM, Hochman DW. Furosemide and mannitol suppression of epileptic activity in the human brain. J Neurophysiol 94:907–18, 2005.

98. Scher MS. Neonatal seizures and brain damage. Pediatr Neurol 29:381–90, 2003.

99. Scher MS. Neonatal seizure classification: a fetal perspective concerning childhood epilepsy. Epilepsy Res 70(Suppl 1):S41–57, 2006.

Chapter 9

Glucose and Perinatal Brain Injury: Questions and Controversies

Jerome Y. Yager, MD • Kenneth J. Poskitt, MD

Hypoglycemia remains a common though controversial problem of the newborn infant (1, 2). Such controversy persists around issues related in the first place to definition and subsequent diagnosis, the relevance of "asymptomatic" versus "symptomatic" hypoglycemia, incidence rates, underlying pathophysiology, treatment, and, of course, neurodevelopmental outcome. Confounding these issues are improved obstetric and neonatal intensive care, which has allowed for the survival of low-birth-weight infants, with their attendant complications of prematurity, respiratory distress, altered metabolism, and higher risks of disorders such as hypoxia-ischemia, seizures, and sepsis.

The adult is completely independent with respect to nutritional requirements. The fetus, in contrast, is fully dependent on the placental transfer of glucose and other nutritional requirements. The newborn is in a transition phase between these two states of complete dependence and independence. For normal cerebral development and consequent function to proceed, an adequate amount of metabolizable substrate must be supplied to the brain during the perinatal period. Glucose is the primary energy substrate for both the adult and newborn brain under physiologic conditions. However, other organic substrates are capable of supplementing glucose during conditions whereby the normal balance of supply and demand for energy production are superseded (3–5).

At birth, the previously consistent supply of maternal glucose is abruptly terminated. Immediately postbirth, hepatic glycogen stores are broken down to maintain reasonable amounts of nutritional support. Glucose-6-phosphatase is the rate-limiting enzyme for this to occur, and is expressed at low levels in the newborn, increasing to adult values within the first few days of life (6). To rapidly adapt, an endocrine stress response involving insulin and glucagon drive hepatic glycogenolysis, lipolysis, and fatty acid oxidation that generate lactate and ketone bodies as alternative fuels important in maintaining cerebral energy metabolism. Estimated rates of glucose metabolism in the 1-day-old newborn are 3-fold greater than older newborns and infants (7). Moreover, measured rates of glucose oxidation suggest that only ~70% of the energy needs of the brain are met through the metabolism of glucose. Hence, the newborn is adapted for utilizing ketone bodies, which can be 5- to 40-fold greater than the adult, and lactate which contributes significantly in the first few hours of life.

Despite the obvious importance of glucose for cerebral energy utilization, particularly during the complex transition from fetal to newborn life, questions remain regarding the role of hypoglycemia, per se, in brain damage and neurodevelopmental outcome. It is therefore the intent of this chapter to provide the reader with a general review of glucose metabolism and its alternative substrates in the newborn brain, to describe the recognized derangements associated with hypoglycemia, and finally to review the clinical aspects of hypoglycemia. Further, we will present case examples that exemplify aspects of neonatal hypoglycemia, highlighting questions and controversies around this complex issue.

GLUCOSE METABOLISM IN THE FETUS AND NEWBORN

In most species studied, including humans, glucose serves as the primary organic fuel for energy production under physiologic circumstances(5, 8). In the fetus, a linear relationship has been observed between the glucose level in the mother and that of the fetus (9–12). At birth, blood glucose concentrations in the newborn are at about 80–90% of that of the mother (13). This linear relation has been seen during all states of maternal euglycemia, hyperglycemia, and hypoglycemia, and is important in that it implies at least a one-to-one relationship between maternal and fetal glucose needs.

At the time of birth, glucose concentrations in the term healthy newborn fall within the first hour of life, recovering and becoming more stable by 3 hours of age, and gradually increasing for at least the first 96 hours, when infants receive exogenous nutrition (13–17). In preparation for birth, a doubling of the glycogen stores occurs at 36 weeks of gestation. At birth, plasma insulin levels fall, together with a marked surge in glucagon levels, leading to a mobilization of glycogen stores, which are rapidly depleted within the first 12–24 hours of life (18, 19). Glucagon levels remain elevated through the first week of life. Subsequent glucose concentrations, in the normal newborn, depend on feeding practices. Though some studies have suggested feeding intervals to be a major determinant of blood glucose concentrations (20), others have not found this to be the case (17). Irrespective, "low" blood glucose concentrations, in appropriately fed term infants, are very rare.

Preterm Infants

It is a generally held belief that blood glucose concentrations in the preterm infant are lower than those of the term infant. Though recent studies suggest that this is not likely the case, given more recent policies of early feeding and intravenous glucose supplementation (20), the theoretical risks certainly apply. In this regard, the preterm infant has not as yet had the opportunity afforded the term infant to build up glycogen stores, typically occurring in the last 4 weeks of gestation. Moreover, the rate-limiting enzyme for glyconeogenesis is significantly lower in the preterm compared to the term infant (6), hence the ability to break down even these stores is limited. The capability of the preterm to mount a response with alternative substrates may also be impaired. Hawdon et al. (20) compared 156 term infants to 62 preterms, and found that, although blood glucose concentrations were not statistically different, preterms were unable to mount a significant ketone body response at the lower end of the blood glucose values. Others have found preterms to variably mount an inadequate glycemic response to glucagons suggesting features of insulin resistance (21).

Intrauterine Growth Restriction

Clearly, intrauterine growth restriction (IUGR) can occur, during which time the fetus is exposed to an environment in which nutrition is restricted either due to placental insufficiency or maternal lack of nutrition. Previous reports (Table 9-1) have certainly indicated a higher prevalence of hypoglycemia in the small baby compared to those within the normal weight range (22, 23). More recent reports are controversial, with some reporting similar glucose concentrations in small for gestational age (SGA) versus appropriate for gestational age (AGA) babies (13, 24), again likely the result of more aggressive nutritional management. Others, however, continue to show differences between the two weight groups, with SGA babies showing lower glucose concentrations compared to appropriately sized babies (25). In either case, IUGR babies display altered metabolic profiles that include reduced glycogen stores, limited oxidation of free fatty acids, and functional hyper-insulinism (18). Combined with a relatively larger brain size, one can see the predisposition of these babies to neurologic injury from a hypoglycemic insult.

CEREBRAL METABOLISM OF GLUCOSE

The ontogeny of regional changes in cerebral glucose utilization has important implications regarding the sensitivity of the immature brain to hypoglycemia.

Table 9-1	Incidence of Hypoglycemia Classified by Birth Weight and Gestational Age	
	Blood glucose concentrations	
	< 1.6 mmol/L (30 mg/dL) (%)	< 1.1 mmol/L (20 mg/dL) (%)
SGA[a]		
Preterm	67	40
Term	25	21
Post-term	18	9
AGA[a]		
Preterm	15	3
Term	10	2
Post-term	5	0
LGA[a]		
Preterm	38	13
Term	4	2
Post-term	7	0
Number of episodes[b]	> 0.6 < 1.6 mmol/L (> 11 < 30 mg/dL)	> 1.6 < 2.6 mmol/L (> 30 < 45 mg/dL)
2–5	30%	58%
More than 6	2%	21%

[a]Modified from the data of Lubchenco and Bard (23).
[b]Modified from the data of Duvanel et al. (22).
SGA, small for gestational age; AGA, appropriate for gestational age; LGA, large for gestational age.

Using the 2-deoxyglucose (2-DG) technique, regional cerebral glucose utilization (rCGU) in the perinatal animal has been shown to be high in brainstem gray matter structures, declining in a caudal to rostral progression to the cerebral cortex (26). Using positron emission tomography (PET) scanning with [^{18}F]-2-deoxyglucose as the isotope, Chugani et al. (27–29) and others (30–32) measured rCGU in humans from birth through adulthood. In infants 5 weeks of age, CGU was highest in the sensorimotor cortex, thalamus, midbrain–brainstem, and cerebellar vermis. By 3 months of age, maximal glucose utilization had shifted to the parietal, temporal, and occipital cortices and in the basal ganglia, with subsequent increases in frontal and various association regions of cerebral cortex occurring by 8 months of age. Little further change in rCGU was observed between 8 and 18 months, with adult values being reached by 2 years old.

Alternative Substrates to Glucose

As previously noted, the perinatal brain is capable of incorporating and metabolizing alternative substrates, most notably lactic acid and the ketone bodies, beta-hydroxy-butyrate and acetoacetate. In vitro studies of regional energy status and the availability of alternative substrates in rats have shown lactate concentrations to be elevated 6-fold in newborn brain compared to adult, and beta-hydroxybutyrate to be double (33).

With respect to the latter, both animal and human studies of the newborn have shown an enhanced capacity for the cerebral extraction of ketone bodies from blood, as compared to older infants and adults. The investigation of ketone body utilization in suckling rats suggests they may account for between 20 and 35% of cerebral energy metabolism in this age group (3, 4, 34). Ketone body utilization peaks at P14, and subsequently diminishes to P21, at a time during which CGU is increasing and glucose becomes the major substrate for energy metabolism. These findings coincide with the capacity of the immature blood–brain barrier to transport ketone bodies at a 3-fold greater rate compared to glucose (35). Furthermore, those enzymes linked to ketone body metabolism in brain display a rapid increase in activity after birth and a subsequent decline after weaning, in contrast to the pattern displayed by the key enzymes of glycolysis whose activity increases with advancing age in an inverse relation to those of ketogenesis (36).

Though ketone bodies appear to play a role in normal energy metabolism of the immature brain, whether they do under pathophysiologic circumstances of glucose deprivation seems unlikely. Data from human infants suggest that the capacity for hepatic ketone synthesis in the neonate is restricted. The findings demonstrate (i) low blood ketone levels, (ii) a failure of ketone bodies to rise with fasting, and (iii) a failure of ketone bodies to rise with hypoglycemia (37, 38). In contrast, lactic acid has been shown to be an important source of energy during hypoglycemia. Elegant studies in the newborn dog (39) during nor-moglycemia show that 95% of cerebral energy requirements are met by glucose with ketone bodies and lactate contributing 1 and 4%, respectively. With insulin-induced hypoglycemia, and a concomitant reduction in CGU, lactate was able to support 58% of cerebral oxidative metabolism. Subsequent experiments showed that, under these conditions, there was no significant decline in brain high-energy phosphate levels (40). Other investigators have shown a preferential utilization of lactate over either glucose or ketone bodies in the newborn rat and dog, and a sparing effect on glucose utilization during hypoglycemia (41–45).

Glucose Transporters

The mechanism by which glucose is transported from blood into brain across cell membranes occurs by a Na$^+$–glucose cotransporter protein that is energy independent. These facilitative glucose transporter proteins are a family of structurally related proteins. Six glucose transporters have been identified and labeled as GLUT 1–5 and GLUT 7. Within the brain, GLUT 1 and 3 are predominant. GLUT 1 is the most prevalent of the glucose transporters, and is highly expressed in all blood–tissue barriers, including the blood–brain barrier. GLUT 3 is the predominant isoform in neurons. GLUT 5 has been detected in the microglia of both humans and rats.

The expression of glucose transporter proteins, not surprisingly, reflects the energy demands of the brain. Hence, analysis of cerebral cortical microvessels and membranes in the newborn rat demonstrates that all GLUT proteins are low during the first week of life. During the second and third postnatal weeks, GLUT proteins increase, particularly in the deep gray matter structures of the thalamus and hypothalamus, coincident with enhanced utilization of glucose as a fuel. Similarly, and in an almost linear fashion, GLUT proteins in the cortex and hippocampus increase from 20 to 100% of adult values between 7 and 30 postnatal days, during a recognized period of rapid neuronal maturation and synaptogenesis (46–48).

DEFINITIONS

Ambiguity surrounding a precise definition of neonatal hypoglycemia continues (49), and was emphasized by the study of Koh et al. (50). Their group surveyed 36 pediatric textbooks and 178 pediatric consultants searching for agreement on the definition of neonatal hypoglycemia. Perhaps not surprisingly, there was none, with definitions ranging from <1 mmol/L to <4 mmol/L. In 1937, Hartmann and Jaudon (8) published a series of 286 neonates and infants with "significant hypoglycemia" as determined by recurrent or persistent low "true" blood sugar values. Only those infants with clinical manifestations were considered. These authors defined hypoglycemia as being "mild" (2.2–2.78 mmol/L); "moderate" (1.11–2.22 mmol/L); or "extreme" (<1.11 mmol/L). Their approach incorporated the important concept that the definition of hypoglycemia must represent a continuum of values which deviate from the biologic norm. This latter concept is particularly relevant today as definitions of "treatable" hypoglycemia take into account gestational age, multisystem organ complications, and neurophysiologic and/or clinical symptomatology.

Difficulty in arriving at an absolute value for hypoglycemia in the newborn stems from the obvious factors that encompass a dynamic and vulnerable biologic process. Hypoglycemia simply refers to an *abnormally low blood sugar concentration.* In this context, the definition of "abnormal" becomes relevant, given that "hypoglycemia" or "euglycemia" for that matter is an evolving, dynamic process, itself dependent on a large number of variables.

Absolute glucose concentrations below which the term hypoglycemia can be applied have been defined based on statistical measures (within 2 standard deviations of the mean). Hence, serial plasma glucose determinations in term healthy newborn infants revealed an initial drop to 55–60 mg/dL (3.05 mmol/L) within the first 2 hours of life, followed by a rise to 70 mg/dL (3.88 mmol/L) from 3 to 72 hours, and levels in excess of 80 mg/dL (4.44 mmol/L) beyond the 3rd day (16). Values below the 5th percentile were therefore considered by these authors as representing "statistical hypoglycemia" (Table 9-1).

Lubchenco and Bard (23) studied the incidence of hypoglycemia as determined by gestational age and birth weight. Their work showed that preterm infants who were of AGA weight displayed a mean glucose concentration of 48 mg/dL (2.6 mmol/L), compared to 54 mg/dL (3.0 mmol/L) in the term AGA infants. In the SGA infants born at term, there was a further shift to the left with mean glucose concentrations being 44 mg/dL (2.4 mmol/L).

In more recent studies that have looked at glucose concentrations in healthy, term infants, Hoseth et al. (14) studied 223 term, breast-fed newborns, serially over the first 96 hours, and found lowest blood sugars to occur within the first hours of life, with an overall range of 1.4 to 5.3 mmol/L (median 3.1). Similar results were reported by a study of over 200 term, healthy newborns (17), where a mean glucose concentration of 2.8 mmol/L was found. In both of the above studies, 12–14% of the children had blood sugars less then 2.6 mmol/L, mostly during the first day of life.

A recent meta-analysis (51) analyzing 10 studies, inclusive of 723 healthy, term AGA babies, suggested parameters that are <5th percentile of norm for the definition of neonatal hypoglycemia. In this regard, thresholds for hypoglycemia would be on a sliding scale based on time after birth and include values of <1.6, 2.2, and 2.67 mmol/L at 1 to 2, 3 to 47, and 48 to 72 hours of age, respectively.

Based on the above findings then, it is reasonable to state that normal glucose concentrations in term, healthy infants have a wide range, with the lowest concentrations occurring during the first few hours of life. Within this range, the risk of neurologic sequelae is remote, and routine testing for blood sugars has been suggested to be unnecessary (49).

Controversy and Question

These data do not, however, direct themselves to the more controversial and clinically relevant questions that remain somewhat unanswered. Hence, the definition of neonatal hypoglycemia remains nonspecific, and is dependent on gestational age, appropriateness of fetal growth, the age of the newborn at the time of sampling, and whether or not the infant has fed. Given these parameters, current data suggest that hypoglycemia is not clinically evident, nor perhaps relevant, until values are <1.1 mmol/L. We therefore need to ask:

1. *Are there other parameters or markers of hypoglycemia that suggest an association with resultant encephalopathy?*

SYMPTOMATIC VERSUS ASYMPTOMATIC HYPOGLYCEMIA

Most common among the features of hypoglycemic encephalopathy is an alteration in the level of consciousness, described as lethargy or somnolescence. Irritability, high-pitched cry, or exaggerated primitive reflexes may also be found. Newborns will often be described as being jittery, and this may progress to seizures, apnea, hypotonia, and coma (52).

In this regard, a number of investigators have shown that perhaps the more "relevant" way to define hypoglycemia is to do so based on whether or not the infant is symptomatic. Koivisto et al. (53) reported on 151 children divided into three groups comprising (i) a symptomatic–convulsive group [$n = 8$], (ii) a symptomatic–nonconvulsive group [$n = 77$], and (iii) an asymptomatic group [$n = 66$]. In this group of patients, feeding was not initiated for the first 24 hours of life. Symptoms were characterized by the presence of tremor, cyanosis, pallor, limpness, irritability, apathy, or tachypnea, which disappeared with glucose therapy. Hypoglycemia was defined as a glucose concentration of <20 mg/dL (1.1 mmol/L). The findings indicated that 50% of the symptomatic convulsive group and 12% of the symptomatic nonconvulsive group had neurologic abnormalities on follow-up compared to only 6% of both the asymptomatic and control groups. In a study by Singh et al. (54), 107 babies with severe hypoglycemia (<25 mg/dL) were evaluated over 15 months. Symptoms were present in 40%. Neurodevelopment in asymptomatic babies was normal.

Moore and Perlman (55) described three cases of profound hypoglycemia in term, breastfed newborns, who developed seizures following discharge from hospital.

All were symptomatic with pallor, jitteriness, poor feeding, but had nevertheless been home on early discharge. All of the patients showed glucose concentrations <1.1 mmol/L. Late follow-up suggested that two of the three were normal, and one was significantly delayed.

Alkalay et al. (56) reviewed reports of hypoglycemia over the last four decades. Their criterion for inclusion, albeit retrospective, was the presence of neurologic sequelae, felt to be directly or primarily the result of hypoglycemia. The study was inclusive of both AGA and SGA babies, as well as preterms. Their findings indicated that, of the study patients reported, over 95% had plasma glucose concentrations of <25 mg/dL (1.4 mmol/L). The incidence in this group with neurologic abnormality was 21%.

In order to correlate a critical threshold of blood glucose concentration with neurologic dysfunction, several studies have evaluated neurophysiologic parameters in association with hypoglycemia. Koh et al. (57) reported abnormalities in sensory-evoked potentials in children when blood glucose concentrations fell below 2.6 mmol/L. Unfortunately, only four of these children were less than 1 month of age. Cowett et al. (58) studying term and preterm infants found no such correlation, and Pryds et al. (59) also found no correlation between hypoglycemic glucose concentrations and BAER and EEG patterns.

DURATION OF HYPOGLYCEMIA

The above study also found that the minimal age that hypoglycemia was detected was 10 hours, suggesting that a prolonged period of "hypoglycemia" is required before neurologic sequelae or symptomatology become evident (56). Others have similarly suggested prolonged hypoglycemia as a prerequisite for damage. Lucas et al. (60) determined the neurologic outcome of 661 preterm infants. Moderate hypoglycemia, defined in their study as <2.6 mmol/L, occurred in 433, of which 104 displayed recurrent events on three or more separate days. A strong correlation existed between the number of separate days in which hypoglycemia was recorded and reduced mental and motor development scores at 18 months corrected age. When hypoglycemia was present on five or more days, the incidence of cerebral palsy or developmental delay was increased by a factor of 3.5.

A more recent study conducted by Duvanel et al. (22) illustrated similar results. Eighty-five SGA preterm newborns were tested for hypoglycemia (defined as <2.6 mmol/L). In their cohort, 73% met the criteria for hypoglycemia, and recurrent episodes were once again strongly correlated with persistent neurodevelopmental and physical growth deficits to 5 years of age.

A primate study determining the effect of prolonged insulin-induced hypoglycemia on outcome (61) also showed that the longer the duration of hypoglycemia, the greater the degree of abnormal behavioral outcome. However, even in those in whom hypoglycemia was produced for 10 hours, the effects were transient, and reversible when training was done for the behavioral task. Blood glucose concentrations were <25 mg/dL. Unfortunately, no neuropathologic examination was reported for this group of animals.

To provide basic guidelines by which to define hypoglycemia, Cornblath et al. (62) issued a consensus statement regarding "operational thresholds" for blood glucose concentrations. They defined operational threshold as that concentration of plasma or blood glucose at which clinicians should consider intervention. In that regard, they felt that healthy, asymptomatic full-term infants need not have routine monitoring of their glucose concentrations. On the other hand, any infant with clinical manifestations compatible with hypoglycemia should be tested, and intervention taken for those with values <45 mg/dL (2.5 mmol/L). For infants "at risk" of hypoglycemia due to alterations in maternal metabolism, intrinsic neonatal problems, or endocrine or metabolic disturbances, glucose monitoring should begin as soon after birth as possible. For values <36 mg/dL (2.0 mmol/L), close surveillance should be maintained and intervention recommended if concentrations remain low, regardless of the presence or absence of symptoms. In those infants in whom very low concentrations are detected (<20–25 mg/dL; 1.1–1.4 mmol/L), therapeutic intervention should be initiated immediately. Newborn infants being fed by continuous parenteral nutrition will have persistently high insulin levels. As a result, their ability to manifest significant ketogenesis and the means by which to utilize alternative substrates will be impaired. Under these circumstances, prudent caution suggests maintaining glucose concentrations in the higher therapeutic ranges (>45 mg/dL; 2.5 mmol/L).

While this consensus certainly addresses many of the concerns regarding under what circumstances clinicians should be vigilant in their approach to the diagnosis and treatment of "hypoglycemia," it does not answer several other important questions regarding the newborn in particular. Before attempting to answer these questions, further understanding of the epidemiology and pathophysiology of hypoglycemia would be in order.

CAUSES OF HYPOGLYCEMIA

Though it is not the intent of this chapter to discuss the underlying causes of hypoglycemia, a list of etiologies is found in Table 9-2.

Incidence

The reported incidence of hypoglycemia depends on those variables also specific to its definition. Sexson (19) found 8.1% of 232 infants had glucose values of <30 mg/dL (1.6 mmol/L) in the first hours of life, with 20.6% having glucose concentrations <40 mg/dL (2.2 mmol/L). When <30 mg/dL was used as a definition, Lubchenco and Bard (23) studied the incidence of hypoglycemia according to gestational age and weight and found the overall incidence to be 32% for SGA infants, and 10% and 11.5% for AGA and LGA infants, respectively. With a definition of <20 mg/dL, the incidence obviously decreases. Of the 73% of SGA infants studied by Duvanel et al. (22) who had hypoglycemia, 30% would have had six or more episodes with glucose values between 1.6 and 2.6 mmol/L (Table 9-1).

Table 9-2	Differential Diagnosis of Severe Recurrent Hypoglycemia

Hyperinsulinism
Beta-cell hyperplasia
Nesidioblastosis
Macrosomia
Beckwith–Weidmann syndrome
Endocrine abnormalities
Panhypopituitarism
Hypothyrodism
Growth hormone deficiency
Cortisol deficiency
Hereditary metabolic disorders
Abnormalities of carbohydrate metabolism
Amino acid disorders (maple syrup urine disease)
Organic acid disorders
Fatty acid oxidation defects
Glucose transporter defects

Pathophysiology of Hypoglycemia

Cerebral Blood Flow, Glucose Utilization, and Cerebral Energy Metabolism

As the major metabolic fuel for cerebral energy production, there is an inextricable link between the demands for energy production and the supply and extraction of substrate. In that regard, studies in newborn dogs (63) displayed an inverse linear relationship between blood glucose concentrations and cerebral blood flow (CBF). Therefore, increases in CBF ranging from 150 to 450% of normal occurred as blood sugar concentrations decreased from 40 to <5 mg/dL (2.2 to <0.3 mmol/L). Increases followed ontogeny and were more predominant in brainstem structures compared to other major regions of the brain. The same phenomenon is seen in human infants. Pryds et al. (59) found CBF to increase by 200% above normal at levels of blood glucose below 30 mg/dL (1.6 mmol/L).

Vannucci's group of collaborators found similar results, and importantly looked at the alterations in white matter glucose utilization during hypoglycemia (64). In this study blood glucose concentrations were reduced to ~1.0 mmol/L. Hypoglycemia was associated with increases in regional CBF ranging from 170% (white matter) to 250% (thalamus). In both of the former studies, there was a direct relation between CBF and mean arterial pressure. Regional CGU was unchanged in 11 of the 16 structures measured, but significantly, was reduced by 30–45% in the occipital white matter structures and cerebellum. Calculations of the extent to which glucose transport into the brain during hypoglycemia was enhanced by the increases in CBF suggested that glucose delivery contributed minimally (<10%) to the maintenance of CGU. Earlier studies had also shown that with hypoglycemia to levels as low as <1.0 mmol/L, cerebral metabolic rate for oxygen ($CMRO_2$) decreased to 50% of normal. At this same level, cerebral metabolic rates for lactate increase 10-fold, and became the dominant fuel for oxidative metabolism in the newborn dog brain (39). Later experiments showed that using a similar experimental paradigm of hypoglycemia, high-energy phosphate reserves (phosphocreatine, ATP) remained within normal concentrations (40). From this group of studies, the authors concluded that CBF autoregulation is lost during hypoglycemia in the newborn, and that rather than glucose delivery, low energy demands serve to maintain glucose homeostasis and preclude tissue glucose deficiencies. They further hypothesized that alternative cerebral energy fuels, predominantly in the form of lactate, substitute for glucose at levels of blood glucose below 1 mmol/L.

Cerebral Biochemical Alterations During Hypoglycemia

Little work has actually been done on the biochemical perturbations that arise as a result of hypoglycemia in the immature brain. Much of what is known in this regard is derived from experiments done in the adult animal exposed to insulin-induced hypoglycemia. However, given the information discussed in the previous section, important comparisons between the adult and newborn brain can be made, and perhaps some tentative conclusions drawn.

As in the newborn, CBF increases during hypoglycemia. In the adult, this is where the similarities end. Hence in adult models of hypoglycemia, cerebral high-energy phosphate levels (ATP, phosphcreatine) plummet to levels less than 20% of normal as blood glucose concentrations fall below 1 mmol/L (<20 mg/dL). In concert with this depletion of high-energy reserves, neurophysiologic monitoring reveals an isoelectric EEG, a marked increase in intracellular Ca^{2+}, and a 10-fold and 4-fold rise in extracellular concentrations of the excitatory amino acids (EAAs) aspartate and glutamate, respectively (65–67). Hence, at least in the adult, it now appears that the mechanism of neuronal death as a result of hypoglycemia is similar

Table 9-3   Comparison of Pathophysiologic Mechanisms Responsible for Brain Damage in Adult versus Newborn Animals

Mechanism	Adult	Newborn
Cerebral blood flow	Increased	Increased
Cerebral uptake of glucose	Increased	Increased
Cerebral energy reserves	Depleted	Maintained
Utilization of alternative substrates	Neutral	Increased
Glucose utilization	Increased	Decreased

to that of hypoxia-ischemia (energy depletion–excitatory amino acid release–Ca^{2+} influx–free radical production–cell death).

As indicated earlier, the preservation of cerebral energy status in the newborn, even at very low concentrations of glucose, is accompanied by a preservation of neurophysiologic function as demonstrated by EEG. A possible underlying cause of cellular injury in the newborn may however be related to the release of EAAs. Silverstein et al. (68) induced hypoglycemia by insulin injection in 7-day-old immature rats. Blood glucose concentrations gradually diminished over time to 30–40 mg/dL in the 1st hour after injection, 20 mg/dL in the 2nd hour, and to <5 mg/dL by 3 to 4 hours after injection. Their results indicated a direct correlation between decreasing glucose levels and increasing concentrations of extracellular glutamate. In hypoglycemic newborn human infants, Aral et al. (69) also reported on their finding of increased concentrations of glutamate and aspartate in the cerebrospinal fluid.

Beyond the above experimental data, there is very little information regarding the underlying mechanisms of hypoglycemic brain injury in the newborn. In comparing the newborn response to hypoglycemia to that of the adult (Table 9-3), several important differences become evident, particularly related to the controversy surrounding hypoglycemic brain injury. In this regard then, the newborn appears to respond to hypoglycemia with physiologic alterations that appear to protect the brain from damage. Hence, CBF increases, glucose utilization decreases, alternative substrates are able to substitute for demands of energy production, and, as a result, cerebral energy reserves are preserved, at least in experimental animals. These metabolic adaptations beg the question as to whether or not hypoglycemia per se does cause brain damage, certainly an area of ongoing controversy.

HYPOGLYCEMIA AND BRAIN DAMAGE

Evidence of pathologic injury to the brain as a result of neonatal hypoglycemia has been particularly difficult to obtain. In this regard, in vitro cell culture studies as well as animal models of pure hypoglycemia have been helpful in documenting the effects of significantly low blood sugars on brain pathology.

In vitro NMR studies on energy metabolism of neurons and astroglia under various pathologic conditions has shown that hypoglycemia per se did not significantly alter the high-energy reserves of either neurons or glia, even at levels as low as 0.1 mmol/L (70). In our own laboratory, immature astrocytes in culture were exposed to a substrate-free medium (absence of glucose and amino acids). Under these circumstances, which do not allow for the utilization of any alternative substrate, the immature cells were able to survive for almost twice as long as the mature astrocytes. Though not strictly an indication of the effects of hypoglycemia, the study clearly points out the resistance of immature cells to substrate deprivation (71).

Brierly et al. (72) investigated the effects of insulin-induced hypoglycemia in a group of adolescent primates. Physiologic parameters were controlled. Six of the 10 animals whose blood sugar was lowered to <20 mg/dL (1.1 mmol/L) for 2 hours or more displayed selective neuronal necrosis throughout the cerebral cortices, with particular vulnerability in the parieto-occipital region, as well as the hippocampus, caudate, and putamen. Similar findings were present in primates exposed to severe (<20 mg/dL) and prolonged hypoglycemia of >6 hours. In these animals neuropathologic alterations primarily occurred in the basal ganglia, cerebral cortex, and the hippocampus (73).

In the adult rat, Auer and colleagues (74–79) have done extensive work defining the neuropathologic consequences of severe hypoglycemia. In a series of papers, this group defined the timing, evolution, and distribution of hypoglycemic brain damage in the rat. These investigators defined severe hypoglycemia as that level of blood glucose which caused electrocerebral silence (80). Their previous studies had shown that glucose concentrations under these circumstances were between 0.12 and 1.36 mmol/L. Over the course of these investigations, they described several important features of hypoglycemic brain damage that distinguishes it from ischemic injury. These include: (i) that infarction of brain tissue does not occur with hypoglycemia, (ii) a superficial to deep gradient in the density of neuronal necrosis is seen in the cerebral cortex, (iii) the caudatoputamen is involved more heavily near the white matter, and near the angle of the lateral ventricle, and (iv) the hippocampus shows dense neuronal necrosis at the crest of the dentate gyrus (which is always spared in ischemia), and a gradient of increasing damage in the medial aspect of CA_1 (75, 76, 81). Interestingly, white matter injury was not particularly dealt with in these latter studies.

In the human neonate, there is clearly a paucity of neuropathologic papers that allow us some insight into the distribution of injury in the newborn brain as a result of hypoglycemia. Anderson et al. (82) described six neonates who had been diagnosed with hypoglycemia and died within the first year of life for other noncentral nervous system-related causes. Blood glucose concentrations were <20 mg/dL in all cases. In four of the six neonates, the duration of hypoglycemia was greater than 36 hours. All infants were symptomatic. Histopathologically, those authors observed widespread necrosis of neuronal and glial cells in the cerebral cortex, hippocampus, and basal ganglia. Within the cortex, the authors commented on a greater degree of involvement in the occipital region than the frontal region. They also noted no predilection for the boundary zones between major blood vessels which often distinguishes ischemic lesions. Larroche (83) emphasized the white matter damaging potential of hypoglycemia, and demonstrated prominent periventricular leukomalacia in her series of newborns expiring of hypoglycemia.

Neuroimaging Abnormalities

The recognition of specific patterns of abnormality on computed tomography (CT) and magnetic resonance imaging (MRI) scans of infants with diagnosed hypoglycemia has been a relatively recent finding in the literature. Spar et al. (84) described a newborn with well-documented hypoglycemia for at least 15 hours. The MRI scan, completed at 19 days of age, demonstrated a predominance of tissue loss in the parenchyma of the occipital lobes, bilaterally. Barkovich et al. (85) described their group of five patients who suffered from hypoglycemia in the newborn period and emphasized the findings of white matter damage in the parietal and occipital lobes. Globus pallidus injury was present in only one of the infants described. Kinnala et al. (86) published the findings of 18 full-term infants with blood sugars <45 mg/dL (2.5 mmol/L). All were symptomatic. Only three of the infants reported had hypoglycemia for greater than 24 hours with the longest duration being 33 hours. The mean blood sugar value was 25 mg/dL (1.4 mmol/L), with only two of the infants displaying sugars below 5 mg/dL (0.3 mmol/L). Four of the infants showed hyperintensity lesions on T1-weighted images either in the occipital periventricular regions, or the thalamus. Ninety-four percent of the infants were developmentally normal at follow-up. Murakami et al. (87) confirmed these latter results in their retrospective review of brain MRI in eight term infants, all of whom were symptomatic and had blood glucose concentrations below 20 mg/dL (1.1 mmol/L). Once again abnormalities were consistently found in the parieto-occipital white matter in all but one of the children.

Within the last decade, a pattern of predominantly parieto-occipital white matter abnormalities, often in association with abnormal signal in the deep gray matter structures of the thalamus and/or basal ganglia, has been identified on follow-up of those neonates who had experienced symptomatic hypoglycemia. Though the number of studies and patients is few overall, the abnormalities appear to be relatively distinct for the syndrome of neonatal hypoglycemia. Alkalay et al. (88) reported a case of term hypoglycemia and reviewed the available reports of associated imaging findings. Blood sugar findings were always <25 mg/dL (1.4 mmol/L); they were generally low for a prolonged period of time; and patients were symptomatic. When neuroimaging was done in this group, it was abnormal, with over 80% showing consistent abnormalities of the occipital lobes, similar to those displayed in Figure 9-1.

Metabolically, these neuroimaging findings are consistent with studies by Mujsce et al. (64) which showed a reduction in cerebral glucose utilization in the occipital white matter of newborn dogs during insulin-induced hypoglycemia. These findings occurred in contrast to the preservation of glucose utilization in other regions of the brain, and an increase in brainstem structures. These data suggest an uncoupling of supply and demand requirements for glucose in this region of the newborn brain, and an outstripping of the available substrate supply for energy production, resulting in the enhanced sensitivity of the occipital regions.

Given the above, several aspects of hypoglycemia and its affect on the newborn brain can be summarized:

1. The definition of hypoglycemia within statistical boundaries has been reasonably consistent as being abnormal if <2.5 mmol/L, and severely so if <1.1 mmol/L.
2. The definition and risk of hypoglycemia is not static, but dependent on the gestational age of the infant at birth, weight of the infant, and timing of the evaluation of glucose as it relates to the age of the infant from birth, and whether or not feeding has been implemented.

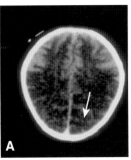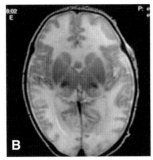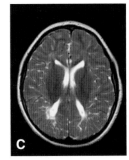

Figure 9-1 Series of images from term infant, normal Apgar scores, and hypoglycemia at 20 hours of age. (A) CT scan on day 3 of life. Note the areas of attenuation bilaterally in the occipital regions. (B) T2-weighted MRI scan on day 10 of life. Loss of cortex in the occipital region and hyperintense putamen are noted. (C) T2-weighted MRI scan at 7 years of age displaying chronic alterations with focal white matter and cortical injury in the occipital regions.

3. A consistent association of "hypoglycemia" and neurologic injury has occurred only when the infant has, in addition to evidence of low blood concentrations of glucose, been symptomatic, and continued to have "hypoglycemia" for a prolonged period of time.

Controversy and Question

While these parameters provide important information regarding the approach to hypoglycemia in the otherwise healthy infant, because glucose is a metabolically active substance in constant flux, confounding factors may influence whether or not hypoglycemia contributes to brain injury, and at what level that might occur. Hence, disorders that the newborn faces alter the metabolic demands of the brain, tipping the balance of supply and demand towards injury. Common examples in the newborn whereby the demand for glucose may outstrip its supply include hypoxia-ischemia and seizures, the latter being a complication of both hypoxia-ischemia and hypoglycemia itself. In these circumstances (89) we ask:

1. *Does hypoglycemia contribute to the brain damage caused by hypoxia-ischemia or seizures in the newborn infant?*

Hypoglycemia and Hypoxia-Ischemia, Seizures

Hypoglycemia is deleterious when superimposed on hypoxia-ischemia. Vannucci and Vannucci (90) subjected newborn rat pups to anoxia in 100% nitrogen. The experimental group was rendered hypoglycemic to 0.75 mmol/L (14 mg/dL) by intraperitoneal insulin injection. Normoglycemic animals survived 10 times as long as those that were hypoglycemic. In newborn dogs made hypoglycemic in combination with asphyxia, brain ATP concentrations fell by 61%, compared to those puppies with hypoglycemia alone, in whom ATP was preserved.

In determining the combined effects of substrate utilization and hypoxia-ischemia in the neonate (5), Yager et al. (91) subjected 7-day-old rat pups to hypoglycemia by either fasting them for 12 hours or subcutaneous injection of insulin. Both control and experimental rat pups underwent hypoxia-ischemia by exposure to 8% oxygen combined with unilateral common carotid artery ligation. Although hypoglycemia was only mild in nature, 5.4, 4.3, and 3.4 mmol/L for control, insulin, and fasted groups, respectively, brain damage was significantly greater in the insulin-treated animals than either of the other two groups. Fasted animals had the least damage, presumably due to the enhanced ketogenesis and alternative substrate utilization displayed by this group.

Seizures are associated with an increase in energy demands, and hence a several-fold increase in glucose utilization. The increased demand produces a decrease in brain glucose stores, placing the brain in a vulnerable position. Hence it is not surprising that during hypoglycemia, supplies of glucose are further depleted and a deficit in energy reserves might be expected. Thus in the newborn puppy, significant depletion of cerebral high-energy phosphate stores, as measured by ^{31}P NMR spectroscopy, occurred when seizures and hypoglycemia were combined, as compared to seizures alone (92). In a model of neonatal hypoxic-ischemic-induced seizures (93), Yager and colleagues concluded that a relative decrease in the concentration of brain glucose, compared to controls, was responsible for the increase in brain damage seen in this model (94). These data serve to highlight the importance of controlling seizures, particularly in the face of hypoglycemia.

In the human newborn, several studies have reviewed the effects of compounding hypoglycemia and perinatal asphyxia. Salhab et al. (95) retrospectively reviewed 185 term infants with perinatal asphyxia defined by a cord pH of <7.00. Fifteen percent (27) of the infants had an initial blood sugar of <40 mg/dL (2.2 mmol/L). These authors found a significant contribution of hypoglycemia to abnormal outcome, compared to those infants with blood sugars >40 mg/dL. The authors did not comment in this paper about the duration of hypoglycemia. Additional complicating features were also present.

ILLUSTRATIVE CASE

Not infrequently medicolegal questions arise surrounding the contribution of perinatal asphyxia to children who have developmental disability (89). Among the confounding factors is often hypoglycemia.

A baby male was born at 42 weeks of gestation following a normal pregnancy. Delivery was forceps assisted. Birth weight was 3.27 kg. Thick meconium was present, and the baby was suctioned for significant amounts. Apgar scores were 2 and 4 at 1 and 5 minutes. Approximately 3.5 hours after birth, the baby, still displaying evidence of a neonatal encephalopathy, developed clinical seizures. Blood sugar was determined to be 54 mg/dL (3.0 mmol/L). Seizures persisted intermittently that day. Blood glucose concentrations measured at 14 and 24 hours after delivery were 20 and 59 mg/dL (1.1 and 3.3 mmol/L), respectively. Electroencephalogram revealed multifocal areas of electrographic seizures. CT revealed bilateral occipital infarcts. In his teens, this young man now has bilateral cortical blindness and mild developmental delay.

Clearly this baby illustrates a number of complexities. Firstly there is some evidence of perinatal asphyxia (though a cord pH was not available), with respect to modestly depressed Apgar scores. Though he has cortical blindness, there is minimal developmental delay, suggesting the majority of injury was, in fact, in the occipital cortical regions. The question is, to what extent, if any, did hypoglycemia contribute to the injury?

Though there was not severe hypoglycemia at birth, certainly depressed glucose levels persisted for at least 24 hours. This occurred concurrently with repetitive seizures, as circumstance of increased metabolic demand, on a background of a diffuse brain insult. Clinically this child did express a neonatal encephalopathy with both altered neurologic status and seizures. Outcome suggests that the injury, however, was relatively restricted to the occipital cortices. Hence in the current scenario, hypoglycemia on the background of perinatal asphyxia not only contributed to the brain damage incurred, but may also have had the greatest effect, despite only one value that would have been categorized as severe hypoglycemia.

The findings are consistent with the available data that suggest that the otherwise normal neonatal brain is relatively tolerant of hypoglycemia. However, when superimposed on a brain that has been compromised by hypoxia-ischemia or seizures or both, it may exact damage, even when the levels of glucose are only borderline for hypoglycemia (93).

OUTCOME

Given the complexities surrounding the definition and diagnosis of hypoglycemia in the newborn period, it is not surprising that there are difficulties in determining the neurologic morbidity surrounding this clinical entity. Several important papers regarding definition (see above) and looking at clinical prognosis allow us to make important observations regarding the thresholds to be assumed for the hypoglycemic neonate. Hence, Lucas et al. (60) detailed the neurologic outcome of a multicenter study of 661 preterm infants weighing less than 1850 g. Developmental outcome was determined at 18 months of age. The authors excluded variables independent of glucose concentrations and found that reduced mental and motor developmental scores were inversely related to the number of days that glucose concentrations were <2.6 mmol/L (47 mg/dL), whereas above this concentration no relationship was found. The relative risk of neurodevelopmental impairment in infants with hypoglycemia compared to those with no hypoglycemia was 3.5 times as great for those with blood sugars <2.6 mmol/L for >5 days.

A more recent study by Stenninger et al. (96) reviewed the long-term neurologic morbidity in 13 children with neonatal hypoglycemia defined as blood glucose concentrations <1.5 mmol/L (27 mg/dL), and compared them to 15 children without neonatal hypoglycemia. Neurodevelopmental assessments were done at approximately 7.75 years of age. These investigators found that children with neonatal hypoglycemia had significantly more difficulties in a screening test for minimal brain dysfunction, and were more likely to be hyperactive, impulsive, and inattentive. These children also had lower developmental scores than did controls.

Brand et al. (97) evaluated 75 healthy term LGA babies of nondiabetic mothers. The value of glucose considered to be significant for hypoglycemia was <2.2 mmol/L. Treatment with intravenous glucose was started if the baby was symptomatic. They concluded that transient neonatal hypoglycemia was not harmful to psychomotor development when evaluated at 4 years of age.

A recent systematic review (98) of neurodevelopment following neonatal hypoglycemia in the first week of life evaluated 18 studies. Sixteen of the studies were felt to be of "poor quality" and two were of high quality, though they could not be pooled for data analysis. Unfortunately, the review concluded that "none of the studies provided a valid estimate of the effect of hypoglycemia on neurodevelopment." A further indication that this topic requires significantly more research regarding the overall outcome of infants experiencing hypoglycemia at birth, in the various scenarios that may occur.

TREATMENT

Despite the issues surrounding neonatal hypoglycemia, a review of the literature, as has been outlined in this chapter, clearly allows for the appropriate recognition of those infants at risk for significant hypoglycemia and the institution of a plan for monitoring and therapeutic intervention. Given the information available to us today, it appears that term infants born without complication and without symptomatology are highly unlikely to be at risk of neurodevelopmental abnormalities unless:

1. Blood glucose concentrations are <1.1 mmol/L.
2. The newborn is symptomatic.
3. Hypoglycemia is prolonged (hours).

In evaluating a newborn whose perinatal course has been complicated by SGA, perinatal asphyxia, seizures, sepsis, or other disorders that suggest an imbalance between substrate supply and demand for cerebral energy production, a broader "definition" of hypoglycemia should be used. Hence, under these circumstances, infants displaying blood glucose concentrations below 40 mg/dL (<2.2 mmol/L), particularly on more than one occasion, should be aggressively treated and followed.

Clearly there are infants who will require specific forms of therapy for their underlying metabolic and endocrinologic abnormalities. In the vast majority of infants, glucose alone will be the predominant therapeutic intervention. Though in the past, relatively large boluses of high concentration glucose have been advised, it is probably best to avoid hyperglycemia, and its attendant risks of rebound hypoglycemia. Lilien et al. (99) have shown that a minibolus of 200 mg/kg (2 mL of 10% glucose over 1 minute) immediately followed by a continuous infusions of 8 mg/kg/min results in the rapid correction of blood glucose concentrations and stable values of between 70 and 80 mg/dL (3.8–4.4 mmol/L). Continuous monitoring is of course required, and after glucose concentrations appear to have stabilized for 12–24 hours the infusion can be decreased by 2 mg/kg/min every 6–12 hours. In rare circumstances in which hypoglycemia does not respond to this regimen, or to infusions of up to 12/mg/kg/min, or it recurs with tapering, hydrocortisone can be administered at a dose of 5 mg/kg every 12 hours.

CONCLUSIONS

Despite the fact that hypoglycemia is an extremely common disorder of the newborn, consensus has been difficult to reach regarding definition, diagnosis, outcome, and treatment. Several important points can be made.

1. The definition of hypoglycemia is not absolute, and is highly dependent on the age, weight, timing of evaluation, whether the baby was fed, and on extenuating and complicating factors. Hence, it should be assessed on a per patient basis.
2. Healthy, term infants of appropriate weight, and who are fed early, are not at risk for hypoglycemic injury.
3. Significant hypoglycemia, with the potential to result in abnormal neurodevelopmental outcome, occurs in those in whom (i) blood sugars are <1.1 mmol/L, (ii) hypoglycemia is prolonged, and (iii) neurologic symptoms are present.
4. A high level of sensitivity for hypoglycemia needs to be applied to all newborns who are compromised by SGA, perinatal asphyxia, seizures, sepsis, or other pathologies that increase metabolic requirements. In these circumstances, a broader "definition" should be applied, and glucose concentrations should be maintained at levels of at least 40 mg/dL or higher.

With improved neuroradiologic techniques such as MRI and PET scanning becoming increasingly available, studies to determine the correlation between hypoglycemia and outcome will help to clarify issues surrounding the effects of hypoglycemia on brain pathology. Long-term epidemiologic studies correlating the severity and duration of hypoglycemia with neurologic consequences are required, and can be complemented by appropriate parallel investigations in animal models of neonatal hypoglycemia.

REFERENCES

1. Aynsley-Green A, Hawdon JM. Hypoglycemia in the neonate: current controversies. Acta Paediatr Jpn 39(Suppl 1):S12–16, 1997.
2. Kalhan S, Peter-Wohl S. Hypoglycemia: what is it for the neonate? Am J Perinatol 17:11–18, 2000.
3. Nehlig A. Respective roles of glucose and ketone bodies as substrates for cerebral energy metabolism in the suckling rat. Dev Neurosci 18:426–33, 1996.
4. Nehlig A, Pereira de Vasconcelos A. Glucose and ketone body utilization by the brain of neonatal rats. Prog Neurobiol 40:163–221, 1993.
5. Vannucci RC, Yager JY. Glucose, lactic acid, and perinatal hypoxic-ischemic brain damage. Pediatr Neurol 8:3–12, 1992.
6. Burchell A, Gibb L, Waddell ID, et al. The ontogeny of human hepatic microsomal glucose-6-phosphatase proteins. Clin Chem 36:1633–7, 1990.
7. Bier DM, Leake RD, Haymond MW, et al. Measurement of "true" glucose production rates in infancy and childhood with 6,6-dideuteroglucose. Diabetes 26:1016–23, 1977.
8. Hartmann A, Jaudon JC. Hypoglycemia. J Pediatr 1–36, 1937.

9. Aynsley-Green A. Metabolic and endocrine interrelations in the human fetus and neonate. Am J Clin Nutr 41:399–417, 1985.

10. Aynsley-Green A, Soltesz G, Jenkins PA, Mackenzie IZ. The metabolic and endocrine milieu of the human fetus at 18–21 weeks of gestation: II. Blood glucose, lactate, pyruvate and ketone body concentrations. Biol Neonate 47:19–25, 1985.

11. Soltesz G, Harris D, Mackenzie IZ, Aynsley-Green A. The metabolic and endocrine milieu of the human fetus and mother at 18–21 weeks of gestation: I. Plasma amino acid concentrations. Pediatr Res 19:91–3, 1985.

12. Bozzetti P, Ferrari MM, Marconi AM, et al. The relationship of maternal and fetal glucose concentrations in the human from midgestation until term. Metabolism 37:358–63, 1988.

13. Heck LJ, Erenberg A. Serum glucose levels in term neonates during the first 48 hours of life. J Pediatr 110:119–22, 1987.

14. Hoseth E, Joergensen A, Ebbesen F, Moeller M. Blood glucose levels in a population of healthy, breast fed, term infants of appropriate size for gestational age. Arch Dis Child Fetal Neonatal Ed 83:F117–19, 2000.

15. Tanzer F, Yazar N, Yazar H, Icagasioglu D. Blood glucose levels and hypoglycaemia in full term neonates during the first 48 hours of life. J Trop Pediatr 43:58–60, 1997.

16. Srinivasan G, Pildes RS, Cattamanchi G, et al. Plasma glucose values in normal neonates: a new look. J Pediatr 109:114–17, 1986.

17. Diwakar KK, Sasidhar MV. Plasma glucose levels in term infants who are appropriate size for gestation and exclusively breast fed. Arch Dis Child Fetal Neonatal Ed 87:F46–8, 2002.

18. Ward Platt M, Deshpande S. Metabolic adaptation at birth. Semin Fetal Neonatal Med 10: 341–50, 2005.

19. Sexson WR. Incidence of neonatal hypoglycemia: a matter of definition. J Pediatr 105:149–50, 1984.

20. Hawdon JM, Ward Platt MP, Aynsley-Green A. Patterns of metabolic adaptation for preterm and term infants in the first neonatal week. Arch Dis Child 67:357–65, 1992.

21. Jackson L, Burchell A, McGeechan A, Hume R. An inadequate glycaemic response to glucagon is linked to insulin resistance in preterm infants? Arch Dis Child Fetal Neonatal Ed 88:F62–6, 2003.

22. Duvanel CB, Fawer CL, Cotting J, et al. Long-term effects of neonatal hypoglycemia on brain growth and psychomotor development in small-for-gestational-age preterm infants. J Pediatr 134:492–8, 1999.

23. Lubchenco LO, Bard H. Incidence of hypoglycemia in newborn infants classified by birth weight and gestational age. Pediatrics 47:831–8, 1971.

24. Hawdon JM, Weddell A, Aynsley-Green A, Ward Platt MP. Hormonal and metabolic response to hypoglycaemia in small for gestational age infants. Arch Dis Child 68:269–73, 1993.

25. Bazaes RA, Salazar TE, Pittaluga E, et al. Glucose and lipid metabolism in small for gestational age infants at 48 hours of age. Pediatrics 111:804–9, 2003.

26. Duckrow RB, LaManna JS, Rosenthal M. Disparate recovery of resting and stimulated oxidative metabolism following transient ischemia. Stroke 12:677–86, 1981.

27. Chugani HT, Phelps ME, Mazziotta JC. Positron emission tomography study of human brain functional development. Ann Neurol 22:487–97, 1987.

28. Chugani HT, Phelps ME. Maturational changes in cerebral function in infants determined by 18FDG positron emission tomography. Science 231:840–3, 1986.

29. Chugani HT, Hovda DA, Villablanca JR, et al. Metabolic maturation of the brain: a study of local cerebral glucose utilization in the developing cat. J Cereb Blood Flow Metab 11:35–47, 1991.

30. Chance B, Leigh JS Jr, Nioka S, et al. An approach to the problem of metabolic heterogeneity in brain: ischemia and reflow after ischemia. Ann NY Acad Sci 508:309–20, 1987.

31. Kinnala A, Nuutila P, Ruotsalainen U, et al. Cerebral metabolic rate for glucose after neonatal hypoglycaemia. Early Hum Dev 49:63–72, 1997.

32. Kinnala A, Suhonen-Polvi H, Aarimaa T , et al. Cerebral metabolic rate for glucose during the first six months of life: an FDG positron emission tomography study. Arch Dis Child Fetal Neonatal Ed 74:F153–7, 1996.

33. Lust WD, Pundik S, Zechel J, et al. Changing metabolic and energy profiles in fetal, neonatal, and adult rat brain. Metab Brain Dis 18:195–206, 2003.

34. Cremer JE. Substrate utilization and brain development. J Cereb Blood Flow Metab 2:394–407, 1982.

35. DeVivo DC, Leckie MP, Agrawal HC. The differential incorporation of beta-hydroxybutyrate and glucose into brain glutamate in the newborn rat. Brain Res 55:485–90, 1973.

36. Booth RF, Patel TB, Clark JB. The development of enzymes of energy metabolism in the brain of a precocial (guinea pig) and non-precocial (rat) species. J Neurochem 34:17–25, 1980.

37. Anday EK, Stanley CA, Baker L, et al. Plasma ketones in newborn infants: absence of suckling ketosis. J Pediatr 98:628–30, 1981.

38. Stanley CA, Anday EK, Baker L, Delivoria-Papadopolous M. Metabolic fuel and hormone responses to fasting in newborn infants. Pediatrics 64:613–19, 1979.

39. Hernandez MJ, Vannucci RC, Salcedo A, Brennan RW. Cerebral blood flow and metabolism during hypoglycemia in newborn dogs. J Neurochem 35:622–8, 1980.

40. Vannucci RC, Nardis EE, Vannucci SJ, Campbell PA. Cerebral carbohydrate and energy metabolism during hypoglycemia in newborn dogs. Am J Physiol 240:R192–9, 1981.

41. Young RS, Petroff OA, Chen B, et al. Preferential utilization of lactate in neonatal dog brain: in vivo and in vitro proton NMR study. Biol Neonate 59:46–53, 1991.

42. Vicario C, Medina JM. Metabolism of lactate in the rat brain during the early neonatal period. J Neurochem 59:32–40, 1992.
43. Miller AL, Kiney CA, Staton DM. Effects of lactate on glucose metabolism of developing rat brain. Brain Res 316:33–40, 1984.
44. Maran A, Cranston I, Lomas J, et al. Protection by lactate of cerebral function during hypoglycaemia. Lancet 343:16–20, 1994.
45. Dombrowski GJ Jr, Swiatek KR, Chao KL. Lactate, 3-hydroxybutyrate, and glucose as substrates for the early postnatal rat brain. Neurochem Res 14:667–75, 1989.
46. Powers WJ, Rosenbaum JL, Dence CS, et al. Cerebral glucose transport and metabolism in preterm human infants. J Cereb Blood Flow Metab 18:632–8, 1998.
47. Vannucci SJ, Maher F, Simpson IA. Glucose transporter proteins in brain: delivery of glucose to neurons and glia. Glia 21:2–21, 1997.
48. Vannucci SJ. Developmental expression of GLUT1 and GLUT3 glucose transporters in rat brain. J Neurochem 62:240–6, 1994.
49. Nicholl R. What is the normal range of blood glucose concentrations in healthy term newborns? Arch Dis Child 88:238–9, 2003.
50. Koh TH, Eyre JA, Aynsley-Green A. Neonatal hypoglycaemia: the controversy regarding definition. Arch Dis Child 63:1386–8, 1988.
51. Alkalay AL, Sarnat HB, Flores-Sarnat L, et al. Population meta-analysis of low plasma glucose thresholds in full-term normal newborns. Am J Perinatol 23:115–9, 2006.
52. Volpe JJ. Neurology of the Newborn, 4th edition. Philadelphia, PA: WB Saunders, 2001.
53. Koivisto M, Blanco-Sequeiros M, Krause U. Neonatal symptomatic and asymptomatic hypoglycaemia: a follow-up study of 151 children. Dev Med Child Neurol 14:603–14, 1972.
54. Singh M, Singhal PK, Paul VK, et al. Neurodevelopmental outcome of asymptomatic and symptomatic babies with neonatal hypoglycaemia. Indian J Med Res 94:6–10, 1991.
55. Moore AM, Perlman M. Symptomatic hypoglycemia in otherwise healthy, breastfed term newborns. Pediatrics 103:837–9, 1999.
56. Alkalay AL, Flores-Sarnat L, Sarnat HB, et al. Plasma glucose concentrations in profound neonatal hypoglycemia. Clin Pediatr (Phila) 45:550–8, 2006.
57. Koh TH, Aynsley-Green A, Tarbit M, Eyre JA. Neural dysfunction during hypoglycaemia. Arch Dis Child 63:1353–58, 1988.
58. Cowett RM, Howard GM, Johnson J, Vohr B. Brain stem auditory-evoked response in relation to neonatal glucose metabolism. Biol Neonate 71:31–6, 1997.
59. Pryds O, Greisen G, Friis-Hansen B. Compensatory increase of CBF in preterm infants during hypoglycaemia. Acta Paediatr Scand 77:632–7, 1988.
60. Lucas A, Morley R, Cole TJ. Adverse neurodevelopmental outcome of moderate neonatal hypoglycaemia. BMJ 297:1304–8, 1988.
61. Schrier A, Wilhelm PB, Church RM, et al. Neonatal hypoglycemia in the rhesus monkey: effect on development and behavior. Infant Behav Dev 13:189–207, 1990.
62. Cornblath M, Hawdon JM, Williams AF, et al. Controversies regarding definition of neonatal hypoglycemia: suggested operational thresholds. Pediatrics 105:1141–5, 2000.
63. Anwar M, Vannucci RC. Autoradiographic determination of regional cerebral blood flow during hypoglycemia in newborn dogs. Pediatr Res 24:41–5, 1988.
64. Mujsce DJ, Christensen MA, Vannucci RC. Regional cerebral blood flow and glucose utilization during hypoglycemia in newborn dogs. Am J Physiol 256:H1659–66, 1989.
65. Butcher SP, Sandberg M, Hagberg H, Hamberger A. Cellular origins of endogenous amino acids released into the extracellular fluid of the rat striatum during severe insulin-induced hypoglycemia. J Neurochem 48:722–8, 1987.
66. Sandberg M, Butcher SP, Hagberg H. Extracellular overflow of neuroactive amino acids during severe insulin-induced hypoglycemia: in vivo dialysis of the rat hippocampus. J Neurochem 47:178–84, 1986.
67. Uematsu D, Greenberg JH, Reivich M, Karp A. Cytosolic free calcium and NAD/NADH redox state in the cat cortex during in vivo activation of NMDA receptors. Brain Res 482:129–35, 1989.
68. Silverstein FS, Simpson J, Gordon KE. Hypoglycemia alters striatal amino acid efflux in perinatal rats: an in vivo microdialysis study. Ann Neurol 28:516–21, 1990.
69. Aral YZ, Gucuyener K, Atalay Y, et al. Role of excitatory aminoacids in neonatal hypoglycemia. Acta Paediatr Jpn 40:303–6, 1998.
70. Alves PM, Fonseca LL, Peixoto CC, et al. NMR studies on energy metabolism of immobilized primary neurons and astrocytes during hypoxia, ischemia and hypoglycemia. NMR Biomed 13:438–48, 2000.
71. Hertz L, Yager JY, Juurlink BH. Astrocyte survival in the absence of exogenous substrate: comparison of immature and mature cells. Int J Dev Neurosci 13:523–7, 1995.
72. Brierly JB, Brown AW, Meldrum BS. The Neuropathology of Insulin Induced Hypoglycemia in Primate. Philadelphia, PA: JB Lippincott, 1971.
73. Myers RE, Kahn KJ. Insulin Induced Hypoglycemia in the Non-human Primate: II. Long Term Neuropathological Consequences. Philadelphia, PA: JB Lippincott, 1971, pp. 195–206.
74. Auer R, Kalimo H, Olsson Y, Wieloch T. The dentate gyrus in hypoglycemia: pathology implicating excitotoxin-mediated neuronal necrosis. Acta Neuropathol (Berl) 67:279–88, 1985.
75. Auer RN, Kalimo H, Olsson Y, Siesjo BK. The temporal evolution of hypoglycemic brain damage: I. Light- and electron-microscopic findings in the rat cerebral cortex. Acta Neuropathol (Berl) 67:13–24, 1985.

76. Auer RN, Kalimo H, Olsson Y, Siesjo BK. The temporal evolution of hypoglycemic brain damage: II. Light- and electron-microscopic findings in the hippocampal gyrus and subiculum of the rat. Acta Neuropathol (Berl) 67:25–36, 1985.

77. Auer RN, Siesjo BK. Biological differences between ischemia, hypoglycemia, and epilepsy. Ann Neurol 24:699–707, 1988.

78. Auer RN, Siesjo BK. Hypoglycaemia: brain neurochemistry and neuropathology. Baillieres Clin Endocrinol Metab 7:611–25, 1993.

79. Auer RN, Wieloch T, Olsson Y, Siesjo BK. The distribution of hypoglycemic brain damage. Acta Neuropathol (Berl) 64:177–91, 1984.

80. Auer RN, Olsson Y, Siesjo BK. Hypoglycemic brain injury in the rat. Correlation of density of brain damage with the EEG isoelectric time: a quantitative study. Diabetes 33:1090–8, 1984.

81. Kalimo H, Auer RN, Siesjo BK. The temporal evolution of hypoglycemic brain damage: III. Light and electron microscopic findings in the rat caudoputamen. Acta Neuropathol (Berl) 67:37–50, 1985.

82. Anderson JM, Milner RD, Strich SJ. Effects of neonatal hypoglycaemia on the nervous system: a pathological study. J Neurol Neurosurg Psychiatry 30:295–310, 1967.

83. Larroche JC. Developmental Pathology of the Neonate. New York: Excerpta Medica, 1977.

84. Spar JA, Lewine JD, Orrison WW Jr. Neonatal hypoglycemia: CT and MR findings. AJNR Am J Neuroradiol 15:1477–8, 1994.

85. Barkovich AJ, Ali FA, Rowley HA, Bass N. Imaging patterns of neonatal hypoglycemia. AJNR Am J Neuroradiol 19:523–8, 1998.

86. Kinnala A, Rikalainen H, Lapinleimu H, et al. Cerebral magnetic resonance imaging and ultrasonography findings after neonatal hypoglycemia. Pediatrics 103:724–9, 1999.

87. Murakami Y, Yamashita Y, Matsuishi T, et al. Cranial MRI of neurologically impaired children suffering from neonatal hypoglycaemia. Pediatr Radiol 29:23–7, 1999.

88. Alkalay AL, Flores-Sarnat L, Sarnat HB, et al. Brain imaging findings in neonatal hypoglycemia: case report and review of 23 cases. Clin Pediatr (Phila) 44:783–90, 2005.

89. Williams AF. Neonatal hypoglycaemia: clinical and legal aspects. Semin Fetal Neonatal Med 10:363–8, 2005.

90. Vannucci RC, Vannucci SJ. Cerebral carbohydrate metabolism during hypoglycemia and anoxia in newborn rats. Ann Neurol 4:73–9, 1978.

91. Yager JY, Heitjan DF, Towfighi J, Vannucci RC. Effect of insulin-induced and fasting hypoglycemia on perinatal hypoxic-ischemic brain damage. Pediatr Res 31:138–42, 1992.

92. Young RS, Cowan BE, Petroff OA, et al. In vivo 31P and in vitro 1H nuclear magnetic resonance study of hypoglycemia during neonatal seizure. Ann Neurol 22:622–8, 1987.

93. Wirrell EC, Armstrong EA, Osman LD, Yager JY. Prolonged seizures exacerbate perinatal hypoxic-ischemic brain damage. Pediatr Res 50:445–54, 2001.

94. Yager JY, Armstrong EA, Miyashita H, Wirrell EC. Prolonged neonatal seizures exacerbate hypoxic-ischemic brain damage: correlation with cerebral energy metabolism and excitatory amino acid release. Dev Neurosci 24:367–81, 2002.

95. Salhab WA, Wyckoff MH, Laptook AR, Perlman JM. Initial hypoglycemia and neonatal brain injury in term infants with severe fetal acidemia. Pediatrics 114:361–6, 2004.

96. Stenninger E, Flink R, Eriksson B, Sahlen C. Long-term neurological dysfunction and neonatal hypoglycaemia after diabetic pregnancy. Arch Dis Child Fetal Neonatal Ed 79:F174–9, 1998.

97. Brand PL, Molenaar NL, Kaaijk C, Wierenga WS. Neurodevelopmental outcome of hypoglycaemia in healthy, large for gestational age, term newborns. Arch Dis Child 90:78–81, 2005.

98. Boluyt N, van Kempen A, Offringa M. Neurodevelopment after neonatal hypoglycemia: a systematic review and design of an optimal future study. Pediatrics 117:2231–43, 2006.

99. Lilien LD, Pildes RS, Srinivasan G, et al. Treatment of neonatal hypoglycemia with minibolus and intraveous glucose infusion. J Pediatr 97:295–8, 1980.

Chapter 10

Neonatal Hypotonia

Keung-kit Chan, MBBS, MRCPCH • Basil T. Darras, MD

Definition of Hypotonia

Physical Examination and Assessment of a Hypotonic Child

Differential Anatomic Diagnosis of Hypotonia

Common Neuromuscular Disorders Presenting Principally With Hypotonia

Approach to Hypotonia

Hypotonia is a common chief complaint listed in referrals to child neurologists in both inpatient and outpatient settings. Neonatal hypotonia, also known as "floppy infant" syndrome, is the main presenting clinical feature of most neuromuscular diseases of early life (1). However, disorders of the central nervous system may also manifest with hypotonia. In this chapter, we will attempt to (i) define hypotonia, (ii) discuss the physical examination and assessment of the hypotonic infant, (iii) discuss the differential anatomic diagnosis of hypotonia, (iv) summarize the most common neuromuscular disorders presenting principally with hypotonia, and (v) present our stepwise diagnostic approach to the diagnostic investigation of infantile hypotonia.

DEFINITION OF HYPOTONIA

Two types of muscle tone can be assessed clinically: postural and phasic. *Postural* (i.e., antigravity) tone is a sustained, low-intensity muscle contraction in response to gravity and is mediated by both the gamma and alpha motor neuron systems in the spinal cord. It is assessed clinically by passive manipulation of the limbs. *Phasic* tone is a brief contraction in response to a high-intensity stretch and is mediated by the alpha motor neuron system only. It is examined clinically by eliciting the muscle stretch reflexes. *Hypotonia* is defined as reduction in postural tone, with or without a change in phasic tone. When postural tone is depressed, the trunk and limbs cannot counteract gravity and the child appears hypotonic or floppy.

Sainte-Anne Dargassies (2) described an approximate caudal–rostral progression in the development of muscle tone. At postconceptional age of 28 weeks, there is minimal resistance to passive manipulation in all limbs; by 32 weeks, flexor tone can be appreciated in the lower extremities; and by 36 weeks, flexor tone is also present in the upper limbs. By term, strong flexor tone in all four limbs can be demonstrated by passive movements.

Table 10-1   Hypotonia: Physical Examination

General physical examination
Appearance/posture (flaccid)
Passive manipulation of the limbs
Traction response (head lag)
Vertical suspension ("slips through")
Horizontal suspension ("drapes over")
"Scarf sign," "heel to ear or chin"
Motility and muscle power
Muscle stretch reflexes
Primary neonatal reflexes
Sensation

PHYSICAL EXAMINATION AND ASSESSMENT OF A HYPOTONIC CHILD

Volpe (3) describes the physical examination of a hypotonic infant in detail. Following a careful general physical examination, the neurologic assessment should include motor examination, evaluation of primary neonatal reflexes, and sensory examination (Table 10-1). *General physical examination* may reveal organomegaly, cardiomyopathy, contractures, abnormalities of the genitalia, respiratory rate or pattern irregularities, or evidence of traumatic injury (e.g., bruising, petechiae); the general examination may be normal also. The *motor examination* includes assessment of posture, muscle tone, motility and muscle power, muscle stretch reflexes, and primary neonatal reflexes. Abnormality of the *primary neonatal reflexes* lies in their persistence. In normal infants, the Moro reflex disappears by 6 months of age (4, 5), the palmar grasp becomes less obvious after 2 months of age, and the tonic neck response becomes less facile at 6–7 months of age (4–6). *Sensation* can be tested by withdrawal from a stimulus (e.g., touching the infant with a small brush). Abnormalities in sensation may be present in some forms of congenital neuropathies, such as hereditary motor-sensory or sensory-autonomic neuropathies, but they are usually difficult to assess in infants.

When assessing muscle tone in young infants, the infant's head should be placed in the midline to eliminate the effect of the tonic neck response. Minimal resistance to passive manipulation of arms or legs is an important clinical feature of hypotonia. Most hypotonic infants demonstrate a classic "frog-like" posture: full abduction and external rotation of the legs as well as a flaccid extension or flexion of the arms. Congenital dislocation of the hips may be noted because poor muscle tone in utero has failed to maintain the femoral head in the acetabulum. Another sign of intrauterine hypotonia and limited fetal movements is arthrogryposis (i.e., contractures of multiple joints). Weak cry, poor suck, and poor respiratory effort may be noticed in some clinically "alert" infants. Spontaneous antigravity movements of limbs may be absent or decreased. Pectus excavatum with a "bell-shaped" chest is sometimes seen, reflecting long-standing weakness of the chest wall muscles. Muscle stretch reflexes may be normal, brisk, or hypoactive (e.g., absent or decreased). In a full-term newborn or older infant, passive movement of the infant's elbow across the midline produces a positive "scarf sign." Similarly, a positive heel-to-ear test is readily demonstrated by opposing the heel to the ear.

Tone can be evaluated further by performing the traction response, vertical suspension, and horizontal suspension maneuvers (7).

Traction Response

To elicit the traction response, the examiner grasps the infant's hands and wrists and slowly raises the infant from supine to sitting. In the normal infant, no significant head lag is expected and the head is maintained in the midline at least for a few seconds when the sitting position is reached. However, the hypotonic infant tends to have significant head lag when pulled up to sitting and does not maintain the head erect when sitting.

Vertical Suspension

The examiner places both hands beneath the infant's armpits and lifts the infant straight up. In a normal infant, the shoulder muscles press down against the examiner's hands and enable him/her to suspend vertically without falling. When the normal infant is in vertical suspension, the head is maintained in the midline and hips, knees, and ankles are in flexion. When this maneuver is performed in the hypotonic infant, the infant slips through the examiner's hands with both legs usually extended.

Horizontal Suspension

The examiner uses one hand to support the infant's trunk in a prone position and observes the resulting posture. A normal infant flexes or fully extends the limbs, straightens the back, and maintains the head in the midline for at least a few seconds. The hypotonic infant's head and limbs hang loosely and the trunk "drapes over" the examiner's hand.

Some clinicians use signs borrowed from the premature infant examination (described above), such as "scarf sign" (i.e., approximation of elbow to opposite shoulder) or "heel to ear or chin," to quantitate muscle tone. We do not use these routinely in the assessment of tone but have found them useful in the diagnosis of congenital laxity of ligaments.

DIFFERENTIAL ANATOMIC DIAGNOSIS OF HYPOTONIA

Hypotonia may be the manifestation of pathology involving the central nervous system (CNS), the peripheral nervous system (i.e., lower motor unit), or both (Table 10-2). In infants with *cerebral or central hypotonia*, who constitute about two-thirds of the cases, the perinatal or prenatal history may be consistent with a CNS insult; there is usually global (rather than an isolated gross-motor) developmental delay, sometimes seizures, microcephaly, dysmorphic features, and malformation of the brain and/or other organs. Infantile reflexes may be brisk and/or persistent and muscle stretch reflexes are normal or brisk. Movement can be triggered via postural reflexes (e.g., Moro or asymmetric tonic neck response) and the degree of weakness noted in the infant is usually less than the degree of hypotonia ("*non-paralytic*" hypotonia) (Table 10-3). In *lower motor unit hypotonia or peripheral*

Table 10-2   **Hypotonia: Differential Anatomic Diagnosis**
Brain
Spinal cord
Anterior horn cell
Peripheral nerve
Neuromuscular junction
Muscle

Table 10-3 Cerebral (Central) versus Lower Motor Unit (Peripheral) Hypotonia

	Cerebral (central)	Lower motor unit (peripheral)
History	Consistent with CNS insult; seizures	
Developmental delay	Global developmental delay	No global delay, delayed gross motor development
General physical examination	Microcephaly, dysmorphic features	Muscle atrophy, fasciculations, joint contractures
Other organ involvement	Malformation of other organs	No abnormalities of other organs besides musculoskeletal
Weakness	Weakness less than degree of hypotonia (*nonparalytic hypotonia*)	Weakness in proportion/excess to degree of hypotonia (*paralytic hypotonia*)
Postural reflexes	Movement through postural reflexes (e.g., tonic neck response)	Failure of movement on postural reflexes
Muscle stretch reflexes	Normal or brisk, clonus, Babinski sign	Absent or depressed
Other	Brisk and/or persistent infantile reflexes (e.g., Moro, palmar grasp)	Decreased antigravity limb movements

hypotonia, the developmental delay is primarily gross-motor and is associated with absent or depressed muscle stretch reflexes and, in some cases, with muscle atrophy and fasciculations of the tongue. In general, antigravity limb movements are decreased and movements cannot be elicited via postural reflexes; notably, the weakness is proportional or in excess to the degree of hypotonia ("*paralytic*" hypotonia) (Table 10-3). Trauma to the high cervical cord due to traction in breech or cervical presentation may initially manifest itself as flaccid paralysis, which may be asymmetric, and absent muscle stretch reflexes; later on, however, upper motor neuron signs develop.

Because muscle tone is also determined by the viscoelastic properties of muscle and joints, connective tissue disorders such as *Marfan, Ehlers–Danlos* syndromes or osteogenesis imperfecta and also benign laxity of the ligaments can present with hypotonia. In addition, there is *combined cerebral and lower motor unit hypotonia* seen in infants and older children with congenital myotonic dystrophy, some of the congenital muscular dystrophies, peroxisomal disorders, mitochondrial encephalo-myopathies, neuroaxonal dystrophy, leukodystrophies (e.g., globoid cell leuko-dystrophy), familial dysautonomia, and asphyxia secondary to motor unit disease (Table 10-4). Further, hypotonia without significant weakness may be a feature of systemic diseases like sepsis, congenital heart disease, hypothyroidism, rickets, renal tubular acidosis, and others.

Neuromuscular diseases in infancy present primarily with *hypotonia* and *weakness*; however, infants with severe hypotonia but only marginal weakness usually do not have a disorder of the lower motor unit (anterior horn cell, periph-eral and cranial nerves, neuromuscular junction, and muscle). These infants may

Table 10-4 Combined Cerebral and Motor Unit Hypotonia

Congenital myotonic dystrophy
Congenital muscular dystrophies
Peroxisomal disorders
Lipid storage diseases
Mitochondrial encephalomyopathies
Neuroaxonal dystrophy
Familial dysautonomia
Asphyxia secondary to motor unit disease

have genetic conditions, metabolic disturbances, or systemic disorders (e.g., congenital heart disease, renal failure). Early on, neonates with central nervous system pathology may present with profound hypotonia, decreased reflexes, and moderate to severe but transient weakness; however, they also tend to have seizures, obtundation, cranial nerve signs, and/or history of perinatal asphyxia. With recovery, they gradually develop better strength, increased muscle stretch reflexes, and muscle tone distally first, in contrast to the asphyxiated infants with disorders of the lower motor unit, in whom the weakness, hypotonia, and hyporeflexia persist. Alternatively, profound weakness and hypotonia without signs of CNS involvement occur in newborn infants with isolated neuromuscular disease and no history of perinatal asphyxia. Muscle stretch reflexes vary depending on the anatomical level of pathology along the motor unit (i.e., prominent hyporeflexia or total areflexia in anterior horn cell disorders and neuropathies, reduced reflexes in proportion to the degree of weakness in myopathies, and almost normal reflexes in neuromuscular junction defects). Again, approximately two-thirds of patients with neonatal hypotonia have cerebral etiologies and one-third have lower motor unit diseases (8).

COMMON NEUROMUSCULAR DISORDERS PRESENTING PRINCIPALLY WITH HYPOTONIA

Next in this chapter, the most frequent genetic and acquired disorders of the lower motor unit (Table 10-5) will be reviewed. Most of these conditions present with hypotonia.

Anterior Horn Cell/Peripheral Nerve Disorders

Spinal Muscular Atrophies

Three clinical variants have been described based on the rate of progression and age at onset of the disease: (i) acute spinal muscular atrophy (SMA), or SMA Type I, or Werdnig–Hoffmann disease; (ii) intermediate SMA, or SMA Type II; and

Table 10-5	**Neuromuscular Diseases in the Hypotonic Infant and Child**	
Anterior horn cell/ peripheral nerve	**Neuromuscular junction**	**Muscle**
Spinal muscular atrophies	Transient neonatal MG	Congenital muscular
Hypoxic-ischemic myelopathy	Congenital myasthenic	dystrophies
Traumatic myelopathy	syndromes	Congenital myotonic
Neurogenic arthrogryposis	Hypermagnesemia	dystrophy
Congenital neuropathies	Aminoglycoside toxicity	Infantile FSHD
Axonal	Infantile botulism	Congenital myopathies
Hypomyelinating		Metabolic myopathies
Dejerine–Sottas		Mitochondrial
HSAN		myopathies
Giant axonal neuropathy		
Metabolic		
Inflammatory		

FSHD, facioscapulohumeral muscular dystrophy; HSAN, hereditary sensory and autonomic neuropathy; MG, myasthenia gravis.

(iii) chronic SMA, or SMA Type III, or Kugelberg–Welander disease (9, 10). Here, we will discuss primarily SMA Type I, which may be seen clinically during infancy.

SMA Type I, Werdnig–Hoffmann Disease

The main signs of *generalized hypotonia* and *weakness* may be noted shortly after birth, and in 95% of the cases before the age of 4 months. *Prenatal* onset has been described and it is experienced by the mother as weakening of fetal movements during the last trimester of the pregnancy. At birth or in the first 6 months of life, weak sucking, difficulty with swallowing, labored breathing, extreme hypotonia, severe weakness, and hyperabduction of the hips ("*frog legs*") become apparent. *Arthrogryposis* multiplex congenita is uncommon in SMA Type I but, nonetheless, has been observed rarely. Type I SMA patients never sit unsupported (9, 11). Examination shows hypotonia, areflexia, and weakness affecting typically the lower extremities earlier and more severely than the upper extremities and the proximal muscles more than the distal ones. The anterior/posterior diameter of the thorax is decreased and there may be pectus excavatum with paradoxical respirations. As the disease advances, there is paralysis of the bulbar muscles, loss of the cough reflex and an inaudible cry. Wasting and fasciculations of the tongue may be observed during wakefulness and sleep but they can be easily confused with simple tongue tremors. Death usually occurs in the first year or less often in the second year of life, most commonly related to aspiration pneumonia. An unusual variety of SMA Type I related to diaphragmatic paralysis (spinal muscular atrophy with respiratory distress Type I, SMARD1) has been described, presenting primarily with respiratory distress in the first 2 months of life before any skeletal muscle involvement. In classic SMA Type I, the respiratory insufficiency is due to intercostal rather than diaphragmatic paralysis (12).

The electromyogram (EMG) may reveal excessive spontaneous activity during the first 3 months of life consisting of multiple discharges at a frequency 5 to 15 Hz in relaxed muscles, which persist during sleep. Fibrillation potentials may also appear later on. Motor unit potentials are increased in duration; many are polyphasic and poorly recruited by voluntary activation. *Muscle biopsy* examination demonstrates small- and large-group atrophy, with intermixed groups of hypertrophic fibers. The *hypertrophic* fibers are histochemically Type I fibers while the atrophic fibers are *Type I* and *Type II* (9). Postmortem histologic examination of the spinal cord shows loss of anterior horn cells. Creatine phosphokinase (CPK) can be mildly to moderate elevated, usually up to 5 times the upper limit of normal. Nowadays, EMG and muscle biopsy are used only rarely in the diagnosis of SMA.

In 1990, all three types of autosomal recessive SMAs were mapped to a single locus on chromosome 5q11.2-13.3 (13); subsequently, in 1995, two groups reported the preferential deletion of two genes, the survival motor neuron (SMN) (14, 15) and the neuronal apoptosis inhibitory protein gene (NAIP) (16) in SMA patients. Homozygous deletions of the telomeric copy of the SMN gene (SMN1) can be detected in 90 to 95% of patients with SMA, regardless of severity (Types I, II, and III) (14). Most of the remaining patients have deletion of SMN1 in one allele and a point mutation in the other; a very small fraction of the deletion-negative patients have rare nonchromosome 5 types of SMA. A commercially available assay for the homozygous loss of telomeric exons 7 and/or 8 of the SMN gene thus provides a highly correlated marker for the prenatal and postnatal diagnosis of SMA Type I. NAIP deletions are seen in over 45% of SMA Type I and less than 20% of Type II and Type III SMA patients (16). Despite the occurrence of NAIP deletions, NAIP has not been proven to be important in the pathogenesis of SMA.

SMA Type II, SMA Type III

Most patients with SMA Type II and III are normal at birth. In a series of 19 infants who were later classified as SMA Type II, all of them were found to be normal at birth (17). The onset of the disease, however, is before the age of 18 months (18). Patients can sit unsupported but never stand. Survival to ages 5 and 25 years is 98.5 and 68.5%, respectively. Many patients with SMA Type III achieve normal gross motor milestones early on and often into later childhood. The onset of symptoms is usually after the age of 18 months and patients can stand alone; lifespan is almost normal. The SMA phenotype is determined, at least in part, by the number of copies of the centromeric copy of the SMN gene, known as SMN2; patients with milder phenotypes tend to have more copies of SMN2. Most SMA1 patients have 1–2 copies of SMN2 (80%), most SMA Type II patients have 2–3 copies (82% have 3 copies), and the vast majority (96%) of SMA Type III patients have 3–4 copies of SMN2 (19).

Congenital Neuropathies

Congenital Hypomyelinating and Axonal Neuropathies

Fourteen infants with neuropathy were reviewed by Sladky (20). He described nine infants with demyelinating neuropathy, including four with hypomyelination, three with steroid-responsive chronic inflammatory demyelinating polyneuropathy (CIDP), and two with a leukodystrophy. Four of five axonal neuropathies in the same sibship were X-linked and one was a sporadic case. Neonates with congenital neuropathies usually present with severe hypotonia, weakness, and hyporeflexia or areflexia closely resembling SMA Type I. However, cerebrospinal fluid protein is elevated in most infants with congenital neuropathies, not a finding in SMA Type I. EMG and *nerve conduction* studies (NCS) are important for confirming the diagnosis and distinguishing between neuropathies and SMA Type I but also between the demyelinating and axonal types. Nevertheless, electrophysiologic studies may be unable to differentiate between inherited noninflammatory and acquired inflammatory neuropathies. Sural nerve biopsy may be helpful in establishing the diagnosis but again it may not exclude CIDP. A number of infants with congenital neuropathies have the early onset of hereditary motor and sensory neuropathy (HMSN) known also as Dejerine–Sottas disease, a metabolic disease such as mitochondrial cytopathy, or a leukodystrophy, hereditary sensory, and autonomic neuropathy (e.g., Riley–Day syndrome), or giant axonal neuropathy.

Disturbances of Neuromuscular Transmission

Transient Neonatal Myasthenia Gravis

This syndrome results from the transplacental transfer of circulating antiacetylcholine receptor antibodies from a myasthenic mother. It develops in about 10 to 20% of infants born to myasthenic mothers. The syndrome usually presents within hours of birth but may be delayed for up to 3 days; the main features are feeding difficulties (87%), generalized weakness (69%), respiratory difficulties (65%), weak cry (60%), facial diplegia (54%), ptosis (50%), and sometimes external ophthalmoplegia. Respiratory failure is uncommon but it may occur. The presence of arthrogryposis, pulmonary hypoplasia, polyhydramnios, weak fetal movements, or stillbirth signify onset in utero. The severity of the disease in infants correlates poorly with clinical severity in mothers and with maternal antibody titer; however, falling antibody titers correlate with clinical improvement. Infants with transient neonatal myasthenia gravis (TNMG) are born to mothers with a relatively high ratio of antibodies directed against the fetal acetylcholine receptor (AChR) versus the adult AChR.

Rarely, TNMG may occur in infants born to seronegative mothers. The mean duration of symptoms is 18 days, with a range of 5 days to 3 months. The diagnosis is confirmed by demonstrating high serum concentration of acetylcholine receptor antibody in newborn infants and also by the reversal of the symptoms with edrophonium chloride (Tensilon), given either as an intramuscular or subcutaneous injection of 0.04 to 0.15 mg/kg or 0.1 mg/kg body weight intravenously delivered in fractional amounts over a number of minutes after a test dose of 0.01 mg/kg. Clinical improvement becomes apparent in a few minutes after the intravenous administration of edrophonium chloride and may last for 10 to 15 minutes. Given the possibility of cardiac bradyarrhythmias subsequent to the intravenous use of edrophonium chloride, however, the intramuscular and subcutaneous routes are preferable in newborn infants. In severely compromised neonates, an exchange transfusion should be attempted. For infants with only feeding and swallowing problems, a longer-lasting effect (1 to 3 hours) may be achieved by the intramuscular or subcutaneous injection of about 0.05 mg/kg per dose neostigmine methyl sulfate 15 to 30 minutes before each feeding; it may, however, induce increased tracheal secretions. The same medication can also be administered through a nasogastric tube at 10 times the parenteral dose (0.5 mg/kg/dose) 45 to 60 minutes prior to feeding.

Acquired Autoimmune Myasthenia Gravis

Only minor differences exist between acquired autoimmune myasthenia gravis in children and adults, but the onset of symptoms is always after age 6 months and in most cases after 2 years.

Congenital Myasthenic Syndromes

Congenital myasthenic syndromes can be classified according to the site of the defect; that is, presynaptic, postsynaptic, synaptic, and mixed (21). These are defects of neuromuscular transmission, and the classification and main features of the most common

Table 10-6	Congenital Myasthenic Syndromes			
Defect	**Inheritance**	**Clinical features**	**Tensilon test**	**Treatment**
Presynaptic				
Familial infantile myasthenia with episodic apnea (ChAT mutations)	AR	Hypotonia Ptosis, apnea, no ophthalmoparesis Generalized weakness	+	AChE inhibitors
Postsynaptic or synaptic				
Congenital end-plate AChE deficiency	AR	Asymmetric ptosis Ophthalmoparesis Distal weakness Delayed pupillary constriction to light	−	No response to AChE inhibitors
Classic slow channel syndrome	AD	Ophthalmoparesis Fluctuating ptosis Head and wrist extensor weakness	−	No response to AChE inhibitors
Congenital AChR deficiency (rapsyn or ε-subunit mutations)	AR	Hypotonia, ptosis Ophthalmoplegia (ε-subunit) Strabismus (rapsyn) Respiratory failure (rapsyn) Feeding difficulties Arthrogryposis (rapsyn)	+	AChE inhibitors

AR, autosomal recessive; AChE, acetylcholinesterase; AChR, acetylcholine receptor; AD, autosomal dominant; ChAT, choline acetyltransferase.

forms are shown in Table 10-6. Congenital myasthenic syndromes usually present in infancy with generalized hypotonia and fluctuating weakness, weak cry and suck, respiratory distress, apnea, and feeding difficulties. Fluctuating ptosis, ophthalmoparesis, and abnormal fatigability on exertion may be present during infancy and childhood. Later on, delayed motor milestones may be noted and in some cases symptoms progress during adolescence and adulthood. Testing for antiacetylcholine receptor antibodies is negative. The diagnosis is based on clinical history and examination, family history (if present), EMG findings, Tensilon test, and the clinical response to acetylcholinesterase inhibitors. In most cases, however, detailed EMG studies, in vitro microphysiologic, ultrastructural, and histochemical studies of intercostal muscle biopsies are required to establish the diagnosis. Edrophonium chloride testing is positive in most types of congenital myasthenic syndromes, except in the classic slow channel syndrome and in congenital end-plate acetylcholinesterase deficiency (see Table 10-6). If clinical response to edrophonium chloride occurs, long-term treatment with neostigmine or pyridostigmine is needed.

Infantile Botulism

Patients developing botulism in infancy are normal at birth but between the age of 10 days to 12 months (median age at presentation is 10 weeks) develop acutely severe weakness, dysphagia, constipation, weak cry, severe hypotonia, and respiratory insufficiency (22). On examination, there is diffuse hypotonia and weakness, ptosis, ophthalmoplegia with pupillary involvement (mydriasis) in some cases, reduced gag reflex, and usually preservation of muscle stretch reflexes (23). Affected infants tend to deteriorate if given aminoglycosides or other neuromuscular blocking agents. On EMG examination, the compound motor unit potential amplitude is low at rest; repetitive stimulation at 2 to 5 Hz typically produces decrement, but with 20 to 50 Hz stimulation, facilitation of 125 to 3000% is seen in almost all cases. To demonstrate the increment, however, a prolonged period of stimulation (10 to 20 seconds) may be required (24). During infancy the pathogenesis of botulism is different. The *C. botulinum* is ingested, colonizes the intestinal tract, and produces toxin in situ, as opposed to older children and adults in whom the disease is related to ingestion of food contaminated by preformed exotoxin (25). The diagnosis in infants is confirmed by isolation of the organism in stool. Infantile botulism is a self-limited disease; the period of profound, severe hypotonia can last from 2 to 6 weeks, so the infant should be observed in the intensive care unit and be supported, if respiratory failure occurs. Botulinum immune globulin (BIG) seems to be safe and reduces the duration of the disease, the cost of the hospitalization, and the severity of illness (26).

Magnesium Intoxication

Generalized weakness, hypotonia, and mental status changes may be seen in infants born to mothers treated with high doses of magnesium sulfate for eclampsia. Since this is a self-limited condition, specialized testing (e.g., EMG/NCS) is not necessary.

Muscle Disorders

The muscle disorders reviewed in this chapter usually present with hypotonia and weakness during infancy; however, a later onset may occur. They are listed in Table 10-7.

Congenital Muscular Dystrophies

In congenital muscular dystrophies (CMDs) the muscle biopsy is abnormal (it shows features often seen in the major muscular dystrophies of later onset); however, there are no unique identifying features.

Table 10-7   Muscle Disorders in the Hypotonic Infant

Classic CMD
Merosin-deficient CMD
  Primary merosin deficiency
  Secondary merosin deficiency
Merosin-positive CMD
  Classic CMD without distinguishing features
  Rigid spine syndrome
  CMD with distal hyperextensibility (Ullrich type)
  CMD with mental retardation or sensory abnormalities
CMDs with central nervous system abnormalities
Fukuyama muscular dystrophy
Muscle–eye–brain disease
Walker–Warburg syndrome
Congenital myotonic dystrophy
Infantile facioscapulohumeral muscular dystrophy
Congenital myopathies
Nemaline myopathy
Central core disease
Centronuclear/myotubular myopathy
Congenital fiber type disproportion
Minicore disease
Other congenital myopathies
Metabolic myopathies
Acid maltase deficiency
Mitochondrial myopathies
  Cytochrome c oxidase deficiency
  Fatty acid oxidation defects
Nonlysosomal glycogenoses

CMD, congenital muscular dystrophy.

CMDs can be classified into two major groups, depending on the association with structural brain abnormalities on neuroimaging studies or autopsy examination (27). The CMDs without structural CNS anomalies, also known as "classic or occidental" CMD, form a heterogeneous group of disorders. In the second group, i.e., those with associated structural CNS abnormalities, concomitant eye involvement and clinical evidence of significant neurologic dysfunction may be evident. The latter group includes the *Fukuyama* muscular dystrophy (FMD), *Walker–Warburg* syndrome (WWS), and *muscle–eye–brain* disease (MEBD) (Tables 10-7 and 10-8).

CONGENITAL MUSCULAR DYSTROPHIES WITHOUT STRUCTURAL CNS ANOMALIES

The CMDs without structural CNS anomalies can be subclassified now on the basis of merosin (laminin α2-chain gene mutation) staining results of their muscle biopsies into merosin-deficient and merosin-positive CMDs (Tables 10-7 and 10-8). Both subgroups can present in early infancy with hypotonia, weakness, elevated serum CPK, and joint contractures. Major feeding and respiratory difficulties are not common. The diagnosis in this group of CMDs rests on head magnetic resonance imaging (MRI), EMG/NCS, CPK testing, and muscle biopsy histology, histochemistry, and merosin immunostaining.

Merosin-deficient Classic Congenital Muscular Dystrophy. All merosin-deficient patients studied with cranial MRI have abnormalities of the white matter on T2-weighted images that were not seen in the merosin-positive group (27). Given the expression of merosin in peripheral nerve and brain, slowing of motor nerve conduction velocities (28) as well as delayed somatosensory evoked potentials have been found. Of interest, both the peripheral nervous system and CNS involvement become more pronounced with age and may be only minimal early in the course of the disease. The *merosin-negative subgroup* is quite unique because of the associated hypomyelination of brain white matter detected by head MRI, the involvement of peripheral nerves (28), and the somewhat severe clinical involvement (29, 30). Despite the white matter changes, most of these patients do not exhibit major neurologic deficits on standard evaluation; nonetheless, patients with seizures have been described. *In general*, the merosin-deficient subgroup comprises a more severe neuromuscular phenotype with relatively high serum CPKs (31); most patients are unable to stand or walk, in contrast to the merosin-positive patients, most of whom will walk independently (32). The phenotype of merosin-deficient CMD seems to be broadening, however. On the one hand, there are patients with mild phenotype who function well into adulthood, whereas, on the other hand, a few patients have been identified with merosin-deficient CMD, who also had evidence of focal cortical dysgenesis (10% occipital agyria) or cerebellar hypoplasia (20%) on brain imaging. An *intermediate phenotype*, with incomplete deficiency and later onset in achievement of ambulation, has also been described. Further, two siblings from a consanguineous family with an internally deleted laminin α2-chain gene, as a result of a splice site mutation in the LAMA2 gene, were reported recently; interestingly, these patients appear mildly affected compared to others who completely lack this protein (33).

Merosin-positive Classic Congenital Muscular Dystrophy. This group of patients with classic CMD, who are merosin positive, may well be quite heterogeneous genetically. As alluded to earlier in the comparative studies with the merosin-deficient patients, it has become apparent that the prognosis for ambulation for the most part appears to be much better in the merosin-positive patients (31, 34–36). However, delayed deterioration has been described in a large study from Japan (37). This would indicate that the underlying dystrophic process is progressive, albeit so slowly that initial motor development outpaces this deterioration.

CONGENITAL MUSCULAR DYSTROPHIES WITH STRUCTURAL CNS ANOMALIES

Fukuyama Muscular Dystrophy. Of the CMDs with structural CNS anomalies, FMD is a major representative (38). Described in 1960, FMD is the second most prevalent form of muscular dystrophy in Japan with a Duchenne muscular dystrophy (DMD)/FMD prevalence ratio of 2.1/1. FMD has been described in non-Japanese Americans and Europeans but, overall, is rare outside Japan. The FMD gene locus has been mapped to chromosome 9q31-33 (39, 40); it appears to be inherited as an autosomal recessive trait; the defective gene has been isolated and the respective protein product has been named fukutin (37).

FMD presents with generalized weakness and hypotonia at birth, joint contractures, and depressed muscle stretch reflexes. Other clinical features include microcephaly and delayed psychomotor development. Convulsions occur in 50% of cases. CPK is usually significantly elevated (10–50 times the upper limit of normal). Muscle biopsy shows myopathic changes consisting of endomysial and perimysial fibrosis, rounded muscle fibers with involvement of both Type I and II fibers, and increased number of Type IIC fibers. Head MRI and autopsy studies usually show diffuse cerebral pachygyria, cerebral and cerebellar polymicrogyria, hydrocephalus ex vacuo, subpial gliosis, and heterotopias. Polymicrogyria is found consistently in the cerebellum. Death usually occurs by 10 years of age.

Walker–Warburg Syndrome. WWS also seems to be inherited as an autosomal recessive trait; although a case of WWS has been described in a family with FMD, linkage to the FMD locus on 9q31-33 has been excluded in at least a number of families. The major features are a severe neonatal phenotype with weakness, hypotonia, hydrocephalus, macrocephaly, and eye abnormalities (41). The muscle biopsy findings are indistinguishable from other disorders in this group; there are major myopathic changes, albeit nonspecific. Deficient laminin α2-chain and α-dystroglycan staining has been described (42).

The neuropathologic features detected by head MRI and autopsy examination vary little from case to case and include hydrocephalus (communicating or ex vacuo), Type II (cobblestone) lissencephaly (43) with or without polymicrogyria, cerebellar hypoplasia, *Dandy–Walker* malformation, small optic nerves and olfactory tracts, absent corpus callosum, colpocephaly, encephalocele(s), and heterotopias. The cortex is composed of two layers separated by an irregular plain layer containing glial fibers and axons. All cerebellar cortical layers can be seen, however. The pathologic changes affecting the eye include optic nerve hypoplasia, retinal detachment and dysplasia, microphthalmia, anterior segment abnormalities, cataract formation, corneal opacities, and shallow anterior chamber. Most WWS patients die in early infancy. A fraction of patients (20%) with WWS have mutations in the gene coding for POMT1 (mannosyltransferase) on chromosome 9q34.1 (Table 10-8) but also in fukutin, fukutin-related protein, and POMT2 genes (42, 44–46).

MEBD (Santavuori Congenital Muscular Dystrophy). The clinical features of this disorder have been described in a number of Finnish families (47), some with a history of consanguinity, suggesting autosomal recessive inheritance. Again, the 9q31-q33 locus of FMD has been excluded in a number of Finnish pedigrees, and although the muscle, eye, and brain findings resemble WWS, the phenotype is much milder. Affected patients can usually sit, stand, and walk but the

Table 10-8   Genetic Loci for Congenital Muscular Dystrophy Identified to Date

Disease	Mode of inheritance	Gene location	Symbol (gene product)
Classic CMD			
Primary merosin deficiency (MDC1A)	AR	6q22-q23	*LAMA2* (laminin α2 chain of merosin)
Secondary merosin deficiency (MDC1B)	AR	1q42	?
Secondary merosin deficiency (MDC1C)	AR	19q13.3	*FKRP* (fukutin-related protein)
Rigid spine syndrome (RSMD)	AR	1p35-p36	*RSMD1* (selenoprotein N)
Ullrich muscular dystrophy (UCMD)	AR	21q22.3	*COL6A1* (collagen VI α1 chain)
	AR	21q22.3	*COL6A2* (collagen VI α2 chain)
	AR	2q37	*COL6A3* (collagen VI α3 chain)
Integrin α7 deficiency	AR	12q13	Integrin α7
CMD with CNS abnormalities			
Fukuyama CMD	AR	9q31-33	*FCMD* (fukutin)
Muscle–eye–brain disease	AR	1p32-p34	*POMGnT1* (glycosyltransferase)
Walker–Warburg syndrome	AR	9q34.1	*POMT1* (mannosyltransferase)
		9q31-33	*FCMD* (fukutin)
		19q13.3	*FKRP* (fukutin-related protein)
		14q24.3	*POMT2* (mannosyltransferase)
LARGE-related CMD (MDC1D)	AR	22q12.3	LARGE (putative glycosyltransferase)

AR, autosomal recessive; CMD, congenital muscular dystrophy; CNS, central nervous system; ?, undetermined. Modified from Jones K, North K. Congenital muscular dystrophies. In Jones HR Jr, De Vivo DC, Darras BT (eds). Neuromuscular Disorders of Infancy, Childhood, and Adolescence: A Clinician's Approach. Philadelphia, PA: Butterworth Heinemann, 2003, pp. 633–47.

subsequent development of spasticity (usually by age 5 years) leads to loss of gross-motor skills. There is *hypotonia* early in life, slow gross-motor development, hydrocephalus, seizures probably related to cortical dysplasia (pachygyria and poly-microgyria) (48), and, of course, eye involvement with optic atrophy, retinal dysplasia, high myopia, progressive failure of vision, and abnormal electroretino-gram (ERG) and visual evoked potentials (VEPs). In the Santavuori variety of CMD, eye involvement is usually not obvious in the newborn period. In fact, the ERG may remain normal until 7 years of age. VEPs become delayed and increased in amplitude. Patients survive beyond age 3 years; death usually occurs between 6 and 16 years. Haltia et al. (48) reported weak immunostaining for merosin with normal laminin β2-chain staining in muscle from patients with MEBD. α-Dystroglycan immunostaining is reduced in MEBD. The gene mutated in MEBD is a glycosyltransferase (POMGnT1) gene and has been mapped at 1p32-p34 (49). Fukutin, POMT1, and POMGnT1 are putative glucotransferases involved in the glycosylation of α-dystroglycan (Table 10-8).

Congenital Myotonic Dystrophy

Myotonic dystrophy, a multisystem disease originally described by Steinert in 1909, is the most prevalent form of muscular dystrophy. The congenital form of the disease occurs in 15 to 25% of infants born to affected mothers. The pregnancy is usually complicated by poor fetal movements and polyhydramnios. Clinical features include hypotonia at birth, respiratory distress, club feet, poor suck and swallow, and myopathic facies. The weakness of facial and jaw muscles produces a "*tented upper lip.*" At birth, respiratory distress is a common occurrence, but myotonia is not present during the neonatal period. In fact, myotonia may not be present until the age of 5 to 8 years. As the child gets older, mental retardation becomes apparent in most cases. Congenital myotonic dystrophy is always transmitted through an affected mother, who may be asymptomatic or only mildly symptomatic.

In *congenital myotonic dystrophy*, the CPK is usually normal. While the infant's EMG may fail to show myotonia, the maternal EMG is always abnormal. Muscle biopsy shows nonspecific abnormalities consisting of increased variability in fiber size with Type I fiber atrophy in some cases. The *genetic defect* in myotonic dystrophy has been identified as an expansion of a trinucleotide CTG repeat located in the 3' untranslated region of a gene, which codes for a serine-threonine protein kinase, also known as myotonin protein kinase (50, 51). In normal individuals the CTG repeat contains between 4 and 49 copies of the CTG repeat; normal individuals with 38–49 copies of the repeat are classified in a borderline category (premutation) because of the small possibility of expansion of the CTG repeat in their offspring (52). Mildly affected individuals or asymptomatic mutation "*carriers*" have 50 to 80 CTG repeats, whereas affected subjects have between 100 to 2000 or more copies (*full mutation*). Infants with congenital myotonic dystrophy usually have more than 750 copies. The CTG copy number increases during successive generations, which explains the phenomenon of genetic anticipation (increasing severity of the disease phenotype and/or earlier onset in successive generations) in myotonic dystrophy families (53). Although for a given number of repeats (above 100) a wide range in disease severity may be observed, infants with severe congenital myotonic dystrophy and their mothers tend to have a greater number of CTG repeats. The greater the CTG repeat expansion in the mother, the higher the probability of myotonic dystrophy offspring being affected with the congenital form of the illness. Unfortunately, these findings do not explain the exclusive maternal inheritance in cases of congenital myotonic dystrophy. Genomic imprinting or the presence of a maternal intrauterine factor have been proposed as possible mechanisms.

If *myotonic dystrophy* is suspected in a hypotonic neonate, the mother should be examined, even if she is asymptomatic, looking for evidence of myotonia or weakness of distal muscles and also neck flexors. Currently, the most sensitive way to confirm the diagnosis in an infant is blood testing for the CTG repeat expansion utilizing PCR and/or Southern blot (54). If the diagnosis of myotonic dystrophy cannot be established in the mother on the basis of clinical presentation and physical examination, EMG sampling of multiple muscles may be necessary to identify myotonia.

Infantile Facioscapulohumeral Muscular Dystrophy

Facioscapulohumeral dystrophy (FSHD) is an autosomal dominant dystrophy with a distinct phenotype (55, 56). The precise genetic defect in this major form of FSHD has yet to be identified. However, the diagnosis in FSHD can be suspected and/or easily made clinically in most patients with this disorder. Typically, these children have prominent facial as well as scapulohumeral muscle weakness; parenthetically, striking asymmetry of muscle involvement is a typical feature of FSHD.

The infantile variety of FSHD, which is often sporadic in inheritance, has a very early onset (usually within the first few years of life) and is rapidly progressive, with wheelchair confinement by the age of 9 to 10 years in most cases (56). There is profound facial weakness, with an inability to close the eyes in sleep, to smile, and to show any evidence of facial expression. The weakness rapidly involves the shoulder and hip girdles with lumbar lordosis, resulting in pronounced forward pelvic tilt, and hyperextension of the knees and the head upon walking. Marked weakness of the wrist extensors may result in a wrist drop. Young children with early onset FSHD and a very small number of chromosome 4q35 repeats often have epilepsy, mental retardation, and severe sensorineural hearing loss (57).

A commercial DNA test is now available for FSH muscular dystrophy (58); most patients with classic FSHD for whom detailed molecular studies have been done carry a chromosomal rearrangement within the subtelomere of chromosome 4q (4q35) (59). A tandem array of 3.3 kb repeated DNA elements (D4Z4) is deleted in patients with FSHD (60). In the general population, the number of repeat units varies from 11 to more than 100; in FSHD patients, an allele of 1–10 residual units is observed because of the deletion of an integral number of these units (61). Most infants with FSHD have only 1–3 copies of the repeat unit. This new diagnostic test is positive in 93% of typical FSHD cases (62). Nonetheless, the exact gene defect is not known yet and thus the sensitivity of the genetic test for atypical cases remains uncertain (63). In typical cases, there is no value in performing a muscle biopsy.

Congenital Myopathies

Shy and Magee introduced the term *congenital myopathy* to describe central core disease and any myopathy present at birth excluding muscular dystrophy (64). Unfortunately, inclusion of conditions like nemaline and centronuclear myopathies, which may be progressive and in some cases lethal, blurred the clinical distinction from the muscular dystrophies. These conditions are, however, distinct at a pathological level. In congenital muscular dystrophies the muscle biopsy findings are dystrophic and nonspecific, whereas in congenital myopathies there are distinct myopathological features without significant fibrosis, muscle fiber degeneration, or replacement with adipose tissue. In congenital myopathies, the specificity of distinguishing pathological features has declined recently with the inclusion of conditions with similar but not identical histological features, such as multicore or minicore disease.

Hypotonia and weakness are the major clinical features. However, other characteristic features of congenital myopathy like scoliosis, ptosis, and ophthalmoplegia may not be apparent at birth. Therefore, despite the frequent history of infantile hypotonia, diagnosis may be delayed until gross-motor developmental delay and associated weakness develop in late infancy or early childhood. In the congenital myopathies, the EMG may be normal or myopathic with small polyphasic motor unit potentials, normal nerve conduction studies, normal repetitive nerve stimulation, and absence of abnormal spontaneous activity. The CPK level is usually normal or slightly elevated. This is a helpful distinction from congenital muscular dystrophies, in which CPK levels are usually moderately to markedly elevated. The diagnosis of congenital myopathies is heavily dependent on the muscle biopsy, which reveals the characteristic features for which the disorder has been named. Table 10-9 summarizes the genetics and main clinical features of congenital myopathies.

Nemaline Myopathy

The term *nemaline* has been used to characterize the presence of rods or thread-like structures (Greek *nema*, "thread") seen in the muscle biopsies of patients with this type of congenital myopathy (65). Of the three different types (neonatal, late infantile/early childhood, late childhood/adult) the neonatal type is the most severe, presenting with hypotonia, diminished spontaneous activity, history of poor fetal movements, and early respiratory distress (66). More commonly, presentation is delayed until after the newborn period when gross-motor delay with proximal weakness develops.

Serum CPK is usually normal or slightly elevated and the EMG may be normal, myopathic, neuropathic, or mixed. The diagnosis is made by the characteristic nemaline bodies on muscle biopsy. These bodies originate from the Z disks and tend to cluster under the sarcolemma. Frequently, Type I fiber predominance is present. Histochemically, α-actinin, myosin, and actin have been detected in nemaline bodies (67). In a large Australian family characterized by relatively late-onset and predominantly distal muscle involvement, close linkage to the 1q22-q23 region (68) was found with subsequent detection of mutations in tropomyosin-3 gene (69). In this family the inheritance was autosomal dominant. This form has been named NEM1. A second type of the autosomal recessive form of the disease (NEM2) has been linked to a locus on chromosome 2q21.2-q22, where the nebulin gene has been mapped; recently, mutations in this gene have been identified in patients with nemaline myopathy. In the autosomal dominant families there is a curious female predominance (70). To date, five genes have been involved in the pathogenesis of nemaline myopathy (α-tropomyosin$_{SLOW}$, nebulin, α-actin, β-tropomyosin, troponin I).

Central Core Disease

The vast majority of patients with central core disease (CCD) present with hypotonia in early infancy and childhood and a subsequent delay in motor milestones (71). Rarely, severe hypotonia and marked contractures are present at birth. More commonly, skeletal abnormalities are present, particularly congenital dislocation of the hips, flat feet, pes cavus, club feet, and kyphoscoliosis. The clinical course varies from nonprogressive to slowly progressive. An association between CCD and malignant hyperthermia has been observed (72). The diagnosis is based primarily on the histologic finding of central cores on muscle biopsy. The cores appear to be packed with myofiber material and depleted of organelles.

CCD is transmitted by autosomal dominant inheritance (73). Linkage analysis in four families with CCD has resulted in mapping of the locus to chromosome 19q12-13.2, and more specifically to the 19q13.1 (74) segment where the ryanodine

Table 10-9 Congenital Myopathies

Disease	Genes	Proteins	Onset	Weakness	Cardiac	Respiratory	Facial	Oculomotor	Prognosis
Centronuclear myopathy, X-linked (myotubular myopathy)	MTM1	Myotubularin	Prenatal–congenital	+++	−	++	+++	+++	Death during infancy, some survive to adulthood
Centronuclear myopathy, classic	?	?	Late infancy–early childhood	+	−	++	++	++	Ambulation until adolescence
Centronuclear myopathy, adult	DNM2	Dynamin 2	Infancy, 2nd–3rd decade	+	−	−	+	+/−	Slowly progressive
Nemaline myopathy, severe (neonatal)	ACTA1 NEM2 TPM3 TNNT1	α-Actin Nebulin α-Tropomyosin$_{SLOW}$ Troponin T type I	Birth	+++	−	++	+++	−	Death in neonatal period
Nemaline myopathy, typical (classic)	ACTA1 NEM2 TPM3 TPM2	α-Actin Nebulin α-Tropomyosin$_{SLOW}$ β-Tropomyosin	1st year	++	+/−	+	+++	−	Many survive to adulthood
Nemaline myopathy, childhood	ACTA1 NEM2 TPM3	α-Actin Nebulin α-Tropomyosin$_{SLOW}$	Prepubertal	+	−	−	−	−	Many survive to adulthood
Central core, classic	RYR1	Ryanodine receptor	Infancy	+	Rare	−	+	−	Adulthood?
Congenital fiber-type disproportion	ACTA1 SEPN1	α-Actin Selenoprotein	1st year	+ to +++	Rare	+ to +++ (30%)	+	+/−	Variable
Multi-minicore disease	SEPN1	Selenoprotein	Infancy–early childhood	++	Rare	++	++	Rare	Variable
Actin myopathy (non-nemaline)	ACTA1	α-Actin	Congenital	+++	+	+++	++	?	High mortality

+++, severe; ++, moderate; +, mild; +/−, mild or absent; −, not reported so far; ?, undetermined.
Courtesy of Dr. Peter Kang, Neuromuscular Program, Children's Hospital Boston.

receptor-1 gene is located. Mutations of ryanodine receptor-1 have been detected in families with susceptibility to malignant hyperthermia and patients with CCD (75). Therefore, it appears that at least some forms of CCD and malignant hyperthermia are allelic disorders of the same genetic defect. Therefore, the expression of CCD may be related to some additional as yet unidentified factor.

Centronuclear/Myotubular Myopathy

The mode of inheritance of the centronuclear/myotubular myopathy has been debated. Two major forms of inheritance have emerged, i.e., an X-linked form seen primarily in congenital, severely affected cases, and an autosomal dominant late-onset form. In some early-onset cases, the inheritance appears to be autosomal recessive. Early-onset cases are the most common form of centronuclear/myotubular myopathy and present with severe hypotonia, weakness, and respiratory distress. Affected infants are very weak and have major feeding difficulties, facial diplegia, bilateral ptosis, and limitation of eye movements (*external ophthalmoplegia*). Frequently, dysmorphic features are evident, such as pectus carinatum, micrognathia, simian creases, high-arched palate, and talipes equinovarus (76). Chest X-ray always shows slender ribs. Despite intensive respiratory support, infants rarely survive and improve their motor function. Survivors have a marfanoid appearance. Focal or generalized seizures, albeit uncommon, have been reported. The muscle biopsy shows central nuclei present in many muscle fibers and Type I fiber predominance (77). A radial pattern of staining is noted with oxidative enzyme stains. The gene defect in the X-linked recessive variety (*MTM1*) was mapped to Xq28 (78) and subsequently isolated. The protein product was designated myotubularin (79). The *myotubularin gene* is highly conserved in evolution (expressed in yeast) and is ubiquitously expressed in human tissue despite the fact that the disease shows muscle specificity. No specific treatment is available and most patients with the neonatal form require intensive respiratory support and gastric feeding. Although some improvement is usually noted with maturation, most neonates remain ventilator dependent. Dynamin 2 mutations have also been described in patients with centronuclear myopathy (80).

Congenital Fiber Type Disproportion

Congenital fiber type disproportion (CFTD) typically presents with hypotonia and weakness at birth or in the neonatal period (81). Contractures of the hands and feet and skeletal abnormalities are common. There is delay in acquisition of motor milestones (82). CPK is normal and EMG may be normal or myopathic. The muscle biopsy shows Type I fiber atrophy, which is a nonspecific finding, noted in other clinically diverse conditions. Therefore, the existence of the CFTD as an entity has been debated. A group of patients with hypotonia and Type I fiber predominance has been described in whom decrease in the size of Type I fibers is not observed. Type I fiber predominance is another nonspecific feature of many myopathies. Despite the debate over the specificity of CFTD, it is not unusual to find Type I fiber atrophy and Type I fiber predominance in muscle biopsies of hypotonic infants. Although these findings do not reliably predict an improving course, many of these infants will have a good outcome and, as such, deserve supportive measures. α-Actin and selenoprotein N (SEPN1) mutations have been described in patients with CFTD (83, 84).

Minicore Myopathy

Minicore myopathy (multi-minicore disease (MmD)) is a recessive congenital myopathy characterized by multiple areas of loss of oxidative activity on muscle biopsy. Its onset is usually at birth or during infancy and sometimes in childhood. It presents with predominantly axial and proximal weakness, hypotonia, and arthrogryposis. Two-thirds of affected children develop scoliosis and respiratory difficulties. The presence of minicores has been linked to four clinical phenotypes: (i) classic phenotype with significant axial weakness, early respiratory impairment, and severe scoliosis; (ii) predominantly hip girdle weakness sometimes associated with arthrogryposis at birth; (iii) classic phenotype with associated external ophthalmoplegia; and (iv) marked distal atrophy and weakness affecting primarily the upper extremities.

Patients with the classic axial presentation of MmD have recessive mutations in the selenoprotein N (SEPN1) gene also causing congenital muscular dystrophy with rigidity of the spine (RSMD1). MmD with predominant hip girdle weakness and the one with distal atrophy and weakness have been linked to mutations in the skeletal muscle ryanodine receptor (RYR1) gene. Recently, RYR1 gene recessive mutations were also identified in the subset of patients with MmD and external ophthalmoplegia (85).

Other Congenital Myopathies

In addition to the four most common congenital myopathies described above, there are uncommon types of congenital myopathies characterized by hypotonia, weakness, delay in motor milestones, and a less well-defined pattern of inheritance. Their names reflect their myopathological features and include: (i) actin myopathy (non-nemaline), (ii) fingerprint body myopathy, (iii) sarcotubular myopathy, (iv) hyaline body myopathy, (v) reducing body myopathy, (vi) cytoplasmic body myopathy, (vii) myopathy with myotubular aggregates, (viii) zebra body myopathy, and (ix) trilaminar myopathy. In all of these conditions, the diagnosis is made by muscle biopsy, which underscores the significance of this procedure in the evaluation of newborns with weakness and hypotonia unrelated to CNS dysfunction or systemic disease.

Metabolic Myopathies

Acid Maltase Deficiency (Glycogen Storage Disease II)

Acid maltase is a lysosomal α-1,4-glucosidase which releases glucose from glycogen, oligosaccharides, and maltose. Acid maltase deficiency (AMD) is separated into three major groups: infantile, childhood, and adult AMD. All types are transmitted by autosomal recessive inheritance.

Infantile Acid Maltase Deficiency (Pompe Disease)

Infantile AMD may present in the newborn period, but the onset is usually during the second or third month of life. The presentation is usually that of rapidly progressive weakness, hypotonia, and enlargement of the heart, tongue, and liver. Storage of glycogen in the brain and spinal cord results in CNS dysfunction with diminished alertness and hyporeflexia. Respiratory and feeding difficulties are common and death, usually from cardiorespiratory failure, commonly occurs before the age of 2 years. The electrocardiogram (EKG) shows a short PR interval, high QRS amplitude, and left ventricular hypertrophy (86). In one infant, a *Wolff–Parkinson–White* syndrome was noted. The diagnosis is supported by an increased CPK, generally less than ten times the upper limit of normal, and a myopathic EMG, with abundant myotonic discharges and occasionally with fibrillation potentials and positive waves. Acid maltase activity is deficient in muscle, liver, heart, leukocytes, and cultured fibroblasts. To confirm the diagnosis the enzyme is usually assayed in lymphocytes and/or muscle tissue, and sometimes in urine (87). The muscle biopsy shows large vacuoles with a high glycogen content (PAS-positive), strongly reactive for acid phosphatase, identifying them as secondary lysosomes. Despite the detection of numerous mutations in the acid α-1,4-glucosidase gene on chromosome 17q23 (88), DNA testing is not yet routinely available. In the past, aside from supportive management of the cardiorespiratory insufficiency, there was no effective treatment for infantile AMD. Recently, enzyme replacement therapy has become available with good results (89).

Mitochondrial Myopathies

CYTOCHROME C OXIDASE (COX) DEFICIENCY

Fatal Infantile Myopathy. This condition presents soon after birth with severe lactic acidosis, profound hypotonia and weakness, and feeding and breathing difficulties. In some cases, myopathy with or without an associated cardiomyopathy may be the only manifestation. More commonly, however, there is an associated renal *deToni–Fanconi–Debre* syndrome. Most of these infants die from cardio-respiratory insufficiency before one year of age. The muscle biopsy shows ragged-red fibers with accumulation of glycogen and lipid in most but not all cases. Histochemical staining for COX activity is undetectable and biochemical analysis of skeletal muscle tissue shows virtual absence of COX activity (90). Recently, a severe depletion of mitochondrial DNA (mtDNA) has been detected in patients with fatal infantile myopathy.

Benign Infantile Myopathy. The benign variety presents at or soon after birth with generalized weakness and hypotonia, respiratory and feeding difficulties, and severe lactic acidosis (91). Unlike the fatal form, this condition is confined to the skeletal muscle. These infants tend to improve spontaneously during the first year of life and are normal by the age of 3 years. Muscle histochemistry and/or standard biochemical assays show almost undetectable COX activity. With age this enzyme activity recovers. Ragged-red fibers have been observed in early muscle biopsies but disappear during childhood. The benign variety is distinguished from the fatal form by the immunological detection (*immunotitration by ELISA*) of the enzyme in muscle tissue (92). In the fatal type of COX deficiency, the enzyme protein is undetectable by ELISA (93). Most cases have been sporadic. This condition is thought to result from mutations in a tissue-specific and developmentally regulated fetal COX isoform. Since the enzymatic deficiency is reversible, aggressive support is advised in infants with COX deficiency.

FATTY ACID OXIDATION DEFECTS

This group of disorders includes: (i) the carnitine deficiency syndromes, (ii) defects in carnitine palmitoyltransferases, CPT I, CPT II, and translocase, and (iii) defects of fatty acid β-oxidation enzymes. Most of these conditions present in infancy with hypotonia, generalized weakness, and in some cases cardiomegaly and/or hepatic failure. There may be associated nonketotic or hypoketotic hypoglycemia, hyperammonemia, reduced total and/or free carnitine (rarely, increased free and total carnitine), elevated serum acylcarnitines, and abnormal urine dicarboxylic acids and acylglycines. Serum CPK may be normal or highly elevated. Affected newborns may be lethargic and/or comatose. Muscle biopsy may reveal accumulation of lipid, primarily in Type I fibers. The diagnosis requires detection of the enzymatic deficiency in cultured skin fibroblasts and/or muscle tissue. In cases of true primary muscle carnitine deficiency, the clinical response to carnitine supplementation may be dramatic. Therefore, a trial of carnitine supplementation is warranted in infants with carnitine transport defects. *Organic acidurias* may also present with weakness, hypotonia, cardiomyopathy, and liver enlargement, probably due to secondary carnitine deficiency. In the secondary syndromes, the muscle biopsy shows lipid but not glycogen accumulation. Abnormal organic acids and acylcarnitines can be demonstrated in urine and serum, respectively, by appropriate testing.

Nonlysosomal Glycogenoses

PHOSPHORYLASE DEFICIENCY

Phosphorylase deficiency may present in early infancy with severe generalized weakness and hypotonia, feeding difficulty, and respiratory insufficiency (94). Areflexia or hyporeflexia is usually present but the child remains alert without evidence of encephalopathy (95). Serum CPK concentration is elevated and the muscle biopsy is diagnostic, showing myopathic changes with subsarcolemmal and intermyofibrillar deposits of glycogen. Phosphorylase activity is undetectable in muscle tissue by either histochemistry or enzymatic methods.

PHOSPHOFRUCTOKINASE DEFICIENCY

A neonatal variety of phosphofructokinase (PFK) deficiency has been described, presenting with congenital weakness, hypotonia, swollen joints, multiple contractures and in some cases seizures, cortical blindness, and corneal opacifications (96). There may be evidence of cardiomyopathy, but none of the infantile cases develop hemolysis. CPK values and uric acid are increased in most patients. The muscle biopsy shows accumulation of glycogen under the sarcolemma and between myofibrils. The diagnosis is confirmed by the *immunohistochemical* demonstration of absent PFK staining in muscle, and diminished muscle PFK activity by enzymatic assay. In infants with PFK deficiency the enzyme is present in red blood cells in normal amounts. The biochemical basis of the infantile variety of PFK deficiency is not clear and is probably heterogeneous.

APPROACH TO HYPOTONIA

The following describes our stepwise approach to the diagnostic investigation of infantile hypotonia.

1. Conduct a detailed history and physical examination (as described above) including tests of muscle stretch reflexes and antigravity limb movements.
2. Exclude systemic illness and congenital laxity of ligaments.
3. If *central hypotonia* is suspected, conduct MRI/MRS studies, metabolic studies, and genetic testing for Prader–Willi syndrome. Also test for very long-chain fatty acids and/or other peroxisomal tests. Consider lumbar puncture for cerebrospinal fluid lactate, glucose, and protein; and, if indicated, cerebrospinal fluid neurotransmitter testing.
4. If *peripheral hypotonia* is suspected, first examine the mother. If she has signs of myotonic dystrophy, perform a DNA test for 19qCTG repeat expansion in the child. Elicit any history of autoimmune myasthenia gravis in the mother.
   - Consider electromyography and nerve conduction studies to evaluate for myasthenia, botulism, neuropathy or anterior horn cell disease, and myopathy. Consider performing a Tensilon test if myasthenic syndrome is suspected.
   - Test the child's electrolytes, CPK, lactate, pyruvate, carnitine, and/or other biochemical tests.
     - If CPK/EMG is normal, conduct a DNA test for Prader–Willi syndrome.
     - If CPK is greater than 10 times the upper limit of normal, electromyography is not crucial. Perform DNA tests for FKRP (fukutin-related protein) gene mutations and/or other muscular dystrophies. Consider brain imaging (MRI). If DNA testing is negative, conduct a muscle biopsy.

– If CPK is elevated less than 10 times the upper limit of normal, conduct electromyography. If the electromyogram is neuropathic, order genetic testing for survival motor neuron (SMN) gene or Charcot–Marie–Tooth/Dejerine–Sottas disease. An electromyogram showing decrement/facilitation indicates a neuromuscular junction defect. If the electromyogram is normal or myopathic, conduct a muscle biopsy (electromyography may be normal in certain myopathies).

REFERENCES

1. Volpe JJ. Neurology of the Newborn, 4th edition. Philadelphia, PA: WB Saunders, 2001.
2. Sainte-Anne Dargassies S. Neurological development in the full-term and premature neonate. New York: Elsevier North Holland, 1979.
3. Volpe JJ. Neonatal hypotonia. In Jones HR Jr, De Vivo DC, Darras BT (eds). Neuromuscular Disorders of Infancy, Childhood, and Adolescence: A Clinician's Approach. Philadelphia, PA: Butterworth Heinemann, 2003, pp. 113–22.
4. Gingold MK, Jaynes ME, Bodensteiner JB, et al. The rise and fall of the plantar response in infancy. J Pediatr 133:568, 1998.
5. Paine RS, Brazelton TB, Donovan DE, et al. Evolution of postural reflexes in normal infants and in the presence of chronic brain syndromes. Neurology 14:1036, 1964.
6. Futagi Y, Tagawa T, Otani K. Primitive reflex profiles in infants: differences based on categories of neurological abnormality. Brain Dev 14:294, 1992.
7. Fenichel GM. The hypotonic infant. In Clinical Pediatric Neurology, a Signs and Symptoms Approach, 5th edition. Philadelphia, PA: Elsevier Saunders, 2005, pp. 149–69.
8. Richer LP, Shevell MI, Miller SP. Diagnostic profile of neonatal hypotonia: an 11-year study. Pediatr Neurol 25:32, 2001.
9. Dubowitz V. Disorders of the lower motor neurone: the spinal muscular atrophies. In Dubowitz V (ed). Muscle Disorders in Childhood. London: WB Saunders, 1995, pp. 325–69.
10. Morrison KE, Harding AE. Disorders of the motor neuron. In Harding AE (ed). Genetics and Neurology. London: Bailliere Tindall, 1994, pp. 431–45.
11. Bundey S. Spinal muscular atrophies (SMAs). In Bundey S (ed). Genetics and Neurology. Edinburgh: Churchill Livingstone, 1985, pp. 172–93.
12. Grohmann K, Varon R, Stolz P, et al. Infantile spinal muscular atrophy with respiratory distress type 1 (SMARD1). Ann Neurol 54:719, 2003.
13. Gilliam TC, Brzustowicz LM. The molecular basis of the spinal muscular atrophies. In Rosenberg RN, Pruisner SB, DiMauro S, et al. (eds). The Molecular and Genetic Basis of Neurological Disease. Philadelphia, PA: Butterworth Heinemann, 1993, pp. 883–87.
14. Hahnen E, Forkert R, Marke C, et al. Molecular analysis of candidate genes on 5q13 in autosomal recessive spinal muscular atrophy: evidence of homozygous deletions of the SMN gene in unaffected individuals. Hum Mol Genet 4:1927, 1995.
15. Lefebvre S, Burglen L, Reboullet S, et al. Identification and characterization of a spinal muscular atrophy-determining gene. Cell 80:155, 1995.
16. Roy N, Mahadevan MS, McLean M. The gene for neuronal apoptosis inhibitor protein (NAIP), a novel protein with homology to baculoviral inhibitors of apoptosis is partially deleted in individuals with Type I, II, and III spinal muscular atrophy (SMA). Cell 80:167, 1995.
17. Byers RK, Banker BQ. Infantile muscular atrophy. Arch Neurol 5:140, 1961.
18. Munsat TL. Workshop report. International SMA collaboration. Neuromusc Disord 1:81, 1991.
19. Feldkotter M, Schwarzer V, Wirth R, et al. Quantitative analyses of SMN1 and SMN2 based on real-time lightCycler PCR: fast and highly reliable carrier testing and prediction of severity of spinal muscular atrophy. Am J Hum Genet 70:358, 2002.
20. Sladky JT. Chronic sensory-motor neuropathies in children. Paper presented at the annual meeting of the American Association of Electrodiagnostic Medicine Course A, New Orleans, LA, 1993.
21. Engel AG, Ohno K, Harper CM. Congenital myasthenic syndromes. In Jones HR Jr, De Vivo DC, Darras BT (eds). Neuromuscular Disorders of Infancy, Childhood, and Adolescence: A Clinician's Approach. Philadelphia, PA: Butterworth Heinemann, 2003, pp. 555–74.
22. Gutmann L, Pratt L. Pathophysiologic aspects of human botulism. Arch Neurol 33:175, 1976.
23. Cherington M. Botulism: clinical, electrical and therapeutic considerations. In Lewis GE (ed). Biomedical Aspects of Botulism. New York: Academic Press, 1981, pp. 327–30.
24. Cornblath DR, Sladky JT, Sumner AJ. Clinical electrophysiology of infantile botulism. Muscle Nerve 6:448, 1983.
25. Sunada Y, Bernier SM, Utani A, et al. Identification of a novel mutant transcript of laminin alpha 2 chain gene responsible for muscular dystrophy and dysmyelination in dy^{2J} mice. Hum Mol Genet 4:1055, 1995.
26. Arnon SS, Schechter R, Maslanka SE, et al. Human botulism immune globulin for the treatment of infant botulism. N Engl J Med 354:462, 2006.
27. Dubowitz V. 41st ENMC international workshop on congenital muscular dystrophy. Neuromusc Disord 6:295, 1996.

28. Shorer Z, Philpot J, Muntoni F, et al. Demyelinating peripheral neuropathy in merosin-deficient congenital muscular dystrophy. J Child Neurol 10:472, 1995.
29. Helbling-Leclerc A, Zhang X, Topaloglu H, et al. Mutations in the laminin alpha 2-chain gene (LAMA2) cause merosin-deficient congenital muscular dystrophy. Nat Genet 11:216, 1995.
30. Tome FM, Evangelista T, Leclerc A, et al. Congenital muscular dystrophy with merosin deficiency. C R Acad Sci III 317:351, 1994.
31. Philpot J, Sewry C, Pennock J, et al. Clinical phenotype in congenital muscular dystrophy: correlation with expression of merosin in skeletal muscle. Neuromusc Disord 5:301, 1995.
32. Kobayashi O, Hayashi Y, Arahata K, et al. Congenital muscular dystrophy: clinical and pathologic study of 50 patients with the classical (occidental) merosin-positive form. Neurology 46:815, 1996.
33. Allamand V, Sunada Y, Salih MAM, et al. Mild congenital muscular dystrophy in two patients with an internally deleted laminin α2-chain. Hum Mol Genet 6:747, 1997.
34. Vainzof M, Marie SKN, Reed UC, et al. Deficiency of merosin (laminin M or α2) in congenital muscular dystrophy associated with cerebral white matter alterations. Neuropediatrics 26:293, 1995.
35. Connolly AM, Pestronk A, Planer GJ, et al. Congenital muscular dystrophy syndromes distinguished by alkaline and acid phosphatase, merosin, and dystrophin staining. Neurology 46:810, 1996.
36. North KN, Specht LA, Sethi RK, et al. Congenital muscular dystrophy associated with merosin deficiency. Neurology 11:291, 1996.
37. Kobayashi K, Nakahori Y, Miyake M, et al. An ancient retrotransposal insertion causes Fukuyama-type congenital muscular dystrophy. Nature 394:388, 1998.
38. Fukuyama Y, Osawa M, Suzuki H. Congenital progressive muscular dystrophy of the Fukuyama type: clinical, genetic and pathological considerations. Brain Dev 3:1, 1981.
39. Toda T, Segawa M, Nomura Y, et al. Localization of a gene for Fukuyama type congenital muscular dystrophy to chromosome 9q31-33. Nat Genet 5:283, 1993.
40. Yoshioka M, Kuroki S. Clinical spectrum and genetic studies of Fukuyama congenital muscular dystrophy. Am J Med Genet 53:245, 1994.
41. Dobyns WB, Pagon RA, Armstrong D, et al. Diagnostic criteria for Walker-Warburg syndrome. Am J Med Genet 32:195, 1989.
42. Beltran-Valero de Bernabe D, Currier S, Steinbrecher A, et al. Mutations in the O-mannosyltransferase gene POMT1 give rise to the severe neuronal migration disorder Walker-Warburg syndrome. Am J Hum Genet 71:1033, 2002.
43. Dobyns WB, Truwit CL. Lissencephaly and other malformations of cortical development: 1995 update. Neuropediatrics 26:132, 1995.
44. de Bernabe DB, van Bokhoven H, van Beusekom E, et al. A homozygous nonsense mutation in the fukutin gene causes a Walker-Warburg syndrome phenotype. J Med Genet 40:845, 2003.
45. Beltran-Valero de Bernabe D, Voit T, Longman C, et al. Mutations in the FKRP gene can cause muscle-eye-brain disease and Walker-Warburg syndrome. J Med Genet 41:e61, 2004.
46. van Reeuwijk J, Janssen M, van den Elzen C, et al. POMT2 mutations cause alpha-dystroglycan hypoglycosylation and Walker-Warburg syndrome. J Med Genet 42:907, 2005.
47. Santavuori P, Somer H, Sainio K, et al. Muscle-eye brain disease (MEB). Brain Dev 11:147, 1989.
48. Haltia M, Leivo I, Sorne RH, et al. Muscle-eye-brain disease: a neuropathological study. Ann Neurol 41:173, 1997.
49. Yoshida A, Kobayashi K, Manya H, et al. Muscular dystrophy and neuronal migration disorder caused by mutations in a glycosyltransferase, POMGnT1. Dev Cell 1:717, 2001.
50. Aslanidis C, Jansen G, Amemiya C, et al. Cloning of the essential myotonic dystrophy region and mapping of the putative defect. Nature 355:548, 1992.
51. Brook JD, McCurrach ME, Harley HG, et al. Molecular basis of myotonic dystrophy: expansion of a trinucleotide (CTG) repeat at the 3′ end of a transcript encoding a protein kinase family member. Cell 68:799, 1992.
52. Harley HG, Rundle SA, Reardon W. Unstable DNA sequence in myotonic dystrophy. Lancet 339:1125, 1992.
53. Suthers GK, Huson SM, Davies KE. Instability versus predictability: the molecular diagnosis of myotonic dystrophy. J Med Genet 29:761, 1992.
54. Brunner HG, Nillesen W, van Oost BA. Presymptomatic diagnosis of myotonic dystrophy. J Med Genet 29:780, 1992.
55. Munsat TL, Piper D, Cancilla P, et al. Inflammatory myopathy with facioscapulohumeral distribution. Neurology 22:335, 1972.
56. Taylor DA, Carroll JE, Smith ME, et al. Facioscapulohumeral dystrophy associated with hearing loss and Coats syndrome. Ann Neurol 12:395, 1982.
57. Funakoshi M, Goto K, Arahata K. Epilepsy and mental retardation in a subset of early onset 4q35-facioscapulohumeral muscular dystrophy. Neurology 50:1791, 1998.
58. Kohler J, Rohrig D, Bathke KD, et al. Evaluation of the facioscapulohumeral muscular dystrophy (FSHD1) phenotype in correlation to the concurrence of 4q35 and 10q26 fragments. Clin Genet 55:88, 1999.
59. Griggs RC, Tawil R, Storvick D, et al. Genetics of facioscapulohumeral muscular dystrophy: new mutations in sporadic cases. Neurology 43:2369, 1993.
60. Hewitt JE, Lyle R, Clark LN, et al. Analysis of the tandem repeat locus D4Z4 associated with facioscapulohumeral muscular dystrophy. Hum Mol Genet 3:1287, 1994.
61. Tawil R, Figlewicz DA, Griggs RC, et al. Facioscapulohumeral dystrophy: a distinct regional myopathy with a novel molecular pathogenesis. FSH Consortium. Ann Neurol 43:279, 1998.

62. Ricci E, Galluzzi G, Deidda G, et al. Progress in the molecular diagnosis of facioscapulohumeral muscular dystrophy and correlation between the number of KpnI repeats at the 4q35 locus and clinical phenotype. Ann Neurol 45:751, 1999.

63. Vitelli F, Villanova M, Malandrini A, et al. Inheritance of a 38-kb fragment in apparently sporadic facioscapulohumeral muscular dystrophy. Muscle Nerve 22:1437, 1999.

64. Shy GM, Magee KR. A new congenital non-progressive myopathy. Brain 79:610, 1956.

65. Shy GM, Engel WK, Somers JE, et al. Nemaline myopathy: a new congenital myopathy. Brain 86:793, 1963.

66. Shafig SA, Dubowitz V, Peterson H, et al. Nemaline myopathy: report of a fatal case with histochemical and electron microscopic studies. Brain 90:817, 1967.

67. Wallgren-Pettersson C, Arjomaa P, Holmberg C. Alpha-actinin and myosin light chains in congenital nemaline myopathy. Pediatr Neurol 6:171, 1990.

68. Laing NG, Majda BT, Akkari PA, et al. Assignment of a gene (NEMI) for autosomal dominant nemaline myopathy to chromosome I. Am J Hum Genet 50:576, 1992.

69. Laing NG, Wilton SD, Akkari PA, et al. A mutation in the alpha tropomyosin gene TPM3 associated with autosomal dominant nemaline myopathy. Nat Genet 9:75, 1995.

70. Scarlato G, Pellegrini G, Moggio M. Familial nemaline myopathy. Neuropediatrics 13:211, 1982.

71. Engel WK, Foster JB, Hughes BP. Central core disease: an investigation of a rare muscle cell abnormality. Brain 84:167, 1961.

72. Denborough MA, Dennett XK, Anderson RM. Central core disease and malignant hyperthermia. Br Med J 1:272, 1973.

73. Byrne E, Blumbergs PC, Hallpike JF. Central core disease. Study of a family with five affected generations. J Neurol Sci 53:77, 1982.

74. Haan EA, Freemantle CJ, McCure JA, et al. Assignment of the gene for central core disease to chromosome 19. Hum Genet 86:187, 1990.

75. Zhang Y, Chen HS, Khanna VK. A mutation in the human ryanodine receptor gene associated with central core disease. Nat Genet 5:46, 1993.

76. Kinoshita M, Cadman TE. Myotubular myopathy. Arch Neurol 18:265, 1968.

77. Spiro AJ, Shy GM, Gonatas NK. Myotubular myopathy: persistence of fetal muscle in an adolescent boy. Arch Neurol 14:1, 1966.

78. Thomas NST, Sarfarazi M, Roberts K, et al. X-linked myotubular myopathy (MTM1) evidence for linkage to Xq28 DNA marker loci. J Med Genet 27:284, 1990.

79. Laporte J, Hu LJ, Kretz C, et al. A gene mutated in X-linked myotubular myopathy defines a new putative tyrosine phosphatase family conserved in yeast. Nat Genet 13:175, 1996.

80. Bitoun M, Maugenre S, Jeannet PY, et al. Mutations in dynamin 2 cause dominant centronuclear myopathy. Nat Genet 37:1207, 2005.

81. Brooke MH. Congenital fiber type disproportion. In Kakulas BA (ed). Clinical studies in myology, Vol. 295. Amsterdam: Excerpta Medica ICS, 1973, p. 147.

82. Lenard HG, Goebel HH. Congenital fibre type disproportion. Neuropediatrics 6:220, 1975.

83. Laing NG, Clarke NF, Dye DE, et al. Actin mutations are one cause of congenital fibre type disproportion. Ann Neurol 56:689, 2004.

84. Clarke NF, Kidson W, Quijano-Roy S, et al. SEPN1: associated with congenital fiber-type disproportion and insulin resistance. Ann Neurol 59:546, 2006.

85. Jungbluth H, Zhou H, Hartley L, et al. Minicore myopathy with ophthalmoplegia caused by mutations in the ryanodine receptor type 1 gene. Neurology 65:1930, 2005.

86. Bulkley BH, Hutchins GM. Pompe's disease presenting as hypertrophic myocardiopathy with Wolff-Parkinson-White syndrome. Am Heart J 92:246, 1978.

87. Salafsky IS, Nadler HL. Deficiency of acid alpha glucosidase in the urine of patients with Pompe disease. J Pediatr 82:294, 1973.

88. Zhong N, Martiniuk F, Tzall S, et al. Identification of a missense mutation in one allele of a patient with Pompe disease, and use of endonuclease digestion of PCR-amplified RNA to demonstrate lack of mRNA expression from the second allele. Am J Hum Genet 49:635, 1991.

89. Kishnani PS, Nicolino M, Voit T, et al. Chinese hamster ovary cell-derived recombinant human acid alpha-glucosidase in infantile-onset Pompe disease. J Pediatr 149:89, 2006.

90. Rimoldi M, Bottacchi E, Rossi L. Cytochrome-c-oxidase deficiency in muscle of a floppy infant without mitochondrial myopathy. J Neurol 227:201, 1982.

91. Zeviani M, Peterson P, Servidei S. Benign reversible muscle cytochrome c oxidase deficiency: a second case. Neurology 37:64, 1987.

92. Tritschler HJ, Bonilla E, Lombes A, et al. Differential diagnosis of fatal and benign cytochrome c oxidase-deficient myopathies of infancy: an immunohistochemical approach. Neurology 41:300, 1991.

93. Bresolin N, Zeviani M, Bonilla E. Molecular defects in cytochrome c oxidase deficiency: decrease of immunologically detectable enzyme in muscle. Neurology 35:802, 1985.

94. DiMauro S, Hartlage P. Fatal infantile form of muscle phosphorylase deficiency. Neurology 28:1124, 1978.

95. Milstein J, Herron T, Haas J. Fatal infantile muscle phosphorylase deficiency. J Child Neurol 4:186, 1989.

96. Servidei S, Bonilla E, Diedrich RG. Fatal infantile form of muscle phosphofructokinase deficiency. Neurology 36:1465, 1986.

Chapter 11

Hyperbilirubinemia and the Risk for Brain Injury

Steven M. Shapiro, MD

Pathogenesis

Approaches: Strategies for Diagnosis and Treatment

Recommendations for Treatment

Gaps in Knowledge

CASE HISTORY

BB is a Caucasian male, born at term gestation weighing 2980 g in August 2005 to a 25-year-old G1P0 blood type B+ mother via spontaneous vaginal delivery. Apgar scores were 8 and 9 at 1 and 5 minutes, respectively. He was blood type A+, had a large cepalohematoma and appeared jaundiced at 24 hours of life. He passed an automated ABR screening and was discharged at 58 hours with a transcutaneous bilirubin level of 13.2 mg/dL and blood bilirubin of 14 mg/dL. One day later at follow-up, the pediatrician said he looked fine. He returned at 6 days of age with a history of lethargy but had regained his birth weight. The pediatrician guessed the bilirubin level was about 5 mg/dL. On day 7 he was more lethargic and feeding was more difficult. On day 8 he was noted to have a high-pitched cry, downward deviation of his eyes, and episodic and then continual extension of arms, legs, neck, and trunk. He was evaluated in an emergency room where a spinal tap was normal except for yellow cerebrospinal fluid. Total bilirubin at 211 hours (8.8 days) of age was 45.6 mg/dL. He was placed under phototherapy lights with blanket underneath, intubated because of low O_2 saturation, and a double volume exchange transfusion was performed at 214 hours of age. Pre- and postexchange total bilirubin values were 35.8 and 20.9 mg/dL. He was intubated and sedated. Five days later, emerging from sedation, he was hypotonic with setting sun sign, and with episodic O_2 desaturation. He was treated with phenobarbital for seizures. An EEG was normal except for some sharp waves over the left temporal region. His episodes improved with treatment for reflux. He was discharged after a 10-day hospitalization. He has subsequently developed feeding issues, incoordination of suck and swallow, hypertonia and dystonia, and delayed motor development. ABRs at 2.5 weeks and 2 months of age were absent, consistent with auditory neuropathy/dyssynchrony, despite normal distortion product otoacoustic emissions (OAEs). Magnetic resonance imaging done at 11 days of age showed increased signal intensity in the globus pallidus bilaterally on both T1- and T2-weighted images, and a resolving cephalohematoma. Because of reflux and failure to thrive, a gastrostomy tube was placed with Nissen fundoplication. Treatment with diazepam was instituted to treat increased tone. Phenobarbital was taped and discontinued. Clonic activity has been noted several times, but video EEG has repeatedly demonstrated that these episodes are not seizures. At 1.5 years of age, he has not developed speech or language, has not responded to amplification, and cannot sit or crawl. A cochlear implant is planned.

This case highlights the risk of visual assessment of jaundice. The bilirubin of 14 at discharge was at the 95th percentile of the Bhutani et al. hour-specific nomogram (1). This and significant cephalohematoma and an A/B blood group abnormality were predictive of a high subsequent bilirubin level. The child had symptoms of acute bilirubin encephalopathy that were not recognized until it was too late to prevent the extreme hyperbilirubinemia, and now the child has all the clinical signs, symptoms, and laboratory findings of kernicterus.

The classic form of brain injury due to hyperbilirubinemia is called kernicterus. Kernicterus was originally a pathological term referring to the yellow staining (*icterus*) of the deep nuclei of the brain (*kern* relating to the basal ganglia), and the terms acute and chronic bilirubin encephalopathy were used to describe the clinical symptoms associated with the neuropathology. In modern times, the use of the term kernicterus has expanded to include clinical bilirubin encephalopathy, and modern testing, such as magnetic resonance imaging (MRI) scans and brainstem auditory evoked potentials (BAEPs; also known as brainstem auditory evoked responses (BAERs) and auditory brainstem responses (ABRs)), has shown objective evidence of both neuropathologic lesions and abnormal neurologic function.

Classic kernicterus is a well-described clinical syndrome which includes: (i) a dystonic or athetoid movement disorder, (ii) an auditory processing disturbance with or without hearing loss, (iii) ocular motor impairment especially impairment of upward gaze, (iv) dysplasia of the enamel of deciduous (baby) teeth, and, perhaps less well known, (v) hypotonia and ataxia due to cerebellar involvement. More subtle forms of brain injury due to excess of hyperbilirubinemia have also been described and termed subtle kernicterus, chronic bilirubin encephalopathy of the subtle type, or, more recently, kernicterus spectrum disorders or bilirubin-induced neurologic disorders (BIND). These describe more subtle neurodevelopmental disorders in children with less than all of the clinical features of classic kernicterus, or with mild or subtle manifestations of the classic abnormalities.

Classic kernicterus is a rare disorder. Its incidence in Denmark has been estimated to be 1 per 110 000 live births, whereas the incidence of extreme hyperbilirubinemia, defined as at or above criteria to perform exchange transfusion (median 28.8 mg/dL, range 22.5–40.3 mg/dL), was 25 per 100 000 (2, 3). A population-based survey in northern California found that 150 per 100 000 developed total serum bilirubin (TSB) $\geq$25 mg/dL, and 10 per 100 000 were $\geq$30 mg/dL (4, 5). The incidence of extreme hyperbilirubinemia and kernicterus is dependent on the care infants receive in the first few weeks of life, the vigilance of screening, and the ability to treat excessive hyperbilirubinemia should it occur. Incidence and prevalence studies are complicated by the lack of specific objective definitions of kernicterus or BIND and the inconsistency of reporting kernicterus or excessive hyperbilirubinemia in most countries. Further, the incidence and prevalence of subtler neurodevelopmental disorders such as auditory processing disorders or visual motor disabilities due to hyperbilirubinemia is a subject of speculation without adequate data or documentation.

Precisely how to determine the risk of brain injury in a hyperbilirubinemic newborn is important not only for determining the level of care but also for determining the optimal allocation of healthcare resources. The precise determination of risk of brain injury will not only allow better guidelines for treatment to prevent brain damage, but also the reduction or elimination of unnecessary treatments. This chapter will discuss new concepts on pathogenesis, approaches or strategies for diagnosis and treatment, gaps in our knowledge, and recommendations for treatment.

PATHOGENESIS

Bilirubin neurotoxicity is highly selective, targeting specific neurons in the central nervous system (CNS). The clinical expression and neuropathology of kernicterus is likewise highly selective. The movement disorders of dystonia and athetosis correspond to lesions in the basal ganglia (globus pallidus and the subthalamic nucleus), cerebellum, and brainstem nuclei having to do with auditory, vestibular, and oculomotor function, and truncal tone. Any explanation of pathogenesis must account for the selective neurotoxicity of bilirubin.

It may be useful to compartmentalize the concept of bilirubin neurotoxicity into (i) what causes the cell to be exposed to excess bilirubin, (ii) what causes the cell to be able to handle or not handle this excess bilirubin, and (iii) what the molecular mechanisms are of cell damage and protection. Bilirubin exposure is a combination of bilirubin production, binding, and excretion. Bilirubin is excreted out of the cell, the CNS, and the circulation. The ability of cells to handle excess bilirubin may vary. Risk factors may be compartmentalized too and, of course, may affect one or more compartments. For example, acidosis decreases binding, increases unbound free bilirubin (Bf), and thus the cell is exposed to more bilirubin. However, pH might also affect cell enzymes, energy production, or transport. Other risk factors, e.g., prematurity, inflammation, isoimmunization, may act in one or more specific compartments. Is important that we start thinking clinically of what is going on at the cellular level in the CNS.

It appears that bilirubin damages cells by both apoptotic and necrotic mechanisms and affects mitochondrial energy metabolism. Recent studies in cultured cells by Brites and colleagues (6–9) have begun to define the role of apoptosis, mitochondria, and other molecular mechanisms of bilirubin neurotoxicity. Purified bilirubin can induce apoptosis in cultured rat brain neurons (7, 8) by triggering the release of cytochrome c from mitochondria with caspase-3 activation and cleavage of poly(ADP-ribose) polymerase, confirming the role of one of the pathways that underlies induction of apoptosis (10). Apoptotic changes are found in cerebellum (10, 11) and brainstem of jaundiced Gunn rats (11) and in the basal ganglia of kernicteric human infants accounting for prominent signs of bilirubin neurotoxicity in each. Furthermore, Brites and colleagues have also raised the possibility that neuroinflammation may be a significant contributor to bilirubin neurotoxicity (12). Recent comprehensive reviews have been published about the molecular mechanism of bilirubin neurotoxicity (9, 13, 14).

The blood–brain barrier (BBB) excludes large molecules including albumin and albumin-bound bilirubin from most of the CNS and transports substances into and out of the CNS (9). The endothelial cells of the BBB restrict diffusion of many toxic compounds to adjacent neurons and astrocytes, but do not restrict the free diffusion of unconjugated bilirubin, which is permeable with single-pass uptake estimated to be as high as 28% in rats (15). Bilirubin rapidly diffuses through lipid membranes (16) and through phosphatidylcholine vesicle membranes as the uncharged diacid (17). The concentration gradient for TSB from plasma to cerebrospinal fluid in humans (18, 19) and jaundiced Gunn rats (20, 21) is thus probably due to the lower concentrations of binding proteins in the cerebrospinal fluid.

Specific transporters for bilirubin, e.g., multidrug resistance protein 1 (MRP1) (9), may protect the CNS from exposure to excessive levels of bilirubin. Tiribelli and colleagues have provided recent evidence that bilirubin is removed from cells via a specific transporter, MRP1, a member of the multidrug-resistance-associated protein subfamily of ATP-binding cassette transporters (9, 13, 22, 23). MRP1 transports bilirubin with an affinity which is 10 times greater that of other substrates (23) and may represent a mechanism by which bilirubin is transported out of the

CNS and excreted into the circulation. They hypothesize that when this transport system is overwhelmed, toxic bilirubin can accumulate in the cell.

We have proposed that bilirubin interferes with intracellular calcium homeostasis and demonstrated decreased activity of calcium and calmodulin-dependent protein kinase II (CaMKII) in our Gunn rat model of kernicterus (24). Bilirubin inhibits CaMKII in vitro (25), and its developmental expression is impaired in jj Gunn rats (26). Further, there is selective decrease in expression of calcium binding proteins (CBPs) in specific brainstem areas susceptible to bilirubin neurotoxicity in the CNS of kernicteric Gunn rats (27, 28). CaMKII regulates neurotransmitter release, calcium-regulated ion conductances, and neuroskeletal dynamics (29) and can trigger programmed cell death (apoptosis).

It has also been proposed that bilirubin and increased calcium damage through an excitotoxic, N-methyl-D-aspartame (NMDA)-dependent mechanism (30–32), though there is also evidence against this hypothesis (33). We have found that MK-801, an NMDA-channel blocker, does not protect against bilirubin neurotoxicity in vitro in hippocampal neurons, nor does it protect against auditory dysfunction in vivo in our Gunn rat model of acute bilirubin encephalopathy (34).

Neurons are susceptible to apoptotic death from oxidative stress. Recent work from the Snyder laboratory has begun to define the role of bilirubin and its precursor, biliverdin, in normal cells (35–39). Bilirubin and heme oxygenase 2, the enzyme that catalyzes its formation, have neuroprotective, antioxidant properties. Depleting cultured HeLA cells and cortical neurons of biliverdin reductase by RNA interference leads to increased oxidative activity and renders cells more susceptible to caspase-dependent death from hyperoxia and hydrogen peroxide toxicity (37). The antioxidant activity is comparable to that of glutathione, long assumed to be the principal cellular antioxidant (37). Hippocampal cultures from heme oxygenase 2 (but not 1) knockout mice are more susceptible to hydrogen peroxide toxicity (35), and heme oxygenase 2 knockout mice are more susceptible to focal cerebral ischemia and excitotoxic injury (40). Bilirubin, despite its extremely low concentration in the cell, is recycled to greatly increase its effect (37). Snyder and colleagues have proposed that the potent physiologic antioxidant action of bilirubin is amplified when the detoxification of reactive oxygen species oxidizes bilirubin back to biliverdin, which is then reduced again by biliverdin reductase to form bilirubin (37). As this redox amplification cycle is repeated, the antioxidant effect of bilirubin is multiplied. While it is proposed that this redox amplification cycle might constitute the principal physiologic function of bilirubin, it should be noted that a protective action of modest levels of bilirubin does not alter the well-established dangers of kernicterus associated with major elevations of serum bilirubin (39).

Windows of developmental susceptibility of the CNS to bilirubin toxicity may exist. Cerebellar neurons undergoing early differentiation at the time of bilirubin exposure are highly susceptible to bilirubin neurotoxicity, whereas slightly more or slightly less mature neurons may show only transient changes (41). Bilirubin-induced cell death, glutamate release, cytokine production, and activation of transcription factors involved in inflammation are enhanced in undifferentiated astrocytes and neurons as compared with more mature cells (12, 42). Falcao et al. have shown that both mRNA and protein levels of Mrp1 increase with cell differentiation, and suggest that the development expression of Mrp1 may explain the susceptibility of premature babies to bilirubin neurotoxicity (43).

It is likely that prolonged exposure of neurons to bilirubin causes cell death and that the developmental stage of the neuron determines whether the cell can handle the bilirubin load. The hyperbilirubinemia must be sufficient to permit Bf to enter the neuron and exceed its capacity to handle it. Neuronal exposure to extremely high bilirubin for relatively short amounts of time probably affects the cell differently than exposure to relatively lower but still excessive levels for a longer time.

The developmental stage of the neuron, for unknown reasons, probably determines in part whether or not the cell can handle the bilirubin load.

APPROACHES: STRATEGIES FOR DIAGNOSIS AND TREATMENT

Strategies for diagnosis and treatment of hyperbilirubinemia are well known. The recent American Academy of Pediatrics (AAP) guidelines for the treatment of hyper-bilirubinemia (44) are a significant improvement over the AAP's 1994 guidelines. Following these guidelines will undoubtedly prevent many cases of kernicterus, though how much and what type of subtle bilirubin encephalopathy (BIND) occurs is unknown. The amount of excessive treatment and its associated cost to the healthcare system is unknown.

However, some concerns with current guidelines should be mentioned. First is the failure to highly recommend a predischarge bilirubin measurement as an indispensable part of risk assessment (rather than saying this is one of two recommended options, the other being risk factor summation). Second is the lack of clear guidelines for bilirubin/jaundice assessment at the first and subsequent follow-up visits. As shown by the pilot kernicterus registry (45) and the author's personal experience, babies that develop severe hyperbilirubinemia and kernicterus are often those whose jaundice at a follow-up visit is not considered severe or extensive enough to warrant a serum bilirubin. This can be the result of forgetting that before a baby becomes pumpkin orange, full body jaundice usually is associated with a clearly deeper yellow in the face and belly than in the legs and feet (Lois Johnson, personal communication). This may lead the observer to assume that full body jaundice is not yet present, and that the bilirubin level is below rather than at or above 15 mg/dL. Third, a level of 11 to 12 mg/dL (jaundice below the umbilicus but not yet to the thighs) also needs to be followed closely and confirmed by a TSB or TcB. This represents a problem, of course, because not all doctors' offices have a TcB meter. Finally, the guidelines fail to take into account new methods of measuring unbound (free) bilirubin and binding, which in the future are likely to lead to better, more effective preventative treatment strategies (46–48). Basing screening and treatment decisions on TSB alone is not likely to improve the sensitivity and specificity of detecting and preventing kernicterus. Using methods to assess individual binding – perhaps a two-step method using TSB and clinical criteria to determine risk category, and then using Bf to determine binding and more precisely TSB action levels for a particular baby – might improve sensitivity and specificity.

Acute Bilirubin Encephalopathy (Acute Kernicterus)

In newborns with acute bilirubin encephalopathy, symptoms progress from lethargy and decreased feeding to variable or fluctuating tone (hypotonia and hypertonia), high-pitched cry, retrocollis and opisthotonus, impairment of upward gaze (setting sun sign), fever, seizures, and death. BAEPs are absent or abnormal (49–51) and reversible with double volume exchange transfusion (52, 53). MRI scans reveal abnormal signal bilaterally in specific subdivisions of the basal ganglia, the globus pallidus, and subthalamic nucleus (54–58). Abnormalities are found within days after the peak total serum bilirubin level (59) and are initially hyper-intense on T1-weighed images, and later become normal or hypointense on T1- and hyperintense on T2-weighted scans (59, 60). The subthalamic nucleus is smaller and is not easily seen in some MRIs, and may be subtle and easily overlooked (59). In some patients, abnormalities may normalize.

The diagnosis of acute encephalopathy can usually be made in term or near-term newborns using clinical examination (mental status, tone, posture, cry, setting sun sign, and late signs of opisthotonus, seizures, and fever) and laboratory values (TSB, unconjugated and conjugated bilirubin, pH, and albumin). Some clinicians feel that hyperbilirubinemia from Rh disease (or hemolysis) is more likely to be damaging than from other causes (perhaps to more rapid rate of rise or rapid rate of bilirubin production). Current illnesses such as sepsis may increase risk. New diagnostic methodology is currently based on BAEP and MRI, both of which give specific diagnostic information in newborns and can usually distinguish encephalopathy due to bilirubin from encephalopathy due to other causes.

Since the auditory system is sensitive to bilirubin neurotoxicity, the BAEP is a sensitive, objective measure of early CNS dysfunction due to bilirubin. Early changes such as increased latency and decreased amplitude of wave III and V herald the onset of bilirubin neurotoxicity, probably at a reversible stage. Wave III arises from the cochlear nuclei in the pons, and wave V arises from the lateral lemniscus in the midbrain, a pathway terminating in the inferior colliculus. The use of interwave intervals, e.g., I–III, III–V, and I–V, reflects conduction time. The earliest BAEP indicators of bilirubin neurotoxicity are I–III and the somewhat more reliably measured I–V. As bilirubin neurotoxicity progresses, BAEP abnormalities progress to absence of wave III and V and, finally, to complete absence of all waves, including I. Clinically, BAEP wave amplitudes are usually too variable to serve as criteria for BAEP normality, though they are useful when serial studies can be compared to a baseline, and the use of amplitude ratios III:I and V:I helps decrease variability.

The automated ABR (AABR) has been used to assess auditory function in hyperbilirubinemic newborns in the neonatal intensive care unit (NICU). The AABR matches the BAEP (also known as ABR) response to a predesigned template and is reported as either present (Pass) or absent (Refer). Absence of AABR in the presence of hyperbilirubinemia, especially in a neonate who has become hyperbilirubinemic and whose AABR has changed from Pass to Refer, is evidence of abnormal auditory function and may reflect significant bilirubin neurotoxicity. Unfortunately, the AABR as opposed to the BAEP does not distinguish CNS from middle or inner ear dysfunction (neither due to bilirubin), and current devices are not able to detect the early changes of bilirubin neurotoxicity. However, the ease of use and availability of AABR at all times in the NICU make it a clinically useful device to consider as part of an evaluation of when to treat sick neonates.

Difficulties in obtaining MRIs in sick neonates in most centers preclude its use for making clinical decisions such as when to intervene, i.e., do an exchange transfusion. However, MRI is useful to establish kernicterus, almost immediately after the fact. If rescue treatments are shown to be neuroprotective after severe hyperbilirubinemia, then MRI may be critically important to select patients and determine response to treatment.

Other neuroimaging techniques such as head computed tomography and ultrasound scans are generally normal in kernicterus, though hyperechogenicity is occasionally seen, and was reported in 1 of 8 preterm and term infants with abnormal MRIs (59). Cerebrospinal fluid measurements of bilirubin and binding, as well as other substances, e.g., indicators of neuroinflammation, may become useful in the future. Magnetic resonance spectroscopy has currently unrealized potential to reveal abnormalities of brain energy metabolism.

New strategies for the diagnosis of acute bilirubin encephalopathy have been proposed. The first is a BIND score, similar to an Apgar score, to be used in babies with significant hyperbilirubinemia. This score, proposed by an ad hoc BIND study group (61), rates neurologic symptoms such as muscle tone, posture, cry, and

Table 11-1	**BIND Score from Zero (Best) to Nine (Worst)**
Mental status (0–3)	0 = Normal 1 = Sleepy, poor feeding 2 = Lethargic, irritable 3 = Semicoma, coma, seizures
Muscle tone (0–3)	0 = Normal 1 = Neck stiffness, mild hypertonia or hypotonia 2 = Arching neck and/or trunk 3 = Opisthotonus
Cry (0–3)	0 = Normal 1 = High pitched 2 = Shrill 3 = Inconsolable

mental status based on Volpe's description of acute bilirubin encephalopathy (62), on a scale of 0–9 in infants with high TSB (Table 11-1) and can be used much like an Apgar score. It has not yet been validated in any study. Though it seems simple to use, it has the problem that cry is difficult to assess objectively and cannot be assessed when the child is intubated.

The BIND score can be used retrospectively to track the clinical progression of acute bilirubin encephalopathy from nonspecific, subtle encephalopathy (score 1–3) through progressive toxicity (score 4–6) to advanced toxicity (score 7–9).

Treatment

Neonatal hyperbilirubinemia with signs of encephalopathy should be considered a neurologic emergency and treated immediately to reduce the duration of exposure to excessive bilirubin and to try to move some bilirubin out of the CNS. Anecdotal evidence suggests that exchange transfusion may in part reverse neurotoxicity. While awaiting blood for exchange transfusion, intense phototherapy (e.g., a double bank of phototherapy lamps overhead as close to the infant as possible, plus intense light from below and, if the infant is not encephalopathic, gavage feedings with preferably elemental formula (63–65) to promote fecal excretion of bilirubin are recommended.

The author's reviews of medical records of children with subsequent kernicterus reveal that treatment mistakes occur both in the emergency room and in the NICU. Mistakes sometimes encountered in the emergency room are: (i) the dose of phototherapy is not considered – it is not recognized that the proximity of phototherapy lights from the baby is important; (ii) babies are made NPO since it is not recognized that oral or nasogastric feeding with elemental formula helps promote bilirubin excretion in healthy, nonencephalopathic babies (65); (iii) unnecessary delay in treatment occurs because treating physicians believe that the initial level "can't be that high"; (iv) initiating phototherapy or preparing for exchange transfusions is delayed until after other investigations, e.g. sepsis work-ups or lumbar punctures, are done; (v) babies with very high total and high conjugated bilirubin levels are not treated in fear of "bronze baby syndrome"; (vi) babies are not treated because the level is so high and the baby so encephalopathic that it is felt to be "too late to treat" (we believe that it is never "too late to treat" acute, symptomatic bilirubin encephalopathy, since the duration of excessive hyperbilirubinemia is related to outcome (66, 67)); and finally (vii) treatment is neglected or forgotten during emergency treatment of critical, life-threatening neonatal illness (we call this "critical illness kernicterus" – e.g., surgical treatment of another urgent, life-threatening illness such as cyanotic congenital heart disease or necrotizing endocarditis with perforation leads to discontinuing phototherapy in the operating and recovery rooms, and subsequent development of kernicterus).

Diagnosis of Chronic Bilirubin Encephalopathy (Chronic Kernicterus)

Examination in older children and adults often involves determining whether cerebral palsy or neurodevelopmental problems are due to neonatal hyperbilirubinemia. Beyond the newborn period, kernicterus is diagnosed by a combination of history, physical examination, and laboratory tests, especially MRI and BAEP (Table 11-2).

In all cases, there should be a history of jaundice and, hopefully, laboratory confirmation of an increased serum bilirubin level, the higher the bilirubin the more significant it is modified by its duration and risk factors. Important is whether the child is neurologically symptomatic at the time of the hyperbilirubinemia. History of neonatal neurologic signs or symptoms such as abnormal tone, cry, posturing, abnormal eye movements, or positions (including sun setting) at the time of, or following, hyperbilirubinemia should be sought. The history should include an estimate of amount and duration of hyperbilirubinemia, other risk factors including gestational age, sepsis, academia, hypoalbuminemia, and a search for etiology such as Rh or ABO isoimmunization, G6PD deficiency, Gilbert's syndrome, Crigler–Najjar syndrome, spherocytosis, or third spacing of blood, for example a large intraventricular hemorrhage, cepalohematoma, caput, or other bruising. A history of muscle cramps, delayed gross or fine motor development, delayed speech, hearing loss, or dental enamel dysplasia is sought. A history of past or present sucking and swallowing dysfunction, gastroesophageal reflux, constipation, and failure to thrive can often be obtained. Inconsistency of hearing or sound localization in a young child raises the suspicion of a subtle auditory neuropathy/dys-synchrony (AN/AD).

History of BAEPs and AABRs obtained early in life should be sought. Note that hearing screening with OAEs detects peripheral auditory problems of the inner ear. OAE screening is unaffected by bilirubin toxicity, and babies with severe AN/AD with deafness have normal OAEs. BAEPs improve in a minority of children with time in our experience; improvement in BAEP does not mean the auditory system has returned to normal. An MRI scan of the brain with abnormal

Table 11-2	Diagnosis of Kernicterus or BIND in Older Children
Neonatal history	Magnitude and duration of hyperbilirubinemia, other risk factors (sepsis, acidosis, Rh isoimmunization), neonatal neurologic signs or symptoms during or following peak hyperbilirubinemia (abnormal tone, cry, posturing/opisthotonus, eye movements/setting sun sign)
Subsequent history	Auditory neuropathy/dys-synchrony (AN/AD); hearing loss; delayed speech; dental enamel dysplasia (or capped teeth); abnormal muscle tone – especially dystonia and/or variable hypotonia/hypertonia; muscle cramps; swallowing problems, gastroesphageal reflux
Examination	Athetosis, dystonia, dystonia and variable hypo-/hypertonia ($\pm$ true velocity-dependent hypertonia, i.e., spasticity), ataxia, impaired upward gaze (may resolve), staining or flaking of baby teeth (enamel hypoplasia) unless capped, hearing impairment
Laboratory	MRI: abnormal signal in globus pallidus $\pm$ subthalamic nucleus, *but* may be normal, and initially abnormal findings may recover Auditory: BAEP abnormal consistent with AN/AD – increased I–III and I–V, absent III and V, or all waves absent with normal cochlear microphonic responses and normal OAEs (though initially normal OAEs may become abnormal, but abnormal BAEPs and AN/AD may recover, in which case central auditory processing disorders may later be found)

globus pallidus with or without an abnormal subthalamic nucleus is nearly pathog-nomonic of kernicterus. Initially T1-weighted scans are hyperintense. Later, T2-weighted images increase in hyperintensity and T1-weighted images normalize or become hypointense. Metabolic disorders such as glutaric academia and mito-chondrial encephalopathies can be excluded by history and specific laboratory tests if necessary.

On physical examination of the older child, one specifically looks for athetosis (slow writhing movements), dystonia (abnormal tone, fixed postures, co-contrac-tion of agonist and antagonist muscles), variable hypo-/hypertonia, spasticity, ataxia, incoordination, impaired upgaze, staining or flaking of deciduous teeth (enamel hypoplasia), dysarthria, hearing impairment, or difficulty localizing sound. Improvement of impaired upward gaze has been described, but it is difficult to examine upward gaze in older infants and young children who have learned to turn their heads to compensate for gaze pareses.

Laboratory evaluation consists of MRI and BAEP (ABR). Other testing may show the presence or absence of other conditions, e.g., seizures, metabolic disor-ders, Gilbert's or Crigler–Najjar syndromes or liver disease if the older child remains jaundiced, G6PD deficiency or partial deficiency, and spherocytosis. The MRI may show abnormal signal in globus pallidus and/or STN, but a normal MRI does not exclude the diagnosis. Abnormal MRIs may or may not improve with time. Few other etiologies cause discrete bilateral lesions in GP and STN, and most of these are metabolic conditions with a different history and onset, e.g., glutaric aciduria with a sudden onset of encephalopathy or abnormal movements during an acute febrile illness or episode of vomiting. In addition, the MRI usually shows more extensive areas of damage in these other conditions. MRI findings consistent with kernicterus may occur with additional lesions in putamen and cortex, or with periventricular leukomalacia, in children with other conditions in addition to kernicterus. We suggest the term "kernicterus plus syndrome" for these children, i.e., kernicterus plus other neonatal encephalopathies, such as hypoxic-ischemia, stroke, encepha-litis, and intraventricular hemorrhage.

The BAEP may be absent or abnormal with an increase of conduction time between waves I and III, and I and V. The cochlear microphonic (CM) response, which can be obtained at the time of BAEP testing, should be present even in the absence of BAEP neural waves (I through V). Occasionally, "giant" CM responses may occur and are often mistaken for BAEP waves by inexperienced readers. Cochlear microphonics can be distinguished from BAEP waves by the fact that they do not change their latencies with intensity (whereas BAEP waves do), and phase reverse with phase reversal of the click stimulus (whereas BAEP waves do not). BAEPs may or may not improve with time. OAEs, initially normal, may disappear with time for unknown reasons, possibly related to overstimulation of the cochlea. A full audiology evaluation is usually advisable. As with MRI, an abnormal BAEP in the presence of AN/AD is consistent with bilirubin neurotoxi-city, but a normal BAEP does not rule out kernicterus.

RECOMMENDATIONS FOR TREATMENT

The concentrations of unconjugated bilirubin (UCB) or TSB, unbound or free bilirubin (Bf), and hydrogen ion (pH) are all important determinants of neuronal injury by bilirubin. Since Bf is not readily available clinically, estimates of binding have been used, e.g., the bilirubin:albumin molar ratio. Wennberg et al. recently concluded that clinical evidence indicates that Bf is better than UCB in discrimi-nating risk for neurotoxicity in patients with severe hyperbilirubinemia (47). Ahlfors argues that the issue is not whether Bf is a *better* measure than UCB (or TcB), but that measuring both UCB and Bf permits a better understanding of the miscible (diffusible) pool of bilirubin, bilirubin binding, the risk of neurotoxicity, and when to treat a particular baby (presentation to Kernicterus Symposium, PAS Annual Meeting, 2006, and personal communication). Ahlfors makes an analogy to blood gases in which both pH and CO_2 are measured because knowing both values, even though they are related, makes for better treatment decisions. He argues that it is not possible to identify a single total bilirubin level at which to intervene for all babies of the same gestation because binding varies from baby to baby. Measuring both Bf and TSB can identify the unique binding in the individual baby, and thus identify the unique TSB at which to intervene for that child. Ahlfors argues that arbitrary TSB cutoffs determined primarily by consensus do not necessarily protect patients, and that measuring Bf in addition to TSB would better determine the total bilirubin level we are trying to avoid in a particular baby. Thinking such as "what bilirubin level is too high?" is like saying "at what pO_2 do we intubate?" – it just is not that simple! We need more information.

Some treatments could be easily implemented with current technology and in the current healthcare delivery system. The first recommendation is to improve the emergency treatment of infants with extremely high bilirubin levels with a "bilirubin crash cart." Both the intensity of treatment and speed in initiating therapy can be improved. There is often delay from the time the child is first identified until a treatment occurs. A protocol for emergency rooms for dealing with children with extreme hyperbilirubinemia should be implemented. We have proposed the idea of a bilirubin crash cart, an incubator outfitted with high-intensity phototherapy lights above and underneath, all the necessary tubes for blood collection, and a protocol for the emergency treatment of all infants admitted with severe jaundice. There is no reason to wait for laboratory results before the yellow- or orange-colored infant is put into high-intensity phototherapy. The first set of laboratories should include all that is necessary to order blood for an exchange transfusion. Nasogastric tubes should be available to administer elemental formula to help with gut elimination of bilirubin in nonencephalopathic babies who can tolerate nasogastric feeding (68). There is no need to withhold treatment while blood is being sent, while abnormal laboratory values are being confirmed, and while other procedures such as spinal taps are being done to rule out other conditions such as meningitis. The patient should be rushed to the NICU without administrative delay for further treatment and line placement. In infants with isoimmune hemolytic disease and TSB rising in spite of intensive phototherapy or within 2–3 mg/dL of exchange level, intravenous immunoglobulin (IVIG) should be administered (44, 64, 69). If babies need to be transferred to another center for an exchange transfusion, then treatment including high-intensity phototherapy should be administered during the transport, and preparations for exchange should be made while the child is being transported.

A second recommendation that could be implemented with current technology is universal bilirubin screening. Current AAP guidelines do not recommend a predischarge bilirubin as an indispensable part of risk assessment, but rather say that this is one of two recommended options, the other being risk factor summation. A comparison of two recommended approaches to identifying newborns at risk of significant hyperbilirubinemia concluded that use of a predischarge bilirubin measurement expressed as a risk zone on an hour-specific bilirubin nomogram is more accurate and generates wider risk stratification than a clinical risk factor score (70). Systems that are not universal or that rely on subjective assessment of jaundice by healthcare providers with different levels of training will allow some preventable cases of kernicterus to "slip through the system." Other recommendations that can be accomplished with existing resources are standardizing laboratory bilirubin measurements and introducing a system of reporting elevated bilirubin levels (e.g., ≥ 25 mg/dL) to get a better idea of the true epidemiology of this problem.

There is also a lack of clear guidelines for bilirubin and jaundice assessments at follow-up visits. Babies who later have kernicterus are often placed at risk because their jaundice was not considered severe or extensive enough to warrant obtaining a transcutaneous or serum bilirubin measurement. Some clinicians and healthcare workers forget that before a baby becomes "pumpkin orange," full body jaundice is often associated with a clearly deeper yellow in the face and belly than in the legs and feet. This leads the observer to assume that full body jaundice is not yet present and the bilirubin level is below, rather than above 15 mg/dL. In addition, levels of 11–12 mg/dL need to be closely followed and confirmed either by TcB or blood measurement.

A TSB level below which the risk of neurotoxicity is minimal has yet to be established (and may never be established for TSB alone – for example, babies with displacers, e.g., sulfonamide (71) or benzyl alcohol (72), may develop kernicterus at extremely low bilirubin levels). Until better information is obtained, the use of the level at which phototherapy is recommended for a particular child can be used as a rough guideline below which hyperbilirubinemia is probably not significant if other clinical factors including other illness, acidosis, or the presence of substances which displace bilirubin from albumin are excluded. The use of BAEPs, especially serial BAEPs that are improving, could be a good guide to the lack of ongoing bilirubin neurotoxicity.

Once the child is stable, consideration should be given to obtaining an MRI scan of the head. Contrast is not necessary. We would currently recommend an MRI scan of the head with special attention to the globus pallidus, and a BAEP with special attention to interwave intervals, cochlear microphonics, and the presence or absence of AN/AD. Often it is not appreciated that OAEs, also known as distortion product otoacoustic emissions (DPOAEs), do not detect the auditory abnormality due to hyperbilirubinemia. Therefore, one must obtain a BAEP (ABR) to obtain diagnostic information. Since the number of children who have abnormalities that then improve is unknown, early testing is important with serial testing if abnormal. A good neurologic examination with special attention to muscle tone and eye movements is important. Serial neurologic evaluations during the first few months of life can be helpful in determining whether brain injury has occurred. Early identification and treatment with physical therapy, occupational therapy, and speech therapy can be helpful. Some children with classic kernicterus have failure to thrive because of swallowing difficulties, gastroesophageal reflux, and excessive metabolic demands of their movement disorders. These children often benefit from placement of nasogastric or gastrostomy tubes though they continue to be fed orally. If severe AN/AD is present or the child acts as if it is deaf or severely impaired, then cochlear implantation has proved beneficial. We agree with current recommendations for this to be done as soon as possible. A large majority of patients with kernicterus who have had this done have had their parents report benefit. In severe cases, medications to treat dystonia and hypertonia are important. Benzodiazepines and baclofen have been useful. Other treatments such as botulinum toxin (Botox) injections and baclofen pumps have been useful in more extreme cases.

GAPS IN KNOWLEDGE

Though there has been significant progress in our understanding of how bilirubin causes brain damage, significant gaps in our knowledge remain. An important gap in basic science knowledge relates to specific cellular and regional selectivity of CNS bilirubin toxicity. The current methods of assessing risk of kernicterus and BIND, i.e., TSB, do not measure the amount of bilirubin in brain tissue. Thus, some infants at relatively "low" TSB values may have BIND, and undoubtedly many at relatively high TSB levels may be treated unnecessarily to prevent kernicterus in a few infants. Research is needed investigate the sensitivity and reliability of new methods to better detect BIND, including clinical examination of newborn infants, additional biochemical measures of bilirubin toxicity such as Bf, and neurophysiology such as BAEP.

Through the decades from the 1950s to the 1980s, clinical practice evolved to essentially eliminate classic kernicterus; however, a reemergence of kernicterus occurred in the 1990s and continues to the present, associated with changes in medical practice and healthcare delivery. Clearly, universal screening of infants combined with close follow-up, monitoring, and aggressive phototherapy treatment at relatively low bilirubin levels could eliminate most of the new cases of kernicterus, but the prevention of a devastating but very rare disorder must be balanced against the costs and possible risks, though minimal with current treatment, of overtreating very large numbers of babies. More precise determination of who is at risk for brain injury is needed to ensure that no baby unnecessarily gets kernicterus, yet the number of babies overtreated is minimized. The concentration of bilirubin when toxicity is increased is a difficult issue for physicians in practice, who must balance the gain in value of an early visit against the worry about whether increased surveillance will result in increased use of resources (phototherapy), more maternal anxiety, and reduced breastfeeding. However, the benefits of an early visit may not only be to screen for and prevent significant hyperbilirubinemia, but also to reduce maternal anxiety and through education increase breastfeeding.

A more precise definition of kernicterus is needed. The definition of classic kernicterus is well established in the literature, but new clinical cases lead to the concept of a spectrum of kernicterus and BIND. Cases of auditory-predominant or motor-predominant kernicterus have been described in which some of the classic features of kernicterus (auditory dysfunction or movement disorders) are prominent, with other features absent or much less pronounced. We have seen a small number of cases of auditory-predominant kernicterus occurring in 30- to 32-week gestation premature infants with TSB levels in the range of 20–25 mg/dL (73, 74).

Precisely which hyperbilirubinemic infant to treat and when they should be treated has not been precisely determined. The role of bilirubin in common neurodevelopmental disorders such as auditory processing disorders, cognitive disorders, sensory motor disorders, autism, or attention deficit hyperactivity disorder (ADHD) has yet to be established. The genetic influences and susceptibilities are not completely known, i.e., why males are more susceptible than females. Precisely when and how bilirubin becomes neurotoxic both on a cellular (molecular) basis and in the whole organism will necessarily preclude understanding better how and when to treat hyperbilirubinemic newborns. Better basic science can thus be expected to lead to a better treatment paradigm for jaundice newborn babies.

Whether total or unconjugated bilirubin levels determine risk when conjugated bilirubin is elevated is not completely resolved. Classic kernicterus was reported in an Rh-sensitized infant with TSB of 45.2 mg/dL, of which 31.6 mg/dL was direct (75), and in a term infant with bronze baby syndrome in which the maximum TSB was 18 mg/dL and direct 4.1 mg/dL (76). Ebbesen found infants with elevated direct bilirubin (6.4–9.9 mg/dL) and bronze baby syndrome had a decrease in reserve albumin binding capacity (77) and suggested that conjugated bilirubin may compete with unconjugated bilirubin for bilirubin binding site to albumin. The AAP recommends that in using guidelines for phototherapy and exchange transfusion, the conjugated bilirubin level should not be subtracted from the total (44). The guidelines go on to state: "In unusual situations in which the direct bilirubin level is 50% or more of the total bilirubin, there are no good data to provide guidance for therapy, and consultation with an expert in the field is recommended." The recommendation of using TSB to determine treatment seems prudent for now.

A significant gap in knowledge is determining when bilirubin neurotoxicity occurs in the premature infant. Guidelines that exist for administration of phototherapy and exchange transfusion are not evidence based. Whether bilirubin encephalopathy contributes to neurodevelopmental disabilities or learning disorders in this population is unknown. We suspect that, if present, bilirubin is likely to cause problems similar to those seen with classic kernicterus, for example auditory process disorders. However, the damage or developmental consequences of excessive bilirubin on the very immature CNS may be fundamentally different from effects on a more mature system.

Following the 2004 AAP guidelines undoubtedly will prevent most kernicterus, though how much potentially preventable BIND occurs by following these guidelines is unknown. The amount of unnecessary treatment and its associated cost to the healthcare system is also unknown. While the emotional cost to children and their families of a lifetime of disability from kernicterus is immeasurable, the financial cost to society of caring for a child with kernicterus over a lifetime is huge, and preventing one case of kernicterus will pay for a lot of preventative screening. The author supports universal screening for hyperbilirubinemia; a systematic screening program will obviously prevent some additional cases of kernicterus, though how many more is currently unknown.

Acknowledgments

The author appreciates suggestions and comments from Drs. Charles Ahlfors, Vinod Bhutani, Thor Hansen, Lois Johnson, M. Jeffrey Maisels, Michael Painter, Ann Rice, Richard Wennberg, Ann Stark, and Jon Watchko.

REFERENCES

1. Bhutani VK, Johnson L, Sivieri EM. Predictive ability of a predischarge hour-specific serum bilirubin for subsequent significant hyperbilirubinemia in healthy term and near-term newborns. Pediatrics 103(1):6–14, 1999.
2. Bjerre JV, Ebbesen F. [Incidence of kernicterus in newborn infants in Denmark.] Ugeskr Laeger 168(7):686–91, 2006.
3. Ebbesen F. Recurrence of kernicterus in term and near-term infants in Denmark. Acta Paediatr 89(10):1213–7, 2000.
4. Newman TB, Escobar GJ, Gonzales VM. Frequency of neonatal bilirubin testing and hyperbilirubinemia in a large health maintenance organization. Pediatrics 104(5 Pt 2):1198–203, 1999.
5. Newman TB, Liljestrand P, Escobar GJ. Infants with bilirubin levels of 30 mg/dL or more in a large managed care organization. Pediatrics 111(6 Pt 1):1303–11, 2003.
6. Rodrigues CM, Sola S, Silva R, Brites D. Bilirubin and amyloid-beta peptide induce cytochrome c release through mitochondrial membrane permeabilization. Mol Med 6(11):936–46, 2000.
7. Silva RF, Rodrigues CM, Brites D. Bilirubin-induced apoptosis in cultured rat neural cells is aggravated by chenodeoxycholic acid but prevented by ursodeoxycholic acid. J Hepatol 34(3):402–8, 2001.
8. Rodrigues CMP, Sola S, Brites D. Bilirubin induces apoptosis via the mitochondrial pathway in developing rat brain neurons. Hepatology 35:1186–95, 2002.
9. Ostrow JD, Pascolo L, Brites D, Tiribelli C. Molecular basis of bilirubin-induced neurotoxicity. Trends Mol Med 10(2):65–70, 2004.
10. Hanko E, Hansen TW, Almaas R, et al. Bilirubin induces apoptosis and necrosis in human NT2-N neurons. Pediatr Res 57(2):179–84, 2005.
11. Conlee JW, Shapiro SM. Morphological changes in the cochlear nucleus and nucleus of the trapezoid body in Gunn rat pups. Hear Res 57(1):23–30, 1991.
12. Falcao AS, Fernandes A, Brito MA, et al. Bilirubin-induced immunostimulant effects and toxicity vary with neural cell type and maturation state. Acta Neuropathol (Berl) 112(1):95–105, 2006.
13. Ostrow JD, Pascolo L, Shapiro SM, Tiribelli C. New concepts of bilirubin encephalopathy. Eur J Clin Invest 33(11):988–997, 2003.
14. Watchko JF. Kernicterus and the molecular mechanisms of bilirubin-induced CNS injury in newborns. Neuromolec Med 8(4):513–30, 2006.
15. Ives NK, Gardiner RM. Blood–brain barrier permeability to bilirubin in the rat studied using intracarotid bolus injection and in situ brain perfusion techniques. Pediatr Res 27(5):436–441, 1990.
16. Hayward D, Schiff D, Fedunec S., et al. Bilirubin diffusion through lipid membranes. Biochim Biophys Acta 860(1):149–53, 1986.

17. Zucker SD, Goessling W, Hoppin AG. Unconjugated bilirubin exhibits spontaneous diffusion through model lipid bilayers and native hepatocyte membranes. J Biol Chem 274(16): 10852–62, 1999.

18. Amatuzio DS, Weber LJ, Nesbitt S. Bilirubin and protein in the cerebrospinal fluid of jaundiced patients with severe liver disease with and without hepatic coma. J Lab Clin Med 41(4):615–18, 1953.

19. Berman LB, Lapham LW, Pastore E. Jaundice and xanthochromia of the spinal fluid. J Lab Clin Med 44(2):273–9, 1954.

20. Sawasaki Y, Yamada N, Nakajima H. Developmental features of cerebellar hypoplasia and brain bilirubin levels in a mutant (Gunn) rat with hereditary hyperbilirubinemia. J Neurochem 27:577–83, 1976.

21. Rodriguez Garay EA, Scremin OU. Transfer of bilirubin-14 C between blood, cerebrospinal fluid, and brain tissue. Am J Physiol 221(5):1264–70, 1971.

22. Gennuso F, Fernetti C, Tirolo C, et al. Bilirubin protects astrocytes from its own toxicity by inducing up-regulation and translocation of multidrug resistance-associated protein 1 (Mrp1). Proc Natl Acad Sci USA 101(8):2470–5, 2004.

23. Rigato I, Pascolo L, Fernetti C, et al. The human multidrug-resistance-associated protein MRP1 mediates ATP-dependent transport of unconjugated bilirubin. Biochem J 383(Pt 2):335–41, 2004.

24. Braun AP, Schulman H. The multifunctional calcium/calmodulin-dependent protein kinase: from form to function. Annu Rev Physiol 57:417–45, 1995.

25. Churn SB. Multifunctional calcium and calmodulin-dependent kinase II in neuronal function and disease. Adv Neuroimmunol 5(3):3, 1995.

26. Conlee JW, Shapiro SM, Churn SB. Expression of the alpha and beta subunits of Ca^{2+}/calmodulin kinase II in the cerebellum of jaundiced Gunn rats during development: a quantitative light microscopic analysis. Acta Neuropathol (Berl) 99(4):393–401, 2000.

27. Shaia WT, Shapiro SM, Heller AJ, et al. Immunohistochemical localization of calcium-binding proteins in the brainstem vestibular nuclei of the jaundiced Gunn rat. Hear Res 173(1–2):82–90, 2002.

28. Spencer RF, Shaia WT, Gleason AT, et al. Changes in calcium-binding protein expression in the auditory brainstem nuclei of the jaundiced Gunn rat. Hear Res 171(1–2):129–41, 2002.

29. Greengard P. Neuronal phosphoproteins. Mediators of signal transduction. Mol Neurobiol 1:51–119, 1987.

30. Hoffman DJ, Zanelli SA, Kubin J, et al. The in vivo effect of bilirubin on the N-methyl-D-aspartate receptor/ion channel complex in the brains of newborn piglets. Pediatr Res 40(6):804–8, 1996.

31. McDonald JW, Shapiro SM, Silverstein FS, Johnston MV. Role of glutamate receptor-mediated excitotoxicity in bilirubin-induced brain injury in the Gunn rat model. Exp Neurol 150(1):21–9, 1998.

32. Grojean S, Koziel V, Vert P, Daval JL. Bilirubin induces apoptosis via activation of NMDA receptors in developing rat brain neurons. Exp Neurol 166(2):334–41, 2000.

33. Warr O, Mort D, Attwell D. Bilirubin does not modulate ionotropic glutamate receptors or glutamate transporters. Brain Res 879(1–2):13–16, 2000.

34. Shapiro SM, Sombati S, Geiger AS, Rice AC. NMDA channel antagonist MK-801 does not protect against bilirubin neurotoxicity. Neonatology 92(4):248–57, 2007.

35. Dore S, Takahashi M, Ferris CD, et al. Bilirubin, formed by activation of heme oxygenase-2, protects neurons against oxidative stress injury. Proc Natl Acad Sci USA 96(5):2445–50, 1999.

36. Dore S, Goto S, Sampei K, et al. Heme oxygenase-2 acts to prevent neuronal death in brain cultures and following transient cerebral ischemia. Neuroscience 99(4):587–92, 2000.

37. Baranano DE, Rao M, Ferris CD, Snyder SH. Biliverdin reductase: a major physiologic cytoprotectant. Proc Natl Acad Sci USA 99(25):16093–8, 2002.

38. Greenberg DA. The jaundice of the cell. Proc Natl Acad Sci USA 99(25):15837–9, 2002.

39. Sedlak TW, Snyder SH. Bilirubin benefits: cellular protection by a biliverdin reductase antioxidant cycle. Pediatrics 113(6):1776–82, 2004.

40. Dore S, Sampei K, Goto S, et al. Heme oxygenase-2 is neuroprotective in cerebral ischemia. Mol Med 5(10):656–63, 1999.

41. Conlee JW, Shapiro SM. Development of cerebellar hypoplasia in jaundiced Gunn rats treated with sulfadimethoxine: a quantitative light microscopic analysis. Acta Neuropathol 93:450–60, 1997.

42. Falcao AS, Fernandes A, Brito MA, et al. Bilirubin-induced inflammatory response, glutamate release, and cell death in rat cortical astrocytes are enhanced in younger cells. Neurobiol Dis 20(2):199–206, 2005.

43. Falcao AS, Bellarosa C, Fernandes A, et al. Role of multidrug resistance-associated protein 1 expression in the in vitro susceptibility of rat nerve cell to unconjugated bilirubin. Neuroscience 144(3):878–88, 2007.

44. American Academy of Pediatrics Subcommittee on Hyperbilirubinemia. Management of hyperbilirubinemia in the newborn infant 35 or more weeks of gestation. Pediatrics 114(1):297–316, 2004.

45. Johnson L, Brown AK. A pilot registry for acute and chronic kernicterus in term and near-term infants. Pediatrics 104(3):736, 1999.

46. Ahlfors CE, Wennberg RP. Bilirubin-albumin binding and neonatal jaundice. Semin Perinatol 28(5):334–9, 2004.

47. Wennberg RP, Ahlfors CE, Bhutani VK, et al. Toward understanding kernicterus: a challenge to improve the management of jaundiced newborns. Pediatrics 117(2):474–85, 2006.

48. Ahlfors CE. Bilirubin-albumin binding and free bilirubin. J Perinatol 21(Suppl 1):S40-2; discussion S59–62, 2001.

49. Wennberg RP, Ahlfors CE, Bickers R, et al. Abnormal auditory brainstem response in a newborn infant with hyperbilirubinemia: improvement with exchange transfusion. J Pediatr 100(4):624–6, 1982.

50. Amin SB, Ahlfors C, Orlando MS, et al. Bilirubin and serial auditory brainstem responses in premature infants. Pediatrics 107(4):664–70, 2001.

51. Funato M, Tamai H, Shimada S, Nakamura H. Vigintiphobia, unbound bilirubin, and auditory brainstem responses. Pediatrics 93(1):50–3, 1994.

52. Nwaesei CG, Van Aerde J, Boyden M, Perlman M. Changes in auditory brainstem responses in hyperbilirubinemic infants before and after exchange transfusion. Pediatrics 74(5):800–3, 1984.

53. Wennberg R. Bilirubin transport and toxicity. Mead Johnson Symp Perinat Dev Med 19:25–31, 1982.

54. Sugama S, Soeda A, Eto Y. Magnetic resonance imaging in three children with kernicterus. Pediatr Neurol 25(4):328–31, 2001.

55. Martich-Kriss V, Kollias SS, Ball Jr WS. MR findings in kernicterus. AJNR Am J Neuroradiol 16(Suppl 4):819–21, 1995.

56. Yilmaz Y, Alper G, Kilicoglu G, et al. Magnetic resonance imaging findings in patients with severe neonatal indirect hyperbilirubinemia. J Child Neurol 16(6):452–5, 2001.

57. Penn AA, Enzmann DR, Hahn JS, Stevenson DK. Kernicterus in a full term infant. Pediatrics 93(6 Pt 1):1003–6, 1994.

58. Johnston MV, Hoon Jr AH. Possible mechanisms in infants for selective basal ganglia damage from asphyxia, kernicterus, or mitochondrial encephalopathies. J Child Neurol 15(9):588–91, 2000.

59. Govaert P, Lequin M, Swarte R, et al. Changes in globus pallidus with (pre)term kernicterus. Pediatrics 112(6 Pt 1):1256–63, 2003.

60. Harris MC, Bernbaum JC, Polin JR, et al. Developmental follow-up of breastfed term and near-term infants with marked hyperbilirubinemia. Pediatrics 107(5):1075–80, 2001.

61. Johnson L, Brown AK, Bhutani VK. BIND: a clinical score for bilirubin induced neurologic dysfunction in newborns. Pediatrics 104(3 Pt 3):746–7, 1999.

62. Volpe JJ. Bilirubin and brain injury. In Volpe JJ (ed). Neurology of the Newborn. Philadelphia, PA: WB Saunders, 2001, pp. 490–514.

63. Hansen TW. Acute management of extreme neonatal jaundice: the potential benefits of intensified phototherapy and interruption of enterohepatic bilirubin circulation. Acta Paediatr 86(8):843–6, 1997.

64. Smitherman H, Stark AR, Bhutan VK. Early recognition of neonatal hyperbilirubinemia and its emergent management. Semin Fetal Neonatal Med 11(3):214–24, 2006.

65. Gourley GR, Kreamer B, Cohnen M, Kosorok MR. Neonatal jaundice and diet. Arch Pediatr Adolesc Med 153(9):1002–3, 1999.

66. Johnson L, Boggs TR. Bilirubin-dependent brain damage: incidence and indications for treatment. In Odell GB, Schaffer R, Sionpoulous AP (eds). Phototherapy in the Newborn: An Overview. Washington, DC: National Academy of Sciences, 1974, pp. 122–49.

67. de Vries LS, Lary S, Dubowitz LMS. Relationship of serum bilirubin levels to ototoxicity and deafness in high-risk, low birth-weight infants. Pediatrics 76(3):351–4, 1985.

68. Gourley GR, Arend RA. Beta-glucuronidase and hyperbilirubinaemia in breast-fed and formula-fed babies. Lancet 1(8482):644–6, 1986.

69. Gottstein R, Cooke RW. Systematic review of intravenous immunoglobulin in haemolytic disease of the newborn. Arch Dis Child Fetal Neonatal Ed 88(1):F6–10, 2003.

70. Keren R, Bhutani VK, Luan X, et al. Identifying newborns at risk of significant hyperbilirubinaemia: a comparison of two recommended approaches. Arch Dis Child 90(4):415–21, 2005.

71. Silverman WA, Andersen DH, Blanc WA, Crozier DN. A difference in mortality rate and incidence of kernicterus among premature infants allotted to two prophylactic antibacterial regimens. Pediatrics 18:614–25, 1956.

72. Jardine DS, Rogers K. Relationship of benzyl alcohol to kernicterus, intraventricular hemorrhage, and mortality in preterm infants. Pediatrics 83(2):153–60, 1989.

73. Shapiro SM, Bhutani VK, Johnson L. Hyperbilirubinemia and kernicterus. Clin Perinatol 33(2):387–10, 2006.

74. Shapiro SM. Definition of the clinical spectrum of kernicterus and bilirubin-induced neurologic dysfunction (BIND). J Perinatol 25(1):54–9, 2005.

75. Grobler JM, Mercer MJ. Kernicterus associated with elevated predominantly direct-reacting bilirubin. S Afr Med J 87(9):1146, 1997.

76. Clark CF, Torii S, Hamamoto Y, Kaito H. The "bronze baby" syndrome: postmortem data. J Pediatr 88(3):461–4, 1976.

77. Ebbesen F. Low reserve albumin for binding of bilirubin in neonates with deficiency of bilirubin excretion and bronze baby syndrome. Acta Paediatr Scand 71(3):415–20, 1982.

Chapter 12

Neonatal Meningitis: Current Treatment Options

David Kaufman, MD • Santina Zanelli, MD • Pablo J. Sánchez, MD

Question 1. What Risk Factors Predispose This Infant to Have Early-onset Bacterial Meningitis?

Question 2. Do Infants With Meningitis Have Positive Blood Cultures?

Question 3. What Is the Optimal Evaluation for Possible Late-onset Sepsis in Preterm Infants in the NICU?

Question 4. What Is the Empirical Antimicrobial Choice for Possible Late-onset Sepsis in the NICU?

Question 5. What Is the Treatment of Meningitis in Neonates, and in Particular That Due to Gram-negative Bacilli?

Question 6. Should Other Therapies Be Considered?

Question 7. What Is the Duration of Treatment for Meningitis in Neonates?

Question 8. When Should Neuroimaging Be Considered and What Type of Examination Is Recommended?

Question 9. Should Other Adjunctive Therapies Be Provided to an Infant With Meningitis?

Question 10. What If the Infant's CSF is Abnormal but Routine Bacterial Cultures of CSF and Blood are Sterile?

Question 11.What Is the Outcome of Meningitis in Neonates?

Conclusions

Bacterial meningitis occurs in approximately 0.4 neonates per 1000 live births. It is defined as inflammation of the meninges that is manifested by an elevated number of white blood cells in the cerebrospinal fluid (CSF). It often is associated with elevated protein content and a low glucose concentration in CSF. Meningitis generally results as a consequence of hematogenous dissemination of bacteria via the choroid plexus and into the central nervous system during a sepsis episode. Invasion of the meninges occurs in about 10 to 20% of infants with bacteremia. Rarely, meningitis develops secondary to extension from infected skin through the

Table 12-1	Causative Agents of Neonatal Meningitis[a]	
1. Bacteria	Aerobic:	
	Gram-positive: group B streptococcus, group A streptococcus, *Enterococcus* spp., viridans streptococci, *Staphylococcus aureus*, coagulase-negative staphylococci, *Listeria monocytogenes*, others[b]	
	Gram-negative: *Escherichia coli, Klebsiella* spp., *Enterobacter* spp., *Serratia* spp., *Proteus* spp., *Citrobacter* spp., *Salmonella* spp., *Pseudomonas aeruginosa, Haemophilus influenzae, Neisseria gonorrhoeae*, others[b]	
	Anaerobic:	
	Gram-positive: *Clostridium* spp., *Peptostreptococcus* spp.	
	Gram-negative: *Bacteroides fragilis*	
	Genital mycoplasmas: *Ureaplasma urealyticum, Mycoplasma hominis*	
	Spirochetes: *Treponema pallidum, Borrelia burgdorferi*	
	Mycobacteria: *Mycobacteria tuberculosis*	
2. Viruses	Herpes simplex virus, cytomegalovirus, enteroviruses, human immunodeficiency virus, varicella-zoster virus, rubella virus, human parvovirus B19, lymphocytic choriomeningitis virus	
3. Fungi	*Candida* spp., *Malassezia* spp., *Aspergillus* spp, *Trichosporon beigelis, Cryptococcus, Coccidiodes immitis*	
4. Protozoa	*Toxoplasma gondii*	

[a]For a more complete listing, see Palazzi DL, Klein JO, Baker CJ. Bacterial sepsis and meningitis. In Remington JS, Klein JO, Wilson CB, Baker CJ (eds). Infectious Diseases of the Fetus and Newborn Infant, 6th edition. Philadelphia, PA: WB Saunders, 2006, pp. 247–95.

[b]For others, see Giacoia GP. Uncommon pathogens in newborn infants. J Perinatol 14:134, 1994.

soft tissues and skull as may occur with an infected cephalohematoma, or direct spread from skin surfaces as in infants with myelomeningoceles or other congenital malformations of the neural tube. In addition, ventriculoperitoneal shunts or ventricular reservoirs may be the primary site of infection. A potential but infrequent complication of meningitis is brain abscess that results from hematogenous spread of bacteria into tissue that has suffered anoxic injury or severe vasculitis with hemorrhage or infarction.

Virtually all organisms that cause neonatal infection or sepsis can result in central nervous disease with severe consequences to the developing brain (1–3). A list of these pathogens is provided in Table 12-1. It is imperative that a correct and timely diagnosis with a specific organism be made since treatment decisions vary by causative agent.

The case of a preterm infant is presented and discussed to illustrate and highlight the multifaceted nature of this disease. It is the objective of this chapter to review the current management of neonatal bacterial meningitis, in the hope of ameliorating the destructive nature of many of these organisms and ultimately improving the outcome of these high-risk infants.

CASE HISTORY

A preterm infant weighing 1004 g was born at 28 weeks' gestation to a 24-year-old mother by caesarean section. The pregnancy was complicated by premature rupture of membranes 2 weeks before delivery, and the mother developed intrapartum fever and was diagnosed with chorioamnionitis. She received antenatal steroids and antimicrobial therapy consisting of ampicillin and gentamicin. At delivery, the infant was floppy with poor respiratory effort, and required intubation and admission to the neonatal intensive care unit (NICU). Apgar scores were 3[1] and 7[5]. The infant's vital signs were stable, and antimicrobial therapy with ampicillin and gentamicin was initiated after blood culture was obtained. Hyaline membrane disease was diagnosed and the infant received exogenous surfactant therapy.

QUESTION 1. WHAT RISK FACTORS PREDISPOSE THIS INFANT TO HAVE EARLY-ONSET BACTERIAL MENINGITIS?

Since meningitis is a complication of bacteremia, the risk factors are similar to those that contribute to neonatal sepsis, namely prematurity, prolonged rupture of fetal membranes of 18 to 24 hours or greater, and maternal intrapartum fever or chorio-amnionitis (4). Likewise, clinical signs suggestive of bacterial meningitis are similar to those of neonatal sepsis. In the full-term infant, fever, lethargy, hypotonia, irritability, apnea, poor feeding, high-pitched cry, emesis, seizures, and bulging fontanel are prominent clinical signs, while in preterm infants, respiratory decompensation consisting of increased number of apneic episodes predominates. Neonates with meningitis are not "asymptomatic" (5).

Maternal antepartum antibiotic use has been associated with early-onset meningitis caused by Gram-negative bacilli (6). The widespread and routine use of intrapartum antimicrobial chemoprophylaxis since 1996 has reduced significantly the rate of early-onset group B streptococcal (GBS) infection by over 70% (7). At the same time, there has not been an increase in early-onset bacterial infections caused by Gram-negative organisms among all newborns in the USA (8, 9). However, among very low birth weight (VLBW) infants with birth weight ≤1500 g, a shift towards more Gram-negative infections has occurred (10). Among the NICUs of the National Institute of Child Health and Human Development (NICHD) Neonatal Research Network centers, intrapartum antimicrobial chemoprophylaxis resulted in a significant decrease in early-onset GBS infection while the rate of infections due to *Escherichia coli* increased significantly from 3 to 7 cases per 1000 live births (10, 11). The majority of *E. coli* isolates were resistant to ampicillin, an antibiotic that is often used for intrapartum GBS chemoprophylaxis.

QUESTION 2. DO INFANTS WITH MENINGITIS HAVE POSITIVE BLOOD CULTURES?

As many as 40% of infants with meningitis who have a gestational age of ≥34 weeks do not have a positive blood culture at the time of their diagnosis (12). Similarly, among VLBW infants, almost one half of cases of meningitis occur with sterile blood cultures (13, 14). Therefore, it is imperative that if sepsis or meningitis is suspected, a lumbar puncture be performed (15, 16). Evaluation of CSF indices and Gram stain not only will establish a diagnosis but also will help guide initial therapy. Normal CSF indices are provided in Table 12-2 (17–24).

Meningitis in preterm infants admitted to the NICU with respiratory distress syndrome is very uncommon (25–28). Therefore, performance of a lumbar puncture in these infants in whom sepsis is not suspected is not mandatory. Similar data are available for full-term infants (5, 29) However, if the blood culture yields a pathogenic organism, then evaluation of CSF should be done (16). Delay in performance of a lumbar puncture because of cardiorespiratory instability, extreme prematurity, or concern for increase in blood pressure due to pain with a lumbar puncture and the risk of intraventricular hemorrhage in extremely preterm infants only delays the diagnosis and leads to prolonged and possibly inappropriate antibiotic use (13).

The infant was extubated and placed on continuous positive airway pressure (CPAP) therapy on the first day of age. Trophic feedings were initiated on the third day of age, and a percutaneous intravenous central venous catheter (PICC) was placed for parenteral nutrition. The infant achieved full enteral feedings on the 20th day. Over the subsequent two days, the infant developed lethargy, hyperglycemia, and increased

Table 12-2 Cerebrospinal Fluid Indices in Neonates

Birth weight (g) / Age (days)	No. of samples	Red blood cells (mm³), mean ± SD (range)	White blood cells (mm³), mean ± SD (range)	Polymorphonuclear leukocytes (%), mean ± SD (range)	Glucose (mg/dL), mean ± SD (range)	Protein (mg/dL), mean ± SD (range)
Preterm neonate (21)						
≤1000						
0–7	6	335 ± 709 (0–1780)	3 ± 3 (1–8)	11 ± 20 (0–50)	70 ± 17 (41–89)	162 ± 37 (115–222)
8–28	17	1465 ± 4062 (0–19 050)	4 ± 4 (0–14)	8 ± 17 (0–66)	68 ± 48 (41–89)	159 ± 77 (95–370)
29–84	15	808 ± 1843 (0–6850)	4 ± 3 (0–11)	2 ± 9 (0–36)	49 ± 22 (41–89)	137 ± 61 (76–260)
1001–1500						
0–7	8	407 ± 853 (0–2450)	4 ± 4 (1–10)	4 ± 10 (0–28)	74 ± 19 (41–89)	136 ± 35 (85–176)
8–28	14	1101 ± 2643 (0–9750)	7 ± 11 (0–44)	10 ± 19 (0–60)	59 ± 23 (41–89)	137 ± 46 (54–227)
29–84	11	661 ± 1198 (0–3800)	8 ± 8 (0–23)	11 ± 19 (0–48)	47 ± 13 (41–89)	122 ± 47 (45–187)
Full-term neonate (17)						
0–30	108	≤1000	7.3 ± 13.9 (0–130), median 4	0.8 ± 6.2 (0–65), median 0	51.2 ± 12.9 (62% of serum glucose)	64.2 ± 24.2

episodes of apnea that resulted in re-initiation of mechanical ventilation. Two blood cultures were obtained, and antimicrobial therapy with nafcillin and gentamicin was initiated.

QUESTION 3. WHAT IS THE OPTIMAL EVALUATION FOR POSSIBLE LATE-ONSET SEPSIS IN PRETERM INFANTS IN THE NICU?

Infants suspected of having late-onset sepsis in the NICU should have a complete evaluation that consists of a complete blood cell count, a urine analysis and culture, and CSF evaluation. Unfortunately, there is no laboratory or clinical finding that has a sensitivity of 100% for the diagnosis of neonatal sepsis (30, 31). Such laboratory tools as complete blood cell (CBC) count, C-reactive protein (CRP), interleukin (IL)-6, IL-8, IL-10, and procalcitonin have suboptimal sensitivity and specificity to replace the blood culture as the gold standard, but these tests may be useful to support a diagnosis of infection when they are abnormal and accompanied by clinical signs of infection (32–34). Polymerase chain reaction (PCR) for detection of bacterial and fungal DNA ultimately may be the answer.

Performance of a CBC with platelets is important for reasons other than diagnosis. Neonatal sepsis may result in neutropenia which is associated with a high mortality rate. The finding of an absolute neutrophil count of $\leq 500/mm^3$ may prompt the administration of immunoglobulin intravenous (IGIV, 750 mg/kg); the use of IGIV has been associated with improvement in the peripheral neutrophil count secondary to neutrophil egression from the bone marrow (35, 36). Granulocyte transfusions also have been found to be beneficial, but lack of timely availability and donor screening has limited its routine use (37). Recombinant granulocyte or granulocyte-macrophage colony-stimulating factors also have been used with some success, and can be considered if IGIV is unsuccessful in improving the neutrophil count (37, 38). Another reason for performance of CBC is evaluation of platelet count since disseminated intravascular coagulation may result in severe thrombocytopenia. In addition, thrombocytopenia may be an early marker of disseminated candidiasis (39).

Debate continues as to whether multiple blood cultures should be performed. Certainly with bacterial organisms that are frequent blood culture contaminants, such as coagulase-negative staphylococci (CoNS), the diagnosis of sepsis is best confirmed by the finding of two or more positive cultures from multiple sites or body fluids that are normally sterile (40, 41). Among infants with PICCs, this means obtaining a blood culture from the PICC and another from a peripheral blood vessel. The isolation of CoNS from only one blood culture when only one is obtained is problematic and of uncertain significance. Since many of these positive cultures represent contamination with skin microflora, the practice of obtaining only one blood culture often leads to prolonged and unnecessary antibiotic therapy. In addition, performance of two blood cultures may increase the likelihood of isolating a causative agent. This practice leads to more prudent antibiotic use – a major goal in the NICU where antimicrobial resistance is an emerging but preventable problem.

Urine culture is an important part of the evaluation since urinary tract infection is relatively common in neonates who are greater than 72 hours of age (42, 43). Urine should be obtained by suprapubic bladder aspiration whenever possible, and the finding of any growth is significant. Alternatively, a catheterized urine specimen may be obtained, recognizing that urethral or perineal bacterial or fungal contamination in these small infants may complicate the assessment of results. In general, growth of a single isolate with a colony count of 10^4 or greater is considered a true pathogen, while lesser colony counts are more indicative of contamination.

Bag specimens should never be obtained for the evaluation of possible urinary tract infection.

Chest radiograph should be obtained if respiratory decompensation is present. A lumbar puncture should always be performed on infants evaluated for possible late-onset sepsis for reasons stated in answer to question 2 above. Risk factors for meningitis in preterm infants include low gestational age and prior bloodstream infection (13). In VLBW infants, the average age of late-onset meningitis is 26 days (median 19 days; range 4–102 days) (13). Therapeutic decisions with regard to antibiotic choices can only be made if one knows whether the central nervous system is involved.

QUESTION 4. WHAT IS THE EMPIRICAL ANTIMICROBIAL CHOICE FOR POSSIBLE LATE-ONSET SEPSIS IN THE NICU?

In general, antimicrobial therapy for neonatal sepsis is dependent upon the agents commonly seen in that particular nursery and their susceptibility pattern. For early-onset sepsis, ampicillin combined with an aminoglycoside, usually gentamicin, has been the empiric therapy of choice since group B streptococcus, other streptococcal species, *Listeria monocytogenes*, and Gram-negative bacilli predominate.

For late-onset sepsis, a penicillinase-resistant, semisynthetic penicillin such as oxacillin or nafcillin in combination with an aminoglycoside is the preferred choice (41, 44). For central nervous system infections, nafcillin is preferred because of improved penetration. Since approximately 50% of all bloodstream infections are due to CoNS, some experts recommend vancomycin instead of a semisynthetic penicillin since CoNS are almost uniformly resistant to these agents. This practice has led to widespread use of vancomycin in NICUs with its attendant risk for emergence of vancomycin-resistant organisms.

The use of a penicillinase-resistant penicillin antibiotic such as nafcillin to treat for possible staphylococcal infection in this infant is based on the goal of reducing vancomycin use in NICUs. Clinical experience suggests that such a practice is safe (44–47). Bloodstream infections due to CoNS are rarely fulminant or fatal, and they are not associated with an increased case-fatality rate over that seen among uninfected VLBW infants (48). The clinical outcome of CoNS bacteremia is similar whether the initial antibiotic therapy is vancomycin or another agent that does not reliably treat CoNS infections (46, 47). In addition, only 1 of 5 evaluations for sepsis yields a causative organism (48). The fact that over 80% of blood cultures that yield CoNS are positive by 24 hours of incubation makes it possible for the clinician to change antibiotic therapy in a timely fashion if needed (49). An additional concern of vancomycin therapy has been the association of prior vancomycin use with subsequent development of Gram-negative bacteremia among hospitalized pediatric patients (50). The emergence of community-associated methicillin-resistant *Staphylococcus aureus* (CA-MRSA) in NICUs may limit the use of such a policy in NICUs where the prevalence of CA-MRSA is high (51, 52). However, by routine screening for MRSA and appropriate isolation precautions for colonized infants, MRSA can be controlled if not eradicated in NICUs (53).

Aminoglycosides have been the time-honored choice for empiric treatment of infections due to Gram-negative bacilli (54). Once daily or extended dosing of gentamicin is used frequently in both full-term and preterm infants based on sound pharmacodynamic and pharmacokinetic considerations (55). Such a dosing schedule may maximize the bactericidal activity of the aminoglycoside while minimizing its potential toxicity. A retrospective review by Jackson et al. (56) reported the occurrence of hypocalcemia in 3.5% of term and near-term newborns who received gentamicin once daily for ≥4 days after a change in dosing regimen from every 12 hours to every 24 hours. While it is known that aminoglycosides enhance urinary calcium excretion, it is not known whether this is potentiated by higher doses of gentamicin.

Aminoglycosides have the distinct advantage of exerting less selective pressure for development of resistance in closed units like the NICU, thus minimizing the risk of emergence of resistant bacteria (57). This is in contrast to the rapid emergence of cephalosporin resistance when these agents are provided routinely for possible late-onset sepsis (58, 59). When used for empirical therapy of early-onset infection, cefotaxime has been associated with neonatal death (60). However, since CSF penetration of aminoglycosides is poor, their use in meningitis is problematic. If a lumbar puncture is not performed as part of the initial evaluation for possible sepsis, and only an aminoglycoside is used, then effective therapy for Gram-negative meningitis is not provided. Delay in the determination of whether a neonate has meningitis will delay optimal therapy for this condition.

Within 24 hours of collection, the blood cultures yielded Gram-negative rods. Cefotaxime was added to the antibiotic regimen. E. coli was subsequently identified from the blood cultures. A lumbar puncture was then performed that demonstrated 4160 white blood cells/mm³ (90% polymorphonuclear cells, 10% mononuclear cells), 8320 red blood cells/mm³, protein of 433 mg/dL and glucose of 84 mg/dL (serum glucose of 180 mg/dL). Culture of CSF yielded E. coli.

QUESTION 5. WHAT IS THE TREATMENT OF MENINGITIS IN NEONATES, AND IN PARTICULAR THAT DUE TO GRAM-NEGATIVE BACILLI?

Table 12-3 provides the recommended antimicrobial treatment for neonatal meningitis based on causative organism (61). The recommended antimicrobial dosages are provided in Table 12-4. The treatment of Gram-negative meningitis initially includes the addition of a third- or fourth-generation cephalosporin such as cefotaxime or cefepime (62, 63), or a carbapenem antibiotic such as meropenem (54, 64, 65). Meningitis caused by Gram-negative enteric bacilli is challenging since eradication of the organism from CSF is often delayed. Moreover, many of these pathogens are now resistant to ampicillin, and aminoglycoside concentrations are typically low in CSF. Cefotaxime has superior in vitro and CSF bactericidal activity, and is the agent of choice. It is combined with an aminoglycoside at least until sterilization of CSF has been achieved. There is no experience or studies using once-daily dosing of aminoglycosides for neonatal meningitis, although from a pharmacodynamic standpoint, such a dosing schedule may be preferred since it should achieve higher CSF concentrations (54). Continued treatment of Gram-negative bacillary meningitis is based on in vitro susceptibility tests. Ampicillin may be used in the infrequent cases where the organism is susceptible.

Of concern is the production by Gram-negative bacteria of both chromosomally determined β-lactamases and plasmid-determined extended-spectrum β-lactamases (ESBLs), both of which can result in resistance to the third-generation cephalosporin antibiotics, even during therapy (66–68). Chromosomally determined β-lactamases are seen in *Enterobacter* spp., *Serratia* spp., *Pseudomonas aeruginosa*, *Citrobacter* spp., and indole-positive *Proteus*, while ESBLs are present in the Enterobacteriaceae, especially *Klebsiella pneumoniae* and *E. coli*. Treatment of infections due to Gram-negative bacteria that produce ESBLs with a third-generation cephalosporin such as cefotaxime has been associated with significantly higher mortality in adults (66). It is therefore recommended that treatment of such infections should be with a carbapenem antibiotic (meropenem or imipenem), possibly in combination with an aminoglycoside (67). Studies on the impact of these

Table 12-3 Recommended Therapy for Neonatal Meningitis

Meningitis	Therapy	Comment
Initial therapy, CSF abnormal but organism unknown	Ampicillin IV AND gentamicin IV, IM AND cefotaxime IV	Cefotaxime is added if meningitis suspected or cannot be excluded Alternatives to ampicillin in nursery-acquired infections: vancomycin or nafcillin
Bacteroides fragilis spp. *fragilis*[a]	Metronidazole IV	Alternative: meropenem
Coliform bacteria[b]	Cefotaxime IV, IM AND gentamicin	Discontinue gentamicin when clinical and microbiologic response documented Alternative: ampicillin if organism susceptible; meropenem or cefepime for mutliresistant organisms Lumbar intrathecal or intraventricular gentamicin usually not beneficial
Chryseobacterium (Flavobacterium) meningosepticum	Vancomycin IV AND Rifampin IV, PO	Alternatives: clindamycin, ciprofloxacin
Gp A streptococcus[c]	Penicillin G or ampicillin IV	
Gp B streptococcus[a]	Ampicillin or penicillin G IV AND gentamicin IV, IM	Discontinue gentamicin when clinical and microbiologic response documented
Enterococcal spp.[c]	Ampicillin IV, IM AND gentamicin IV, IM; for ampicillin-resistant organisms: vancomycin AND gentamicin	Gentamicin only if synergy documented
Other streptococcal species[c]	Penicillin or ampicillin IV, IM	
Gonococcal[d]	Ceftriaxone IV, IM OR cefotaxime IV, IM	Duration of therapy uncertain (5 to 10 days?)
Haemophilus influenzae[c]	Cefotaxime IV, IM	Ampicillin if beta-lactamase negative
Listeria monocytogenes[c]	Ampicillin IV, IM AND gentamicin IV, IM	Gentamicin is synergistic in vitro with ampicillin but can be discontinued when sterilization achieved
Staphylococcus epidermidis (or any coagulase-negative staphylococci)[d]	Vancomycin IV	Add rifampin if cultures persistently positive Alternative: linezolid
Staphylococcus aureus[b]	MSSA: nafcillin IV; MRSA: vancomycin IV	Gentamicin may provide synergy; rifampin if cultures persistently positive
Pseudomonas aeruginosa[b]	Ceftazidime IV, IM AND aminoglycoside IV, IM	Meropenem OR cefepime AND aminoglycoside are suitable alternatives
Candida spp.[e]	Amphotericin B deoxycholate (AmB-D) X 3–6 wks	Alternatives: AmB-lipid complex, AmB-liposomal, fluconazole (for susceptible strains (Candida krusei usually resistant))

(continued)

Table 12-3   Recommended Therapy for Neonatal Meningitis—cont'd

Meningitis	Therapy	Comment
		Addition of fluconazole to amphotericin if cultures persistently positive
Ureaplasma urealyticum[c]	Doxycycline IV OR Azithromycin IV	Alternatives: chloramphenicol; ciprofloxacin
Mycoplasma hominis[c]	Clindamycin OR Doxycycline IV	Alternatives: chloramphenicol; ciprofloxacin

[a]Minimum duration of therapy: 14 days.
[b]Minimum duration of therapy: 21 days; for Gram-negative meningitis, at least 14 days after CSF is sterilized, whichever is longer.
[c]Minimum duration of therapy: 10 days.
[d]Minimum duration of therapy: 7 to 10 days.
[e]Minimum duration of therapy: 4 weeks (or 30 mg/kg total dose of amphotericin deoxycholate).
MSSA, methicillin-susceptible *S. aureus*; MRSA, methicillin-resistant *S. aureus*.
Adapted from Bradley JS, Nelson JD. 2006–2007 Nelson's Pocket Book of Pediatric Antimicrobial Therapy, 16th edition. Buenos Aires: Alliance for World Wide Editing, 2006.

organisms in NICUs and the appropriate antimicrobial therapy of neonatal infections with these organisms are needed.

The treatment of GBS meningitis is ampicillin or penicillin G. No GBS resistance to penicillin G in the USA has been documented despite its extensive use in mothers and neonates. However, a recent report from Japan notes the emergence of penicillin resistance among some isolates of group B streptococci (69). Despite the in vitro resistance of GBS to aminoglycosides, the addition of gentamicin to a penicillin agent provides synergy. In general, gentamicin can be discontinued once CSF sterilization is documented by a repeat lumbar puncture performed 24 to 48 hours after initiation of therapy. With more severe cases of meningitis, some experts continue gentamicin for about 1 week; the benefit of such an approach is unproven.

Similar considerations are applicable in the preterm infant who develops meningitis while in the NICU. Potential pathogens include *Staphylococcus aureus*, coagulase-negative staphylococci, enterococci, and multiply-resistant pathogens such as MRSA and gentamicin- or cephalosporin-resistant Gram-negative enteric bacilli. Empirical therapy may include a combination of ampicillin, nafcillin, or vancomycin and an aminoglycoside, cefotaxime, or even meropenem, depending on the predominant pathogens seen in that NICU. Ceftazidime or meropenem in combination with an aminoglycoside should be used for *P. aeruginosa* meningitis. *Chryseobacterium* (formerly *Flavobacterium*) *meningosepticum*, a multiply-resistant Gram-negative bacillus, is a rare cause of meningitis that requires treatment with vancomycin and rifampin, or even ciprofloxacin.

Meningitis due to anaerobic bacteria is infrequent, and is usually caused by *Bacteroides fragilis* and *Clostridium* spp., mostly *C. perfringens* (70). The mortality rate is high. Penicillin, ampicillin, cephalosporins, and vancomycin are active against many Gram-positive anaerobes. They have little if any activity against most anaerobic Gram-negative bacilli; metronidazole is the agent of choice for meningitis secondary to these organisms. Carbapenem antibiotics such as meropenem and imipenem have excellent anaerobic activity against both Gram-positive and negative organisms and also can be used.

The treatment of neonatal infections caused by *Ureaplasma urealyticum* and *Mycoplasma hominis* is complicated by the susceptibility patterns of these organisms since they usually are resistant to most antibiotics commonly used in neonates (71). For infections due to *U. urealyticum*, doxycycline is recommended, with azithromycin as an alternative. For *M. hominis*, clindamycin or doxycycline is preferred, with ciprofloxacin as an alternative. Although the exact duration of therapy is not known,

Table 12-4 Antimicrobial Dosages for Neonates with Meningitis

(A) Drugs Dosed by Weight and Age

Antibiotic	Route	Dosages (mg/kg/day) and intervals of administration				Chronologic age > 28 days
		Chronologic age < 28 days				
		Body weight ≤ 2000 g		Body weight > 2000 g		
		0–7 d old	8–28 d old	0–7 d old	8–28 d old	
Amphotericin B						
deoxycholate	IV	1 q24h	1 q24h	1 q24h	1 q24h	1 q24h
lipid complex	IV	5 q24h	5 q24h	5 q24h	5 q24h	5 q24h
liposomal	IV	5 q24h	5 q24h	5 q24h	5 q24h	5 q24h
Ampicillin	IV, IM	100 div q12h	150 div q8h	150 div q8h	200 div q6h	200 div q6h
Azithromycin	IV	10 q24h	10 q24h	10 q24h	10 q24h	10 q24h
Cefepime[a]	IV, IM	90 div q8h	90 div q8h	90 div q8h	90–150 div q8h[a]	150 div q8h
Cefotaxime	IV, IM	100–200 div q12h	150–300 div	100–200 div q12h	150–300 div	150–300 div q6–8h
Ceftazidime	IV, IM	100–200 div q12h	150–300 div q8h	100–200 div q12h	150–300 div q8h	150–300 div q8h
Ceftriaxone	IV, IM	50 q24h	80–100 q24h	50 q24h	80–100 q24h	100 q24h
Clindamycin	IV, IM	15 div q12h	20–30 div q8h	20–30 div q8h	20–30 div q8h	30 div q6h
Fluconazole	IV	12 q72h	12 q48h	12 q24h	12 q24h	12 q24h
Linezolid	IV	20 div q12h	30 div q8h	30 div q8h	30 div q8h	30 div q8h
Meropenem	IV	80 div q12h	120 div q8h	80 div q8h	120 div q8h	120 div q8h
Metronidazole	IV, PO	7.5 div q24h	15 div q12h	15 div q12h	30 div q12h	30 div q6h
Nafcillin, oxacillin	IV	100 div q12h	150–200 div q8h	150 div q8h	150–200 div q6h	150–200 div q6h
Penicillin G, crystalline	IV	200,000 U div q12h	300,000 U div q8h	300,000 U div q8h	400,000 U div q6h	400,000 U div q6h
Piperacillin	IV	200 div q12h	300 div q8h	200 div q12h	300 div q8h	400 div q6h
Rifampin	IV, PO	10–20 q24h	10–20 q24h	10–20 q24h	10–20 q24h	10–20 q24h
Ticarcillin	IV	200 div q12h	300 div q8h	300 div q8h	300 div q6h	300 div q6h
Voriconazole	IV, PO	8–20 div q12h	8–20 div q12 h	8–20 div q12 h	8–20 div q12 h	8–20 div q12 h

(continued)

Table 12-4   Antimicrobial Dosages for Neonates with Meningitis—cont'd

(B) Drugs Dosed According Only to Age

Drug	Route of administration	Dosage (mg/kg/dose) by gestational age plus weeks of age			
		< 26 wks	27–34 wks	35–42 wks	≥ 43 wks
Acyclovir	IV	20 q12h	20 q12h	20 q8h	20 q8h
Amikacin[b]	IV, IM	7.5 q24h	10 q24	15 q24h	15 q24h
Ganciclovir	IV	6 q24h	6 q18h	6 q12h	6 q12h
Gentamicin[c]	IV, IM	2.5 q24h	3 q18h	4 q24h	4 q24h
Tobramycin[c]	IV, IM	2.5 q24h	3 q18h	4 q24h	4 q24h
Vancomycin[d]	IV	15 q24h	15 q18h[e]	15 q12h[e]	15 q8h[e]

[a]Cefepime for severe infections (e.g., meningitis or pseudomonas infections) should be given at 90 mg/kg/day div q8h for the first 2 weeks of age, after which the dosing increases to 150 mg/kg/day q8h.

[b]Desired serum concentrations: 20–30 μg/mL (peak), < 10 μg/mL (trough).

[c]Desired serum concentrations: 5–12 μg/mL (peak), < 2.0 μg/mL (trough).

[d]Desired serum concentrations: 20–40 μg/mL (peak), < 10–15 μg/mL (trough).

[e]At 28 days of age (4 weeks), vancomycin is dosed at 20 mg/kg/dose. The interval remains the same.

Adapted from Bradley JS, Nelson JD. 2006–2007 Nelson's Pocket Book of Pediatric Antimicrobial Therapy, 16th edition. Buenos Aires: Alliance for World Wide Editing, 2006.

a 10- to 14-day course seems reasonable when there is associated clinical improvement and microbiologic eradication during that period.

Neonatal fungal infection of the central nervous system is usually caused by *Candida* spp. (72). Amphotericin deoxycholate remains the treatment of choice (73), and it has been used successfully as monotherapy (74). Amphotericin B lipid formulations may be used if renal toxicity occurs while the infant is receiving the deoxycholate preparation. Fluconazole has excellent central nervous system penetration and is frequently added to amphotericin therapy in cases of persistent fungemia or poor clinical response (75, 76). There is limited experience in neonates with the use of newer azoles such as voriconazole that are active against more resistant fungi such as *C. krusei* and *C. glabrata* (77, 78). Echinocandins such as casponfungin and micafungin do not penetrate well into the central nervous system (79, 80).

A lumbar puncture was repeated 24 hours after diagnosis of meningitis and the CSF showed 6900 white blood cells/mm^3 (90% polymorphonuclear cells, 10% mononuclear cells), 2400 red blood cells/mm^3, protein of 550 mg/dL and glucose of 21 mg/dL. Culture of CSF again yielded E. coli that was resistant to ampicillin but susceptible to cefotaxime, ceftazidime, and gentamicin with MICs of 2 μg/mL.

QUESTION 6. SHOULD OTHER THERAPIES BE CONSIDERED?

Meningitis secondary to Gram-negative bacilli is associated with persistently positive CSF cultures despite appropriate therapy. The median duration of positive CSF cultures is 3 days, and the duration of positivity has correlated with long-term prognosis. In addition, duration of positive CSF culture will impact total length of therapy. For these reasons, it is recommended that daily or every other day lumbar punctures be performed in order to determine both occurrence and timing of CSF sterilization.

Both lumbar intrathecal and intraventricular gentamicin have been used for treatment of Gram-negative meningitis (81, 82). Ventriculitis occurs in at least 70% of cases, and the ventricular fluid is poorly accessible to systemically administered antibiotics. However, among infants who received parenteral drug alone or parenteral plus intrathecal therapy (1 mg/day for at least 3 days), no differences in either case-fatality rate or neurologic residua were observed by the Neonatal Meningitis Cooperative Study Group (81). These investigators subsequently studied the use of intraventricular gentamicin (2.5 mg); there was higher mortality among infants who received intraventricular gentamicin (43%) in combination with ampicillin and gentamicin than in those who received systemic antibiotics alone (13%) (82). Subsequent evaluation of ventricular fluid from infants who received intraventricular gentamicin showed significantly greater concentrations of tumor necrosis factor and interleukin 1-β in their CSFs, indicating that greater inflammatory injury may result from this form of therapy (83). In general, intraventricular therapy is not recommended, although it remains an option in those infants who already have a ventricular drain in place and persistently positive CSF cultures.

A cranial ultrasound performed on day 2 and day 7 after presentation did not demonstrate abscess formation or new intracranial hemorrhage, but did show mild ventricular dilatation, and echogenic debris and septations were visualized within the ventricular system (Fig. 12-1). The infant continued to receive cefotaxime and was nearing 21 days of therapy.

QUESTION 7. WHAT IS THE DURATION OF TREATMENT FOR MENINGITIS IN NEONATES?

Unfortunately, there are no randomized studies of duration of antibiotic therapy for neonatal meningitis. In general, duration of therapy is dependent on the

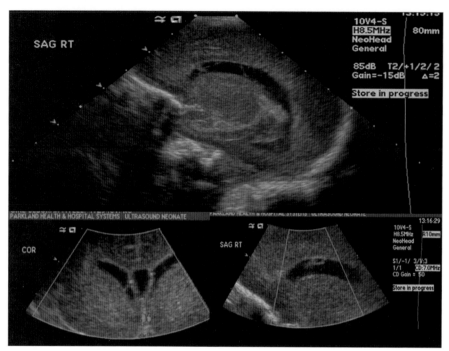

Figure 12-1 Cranial ultrasound performed on a 2-week-old extremely low birth weight infant with meningitis caused by *Escherichia coli*. There is echogenic debris and septation consistent with purulent material within the dilated lateral ventricle.

causative organism, site(s) of infection, clinical severity, and course. This is usually 7 days for uncomplicated bacteremia, 7 to 10 days for sepsis and pneumonia, and 14 to 21 days for meningitis, depending on the causative agent. Normalization of the CRP or other inflammatory markers such as IL-8 or IL-10 has been utilized to discontinue antibiotic therapy (84, 85). Although this approach seems reasonable, more studies involving high-risk neonates with serious infections such as meningitis are needed before such a strategy can be recommended routinely.

For meningitis due to Gram-negative bacilli, the duration of antimicrobial therapy is a minimum of 21 days or 2 weeks after the first sterile CSF culture, whichever is longest. Earlier discontinuation of antimicrobial therapy may result in bacterial relapse. Performance of another lumbar puncture after 21 days of treatment in infants with Gram-negative enteric meningitis and before discontinuation of antibiotic therapy is useful to determine the adequacy of therapy. Markedly abnormal CSF findings, such as glucose concentration <25 mg/dL, protein content >300 mg/dL, or >50% polymorphonuclear cells, without other explanation warrant continued antimicrobial therapy in order to prevent relapse.

For meningitis due to group B streptococcus, a minimum of 14 days of antimicrobial therapy is recommended. The decision of whether to perform an "end of therapy" lumbar puncture in these neonates can be based on clinical course: if the infant has experienced such complications as seizures, significant hypotension, or prolonged positive CSF cultures, or if neuroimaging is abnormal, then it is probably prudent to do it.

The optimal duration of therapy for meningitis due to other microorganisms is not known. Meningitis secondary to *S. aureus* should be treated with at least 3 weeks of antibiotic therapy. In general, cerebral abscess requires more prolonged therapy of 4 to 6 weeks, depending on whether it is surgically drained or there is persistence of abnormalities on neuroimaging.

QUESTION 8. WHEN SHOULD NEUROIMAGING BE CONSIDERED AND WHAT TYPE OF EXAMINATION IS RECOMMENDED?

The timing and the reason for performing neuroimaging studies are important considerations in the decision as to which type of study should be performed. Cranial ultrasonography is safe, convenient, and readily available; it can be done at the bedside and does not require sedation. It provides rapid and reliable information on ventricular size and whether there is development of hydrocephalus (86). It is therefore useful to perform an ultrasound early in the course when the infant is too critical to transport to radiology. Cranial ultrasonography also will provide information on periventricular white matter injury; initially, ischemia may be manifested by increased periventricular echogenicity, which may progress to cystic periventricular leukomalacia in later studies (Fig. 12-2) (87, 88). Ultrasonography, however, does not allow for optimal evaluation of parenchymal abnormalities such as infarct or abscess nor of presence of subdural empyema, all known complications of neonatal meningitis.

Computed tomography (CT) will provide information on whether the course of meningitis has been complicated by a cerebral abscess, hydrocephalus, or subdural collections. In general, however, CT scans should be avoided except if neuroimaging is required on an emergent basis since its use has been associated with subsequent neurodevelopmental impairment and increased risk for cancer (89, 90).

Magnetic resonance imaging (MRI) is the best currently available modality for evaluation of the neonatal brain. It provides excellent information on the status of the white matter, cortex, subdural and epidural spaces, and even the posterior fossa in cases of tuberculous meningitis (Fig. 12-3). In addition, it has been used in preterm infants to predict neurodevelopmental outcome (91). For these reasons, infants with suspected cerebral injury either because of abnormalities on ultrasonography, seizures, persistent CSF abnormalities, or meningitis due to organisms such as *Citrobacter koseri* (formerly *C. diversus*) or fungi that are associated with abscess formation should have brain MRI performed. Cerebral abscess complicates the course of about 70% of cases of *C. koseri* meningitis, whereas it occurs in <10% of meningitis due to other Gram-negative enteric bacilli (Fig. 12-4) (92, 93). Microabscesses also are not infrequent with neonatal fungal meningitis. For these reasons, many experts recommend that at least one brain MRI be performed on every case of neonatal meningitis. In addition, all infants with meningitis require hearing evaluation.

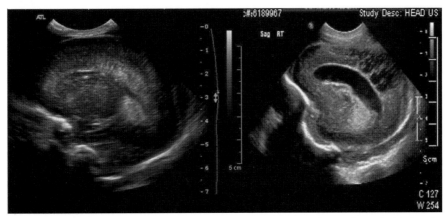

Figure 12-2 Cranial ultrasound performed on an extremely low birth weight infant with meningitis that demonstrates echogenic periventricular white matter (left) with subsequent progression to cystic periventricular leukomalacia (right).

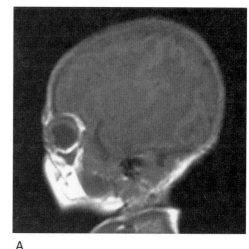

A

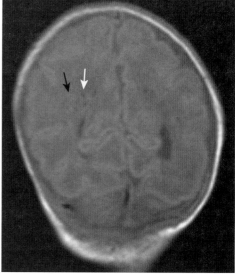

B

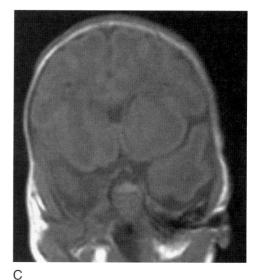

C

Figure 12-3 Magnetic resonance imaging of the brain of an infant who 4 weeks earlier had *Pseudomonas aeruginosa* sepsis and meningitis. (A) On the T2-weighted images, small foci of high signal are seen in the periventricular white matter in the frontoparietal and occipital regions. These represent areas of cystic encephalomalacia, consistent with periventricular leukomalacia. (B) Small foci of hemosiderin deposition (black arrow) are seen in the posterior right temporo-occipital region along with cystic encephalomalacia changes (white arrow). (C) Coronal image of periventricular white matter.

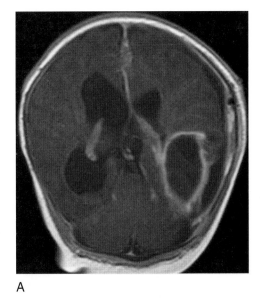

A

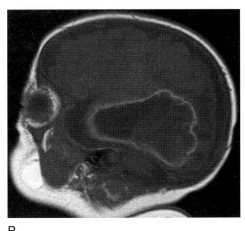

B

Figure 12-4 Magnetic resonance image of the brain of a 3-week-old full-term infant with meningitis and cerebral abscess caused by *Serratia marcescens*. Following gadolinium administration, a large ring-enhancing lesion is seen that extends from the posterior aspect of the temporal lobe into the adjacent parietal and occipital white matter.

QUESTION 9. SHOULD OTHER ADJUNCTIVE THERAPIES BE PROVIDED TO AN INFANT WITH MENINGITIS?

Dexamethasone has been shown in some studies to decrease neurological morbidity in older infants and children with meningitis (94–96). No studies are available in neonates, and its use is not recommended. In a rabbit model of *E. coli* meningitis, the addition of dexamethasone to standard antibiotic therapy was associated with an increase in hippocampal neuronal apoptosis (97).

The prolonged use of broad-spectrum antimicrobial agents, especially third-generation cephalosporins and carbapenems, has been associated with development of systemic candidiasis in preterm infants with birth weight less than 1000 g (98). Prophylactic fluconazole has been shown to decrease the incidence of candidiasis in these infants (99), and it use should be considered in preterm infants with meningitis who require prolonged broad-spectrum antimicrobial therapy (100).

No data from randomized controlled clinical trials are available in infants with birth weight greater than 1000 g.

QUESTION 10. WHAT IF THE INFANT'S CSF IS ABNORMAL BUT ROUTINE BACTERIAL CULTURES OF CSF AND BLOOD ARE STERILE?

The most frequent reason for a sterile CSF culture despite CSF changes indicative of meningitis is previous antimicrobial therapy. However, intraventricular hemorrhage can result in inflammatory changes such as pleocytosis with predominance of poly-morphonuclear cells, elevated protein concentration, and hypoglycorrhachia in the absence of an infectious process, making the performance of a lumbar puncture before initiation of antimicrobial therapy important.

When an infant suspected of having sepsis and meningitis has abnormal CSF indices but routine bacterial cultures are sterile, a repeat lumbar puncture should be performed. Pathogens that can produce aseptic meningitis should be excluded (Table 12-1), especially since specific therapy is available for some of them. CSF should be sent for anaerobic, mycoplasma, fungal, and viral cultures, as well as tests for herpes and enteroviruses by polymerase chain reaction (PCR).

The infant's CSF evaluation was markedly improved after 21 days of cefotaxime, and MRI examination revealed only mild ventriculomegaly. At discharge to home at 3 months of age, the infant passed an automated auditory brainstem response test. At 22 months of corrected gestational age, the infant had mild impairment in both mental and psychomotor development indexes by Bayley Scales of Infant Development.

QUESTION 11. WHAT IS THE OUTCOME OF MENINGITIS IN NEONATES?

Despite improvements in neonatal care and antibiotic therapy, significant morbidity and mortality persist (101). Among preterm infants with birth weight ≤1000 g, infants with meningitis are more likely to have low (<70) mental and psychomotor indexes, cerebral palsy, vision impairment, and head circumference <10% compared with uninfected infants of similar birth weight and gestation (102).

Among infants with Gram-negative enteric meningitis, the case-fatality rate and morbidity remain high. Approximately 20–30% of affected infants die, and neurologic sequelae are found in 35–50% of survivors (81, 82, 103). These include hydrocephalus (30%), seizure disorder (30%), developmental delay (30%), cerebral palsy (25%), and hearing loss (15%). Ten per cent have severe sequelae defined as failure to develop beyond the age at which the disease occurred or required custodial care. It is hoped that prediction of late morbidity will be aided by the use of brain MRI performed towards the end of therapy.

Among infants with GBS meningitis, the mortality is about 25%, and among survivors, another 25 to 30% of children have major neurologic sequelae such as spastic quadriplegia, profound mental retardation, hemiparesis, deafness, or cortical blindness, while 15 to 20% have mild-to-moderate sequelae, and 50 to 60% are normal when compared with sibling controls (104, 105). The occurrence of seizures during the acute illness has been associated with a poor prognosis; these children were more likely to die or sustain major sequelae. On the other hand, children not identified early as having major sequelae performed intellectually, socially, and academically in a manner similar to other family members.

CONCLUSIONS

Meningitis is a serious infection where early therapy is mandatory to improve both short- and long-term outcomes. This is possible only by the timely recognition of its occurrence, thus making performance of a lumbar puncture for CSF analysis and culture the key to rapid institution of effective antimicrobial therapy. Ultimately, however, its prevention will be achieved when neonatal sepsis is controlled, an elusive but not impossible goal in neonatal medicine today.

REFERENCES

1. Kaufman D, Fairchild KD. Clinical microbiology of bacterial and fungal sepsis in very-low-birth-weight infants. Clin Microbiol Rev 17(3):638–80, table of contents, 2004.
2. Palazzi DL, Klein JO, Baker CJ. Bacterial sepsis and meningitis. In Remington JS, Wilson CB, Baker CJ (eds). Infectious Diseases of the Fetus and Newborn Infant, 6th edition. Philadelphia, PA: WB Saunders, 2006, 247–95.
3. Giacoia GP. Uncommon pathogens in newborn infants. J Perinatol 14(2):134–44, 1994.
4. Schrag S, Gorwitz R, Fultz-Butts K, Schuchat A. Prevention of perinatal group B streptococcal disease. Revised guidelines from CDC. MMWR Recomm Rep 51(RR-11):1–22, 2002.
5. Johnson CE, Whitwell JK, Pethe K, et al. Term newborns who are at risk for sepsis: are lumbar punctures necessary? Pediatrics 99(4):E10, 1997.
6. Smith PB, Cotten CM, Garges HP, et al. A comparison of neonatal Gram-negative rod and Gram-positive cocci meningitis. J Perinatol 26(2):111–14, 2006.
7. Schrag SJ, Zywicki S, Farley MM, et al. Group B streptococcal disease in the era of intrapartum antibiotic prophylaxis. N Engl J Med 342(1):15–20, 2000.
8. Schrag SJ, Hadler JL, Arnold KE, et al. Risk factors for invasive, early-onset Escherichia coli infections in the era of widespread intrapartum antibiotic use. Pediatrics 118(2):570–6, 2006.
9. Baltimore RS, Huie SM, Meek JI, et al. Early-onset neonatal sepsis in the era of group B streptococcal prevention. Pediatrics 108(5):1094–8, 2001.
10. Stoll BJ, Hansen N, Fanaroff AA, et al. Changes in pathogens causing early-onset sepsis in very-low-birth-weight infants. N Engl J Med 347(4):240–7, 2002.
11. Stoll BJ, Hansen NI, Higgins RD, et al. Very low birth weight preterm infants with early onset neonatal sepsis: the predominance of gram-negative infections continues in the National Institute of Child Health and Human Development Neonatal Research Network, 2002–2003. Pediatr Infect Dis J 24(7):635–9, 2005.
12. Garges HP, Moody MA, Cotten CM, et al. Neonatal meningitis: what is the correlation among cerebrospinal fluid cultures, blood cultures, and cerebrospinal fluid parameters? Pediatrics 117(4):1094–100, 2006.
13. Stoll BJ, Hansen N, Fanaroff AA, et al. To tap or not to tap: high likelihood of meningitis without sepsis among very low birth weight infants. Pediatrics 113(5):1181–6, 2004.
14. Cohen-Wolkowiez M, Smith PB, Mangum B, et al. Neonatal candida meningitis: significance of cerebrospinal fluid parameters and blood cultures. J Perinatol 27(2):97–100, 2007.
15. Wiswell TE, Baumgart S, Gannon CM, Spitzer AR. No lumbar puncture in the evaluation for early neonatal sepsis: will meningitis be missed? Pediatrics 95(6):803–6, 1995.
16. Malbon K, Mohan R, Nicholl R. Should a neonate with possible late onset infection always have a lumbar puncture? Arch Dis Child 91(1):75–6, 2006.
17. Ahmed A, Hickey SM, Ehrett S, et al. Cerebrospinal fluid values in the term neonate. Pediatr Infect Dis J 15(4):298–303, 1996.
18. Bonadio WA. The cerebrospinal fluid: physiologic aspects and alterations associated with bacterial meningitis. Pediatr Infect Dis J 11(6):423–31, 1992.
19. Pappu LD, Purohit DM, Levkoff AH, Kaplan B. CSF cytology in the neonate. Am J Dis Child 136(4):297–8, 1982.
20. Portnoy JM, Olson LC. Normal cerebrospinal fluid values in children: another look. Pediatrics 75(3):484–7, 1985.
21. Rodriguez AF, Kaplan SL, Mason EO Jr. Cerebrospinal fluid values in the very low birth weight infant. J Pediatr 116(6):971–4, 1990.
22. Sarff LD, Platt LH, McCracken GH Jr. Cerebrospinal fluid evaluation in neonates: comparison of high-risk infants with and without meningitis. J Pediatr 88(3):473–7, 1976.
23. Naidoo BT. The cerebrospinal fluid in the healthy newborn infant. S Afr Med J 42(35):933–5, 1968.
24. O'Shea TM, Klinepeter KL, Meis PJ, Dillard RG. Intrauterine infection and the risk of cerebral palsy in very low-birthweight infants. Paediatr Perinat Epidemiol 12(1):72–83, 1998.
25. Eldadah M, Frenkel LD, Hiatt IM, Hegyi T. Evaluation of routine lumbar punctures in newborn infants with respiratory distress syndrome. Pediatr Infect Dis J 6(3):243–6, 1987.
26. Hendricks-Munoz KD, Shapiro DL. The role of the lumbar puncture in the admission sepsis evaluation of the premature infant. J Perinatol 10(1):60–4, 1990.
27. MacMahon P, Jewes L, de Louvois J. Routine lumbar punctures in the newborn: are they justified? Eur J Pediatr 149(11):797–9, 1990.

28. Weiss MG, Ionides SP, Anderson CL. Meningitis in premature infants with respiratory distress: role of admission lumbar puncture. J Pediatr 119(6):973–5, 1991.

29. Isaacs D, Dobson S. When to do a lumbar puncture in a neonate. Arch Dis Child 64(10):1513–14, 1989.

30. Laborada G, Rego M, Jain A, et al. Diagnostic value of cytokines and C-reactive protein in the first 24 hours of neonatal sepsis. Am J Perinatol 20(8):491–501, 2003.

31. Verboon-Maciolek MA, Thijsen SF, Hemels MA, et al. Inflammatory mediators for the diagnosis and treatment of sepsis in early infancy. Pediatr Res 59(3):457–61, 2006.

32. Manroe BL, Weinberg AG, Rosenfeld CR, Browne R. The neonatal blood count in health and disease: I. Reference values for neutrophilic cells. J Pediatr 95(1):89–98, 1979.

33. Mouzinho A, Rosenfeld CR, Sanchez PJ, Risser R. Revised reference ranges for circulating neutrophils in very-low-birth-weight neonates. Pediatrics 94(1):76–82, 1994.

34. Engle WD, Rosenfeld CR, Mouzinho A, et al. Circulating neutrophils in septic preterm neonates: comparison of two reference ranges. Pediatrics 99(3):E10, 1997.

35. Christensen RD, Brown MS, Hall DC, et al. Effect on neutrophil kinetics and serum opsonic capacity of intravenous administration of immune globulin to neonates with clinical signs of early-onset sepsis. J Pediatr 118(4 Pt 1):606–14, 1991.

36. Christensen RD, Calhoun DA, Rimsza LM. A practical approach to evaluating and treating neutropenia in the neonatal intensive care unit. Clin Perinatol 27(3):577–601, 2000.

37. Cairo MS, Worcester CC, Rucker RW, et al. Randomized trial of granulocyte transfusions versus intravenous immune globulin therapy for neonatal neutropenia and sepsis. J Pediatr 120(2 Pt 1):281–5, 1992.

38. Shaw CK, Thapalial A, Shaw P, Malla K. Intravenous immunoglobulins and haematopoietic growth factors in the prevention and treatment of neonatal sepsis: ground reality or glorified myths? Int J Clin Pract 61(3):482–7, 2007.

39. Benjamin DK Jr, DeLong ER, Steinbach WJ, et al. Empirical therapy for neonatal candidemia in very low birth weight infants. Pediatrics 112(3 Pt 1):543–7, 2003.

40. Struthers S, Underhill H, Albersheim S, et al. A comparison of two versus one blood culture in the diagnosis and treatment of coagulase-negative staphylococcus in the neonatal intensive care unit. J Perinatol 22(7):547–9, 2002.

41. Rubin LG, Sanchez PJ, Siegel J, et al. Evaluation and treatment of neonates with suspected late-onset sepsis: a survey of neonatologists' practices. Pediatrics 110(4):e42, 2002.

42. Bauer S, Eliakim A, Pomeranz A, et al. Urinary tract infection in very low birth weight preterm infants. Pediatr Infect Dis J 22(5):426–30, 2003.

43. American Academy of Pediatrics. Committee on Quality Improvement. Subcommittee on Urinary Tract Infection. Practice parameter: the diagnosis, treatment, and evaluation of the initial urinary tract infection in febrile infants and young children. Pediatrics 103(4 Pt 1):843–52, 1999.

44. Sanchez PJ. Bacterial and fungal infections in the neonate: current diagnosis and therapy. Adv Exp Med Biol 549:97–103, 2004.

45. Karlowicz MG, Buescher ES, Surka AE. Fulminant late-onset sepsis in a neonatal intensive care unit, 1988–1997, and the impact of avoiding empiric vancomycin therapy. Pediatrics 106(6):1387–90, 2000.

46. Krediet TG, Jones ME, Gerards LJ, Fleer A. Clinical outcome of cephalothin versus vancomycin therapy in the treatment of coagulase-negative staphylococcal septicemia in neonates: relation to methicillin resistance and mec A gene carriage of blood isolates. Pediatrics 103(3):E29, 1999.

47. Lawrence SL, Roth V, Slinger R, et al. Cloxacillin versus vancomycin for presumed late-onset sepsis in the neonatal intensive care unit and the impact upon outcome of coagulase negative staphylococcal bacteremia: a retrospective cohort study. BMC Pediatr 5:49, 2005.

48. Stoll BJ, Hansen N, Fanaroff AA, et al. Late-onset sepsis in very low birth weight neonates: the experience of the NICHD Neonatal Research Network. Pediatrics 110(2 Pt 1):285–91, 2002.

49. Garcia-Prats JA, Cooper TR, Schneider VF, et al. Rapid detection of microorganisms in blood cultures of newborn infants utilizing an automated blood culture system. Pediatrics 105(3 Pt 1):523–7, 2000.

50. Van Houten MA, Uiterwaal CS, Heesen GJ, et al. Does the empiric use of vancomycin in pediatrics increase the risk for Gram-negative bacteremia? Pediatr Infect Dis J 20(2):171–7, 2001.

51. Healy CM, Hulten KG, Palazzi DL, et al. Emergence of new strains of methicillin-resistant Staphylococcus aureus in a neonatal intensive care unit. Clin Infect Dis 39(10):1460–6, 2004.

52. Chuang YY, Huang YC, Lee CY, et al. Methicillin-resistant Staphylococcus aureus bacteraemia in neonatal intensive care units: an analysis of 90 episodes. Acta Paediatr 93(6):786–90, 2004.

53. Haley RW, Cushion NB, Tenover FC, et al. Eradication of endemic methicillin-resistant Staphylococcus aureus infections from a neonatal intensive care unit. J Infect Dis 171(3):614–24, 1995.

54. de Hoog M, Mouton JW, van den Anker JN. New dosing strategies for antibacterial agents in the neonate. Semin Fetal Neonatal Med 10(2):185–94, 2005.

55. Nestaas E, Bangstad HJ, Sandvik L, Wathne KO. Aminoglycoside extended interval dosing in neonates is safe and effective: a meta-analysis. Arch Dis Child Fetal Neonatal Ed 90(4):F294–300, 2005.

56. Jackson GL, Sendelbach DM, Stehel EK, et al. Association of hypocalcemia with a change in gentamicin administration in neonates. Pediatr Nephrol 18(7):653–6, 2003.

57. de Man P, Verhoeven BA, Verbrugh HA, et al. An antibiotic policy to prevent emergence of resistant bacilli. Lancet 355(9208):973–8, 2000.

58. Acolet D, Ahmet Z, Houang E, et al. Enterobacter cloacae in a neonatal intensive care unit: account of an outbreak and its relationship to use of third generation cephalosporins. J Hosp Infect 28(4):273–86, 1994.

59. Bryan CS, John JF Jr, Pai MS, Austin TL. Gentamicin vs cefotaxime for therapy of neonatal sepsis. Relationship to drug resistance. Am J Dis Child 139(11):1086–9, 1985.

60. Clark RH, Bloom BT, Spitzer AR, Gerstmann DR. Empiric use of ampicillin and cefotaxime, compared with ampicillin and gentamicin, for neonates at risk for sepsis is associated with an increased risk of neonatal death. Pediatrics 117(1):67–74, 2006.

61. Bradley J, Nelson J. 2006–2007 Nelson's Pocket Book of Pediatric Antimicrobial Therapy, 16th edition. Buenos Aires: Alliance for World Wide Editing, 2006.

62. Ellis JM, Rivera L, Reyes G, et al. Cefepime cerebrospinal fluid concentrations in neonatal bacterial meningitis. Ann Pharmacother 41:900–1, 2007.

63. Capparelli E, Hochwald C, Rasmussen M, et al. Population pharmacokinetics of cefepime in the neonate. Antimicrob Agents Chemother 49(7):2760–6, 2005.

64. Shah D, Narang M. Meropenem. Indian Pediatr 42:443–50, 2004.

65. Odio CM, Puig JR, Feris JM, et al. Prospective, randomized, investigator-blinded study of the efficacy and safety of meropenem vs. cefotaxime therapy in bacterial meningitis in children. Meropenem Meningitis Study Group. Pediatr Infect Dis J 18(7):581–90, 1999.

66. Wong-Beringer A, Hindler J, Loeloff M, et al. Molecular correlation for the treatment outcomes in bloodstream infections caused by Escherichia coli and Klebsiella pneumoniae with reduced susceptibility to ceftazidime. Clin Infect Dis 34(2):135–46, 2002.

67. Patterson JE. Extended spectrum beta-lactamases: a therapeutic dilemma. Pediatr Infect Dis J 21(10):957–9, 2002.

68. Sinha AK, Kempley ST, Price E, et al. Early onset Morganella morganii sepsis in a newborn infant with emergence of cephalosporin resistance caused by depression of AMPC beta-lactamase production. Pediatr Infect Dis J 25(4):376–7, 2006.

69. Kimura KWJ, Kurokawa H, Suzuki S, et al. Emergence of penicillin-resistant group B streptococci. In 46th Annual Interscience Conference on Antimicrobial Agents and Chemotherapy (ICAAC™), San Francisco, CA, September 27–30, 2006.

70. Brook I. Anaerobic infections in the neonate. Adv Pediatr 41:369–83, 1994.

71. Cassell GH, Waites KB, Watson HL, et al. Ureaplasma urealyticum intrauterine infection: role in prematurity and disease in newborns. Clin Microbiol Rev 6(1):69–87, 1993.

72. Fernandez M, Moylett EH, Noyola DE, Baker CJ. Candidal meningitis in neonates: a 10-year review. Clin Infect Dis 31(2):458–63, 2000.

73. Frattarelli DA, Reed MD, Giacoia GP, Aranda JV. Antifungals in systemic neonatal candidiasis. Drugs 64(9):949–68, 2004.

74. Butler KM, Rench MA, Baker CJ. Amphotericin B as a single agent in the treatment of systemic candidiasis in neonates. Pediatr Infect Dis J 9(1):51–6, 1990.

75. Gurses N, Kalayci AG. Fluconazole monotherapy for candidal meningitis in a premature infant. Clin Infect Dis 23(3):645–6, 1996.

76. Black KE, Baden LR. Fungal infections of the CNS: treatment strategies for the immunocompromised patient. CNS Drugs 21(4):293–318, 2007.

77. Steinbach WJ, Benjamin DK. New antifungal agents under development in children and neonates. Curr Opin Infect Dis 18(6):484–9, 2005.

78. Santos RP, Sanchez PJ, Mejias A, et al. Successful medical treatment of cutaneous aspergillosis in a premature infant using liposomal amphotericin B, voriconazole and micafungin. Pediatr Infect Dis J 26(4):364–6, 2007.

79. Odio CM, Araya R, Pinto LE, et al. Caspofungin therapy of neonates with invasive candidiasis. Pediatr Infect Dis J 23(12):1093–7, 2004.

80. Heresi GP, Gerstmann DR, Reed MD, et al. The pharmacokinetics and safety of micafungin, a novel echinocandin, in premature infants. Pediatr Infect Dis J 25(12):1110–15, 2006.

81. McCracken GH Jr, Mize SG. A controlled study of intrathecal antibiotic therapy in gram-negative enteric meningitis of infancy. Report of the Neonatal Meningitis Cooperative Study Group. J Pediatr 89(1):66–72, 1976.

82. McCracken GH Jr, Mize SG, Threlkeld N. Intraventricular gentamicin therapy in gram-negative bacillary meningitis of infancy. Report of the Second Neonatal Meningitis Cooperative Study Group. Lancet 1(8172):787–91, 1980.

83. McCracken GH Jr, Mustafa MM, Ramilo O, et al. Cerebrospinal fluid interleukin 1-beta and tumor necrosis factor concentrations and outcome from neonatal gram-negative enteric bacillary meningitis. Pediatr Infect Dis J 8(3):155–9, 1989.

84. Franz AR, Steinbach G, Kron M, Pohlandt F. Reduction of unnecessary antibiotic therapy in newborn infants using interleukin-8 and C-reactive protein as markers of bacterial infections. Pediatrics 104(3 Pt 1):447–53, 1999.

85. Franz AR, Bauer K, Schalk A, et al. Measurement of interleukin 8 in combination with C-reactive protein reduced unnecessary antibiotic therapy in newborn infants: a multicenter, randomized, controlled trial. Pediatrics 114(1):1–8, 2004.

86. Perlman JM, Rollins N, Sanchez PJ. Late-onset meningitis in sick, very-low-birth-weight infants. Clinical and sonographic observations. Am J Dis Child 146(11):1297–301, 1992.

87. Faix RG, Donn SM. Association of septic shock caused by early-onset group B streptococcal sepsis and periventricular leukomalacia in the preterm infant. Pediatrics 76(3):415–19, 1985.

88. Perlman JM. White matter injury in the preterm infant: an important determination of abnormal neurodevelopment outcome. Early Hum Dev 53(2):99–120, 1998.

89. Brenner DJ. Estimating cancer risks from pediatric CT: going from the qualitative to the quantitative. Pediatr Radiol 32(4):228-31; discussion 242-4, 2002.

90. Frush DP, Donnelly LF, Rosen NS. Computed tomography and radiation risks: what pediatric health care providers should know. Pediatrics 112(4):951–7, 2003.

91. Woodward LJ, Anderson PJ, Austin NC, et al. Neonatal MRI to predict neurodevelopmental outcomes in preterm infants. N Engl J Med 355(7):685–94, 2006.

92. Graham DR, Band JD. Citrobacter diversus brain abscess and meningitis in neonates. JAMA 245(19):1923–5, 1981.

93. Doran TI. The role of citrobacter in clinical disease of children: review. Clin Infect Dis 28(2):384–94, 1999.

94. Lebel MH, Freij BJ, Syrogiannopoulos GA, et al. Dexamethasone therapy for bacterial meningitis. Results of two double-blind, placebo-controlled trials. N Engl J Med 319(15):964–71, 1988.

95. Schaad UB, Kaplan SL, McCracken GH Jr. Steroid therapy for bacterial meningitis. Clin Infect Dis 20(3):685–90, 1995.

96. Wald ER, Kaplan SL, Mason EO Jr, et al. Dexamethasone therapy for children with bacterial meningitis. Meningitis Study Group. Pediatrics 95(1):21–8, 1995.

97. Spreer A, Gerber J, Hanssen M, et al. Dexamethasone increases hippocampal neuronal apoptosis in a rabbit model of Escherichia coli meningitis. Pediatr Res 60(2):210–15, 2006.

98. Cotten CM, McDonald S, Stoll B, et al. The association of third-generation cephalosporin use and invasive candidiasis in extremely low birth-weight infants. Pediatrics 118(2):717–22, 2006.

99. Kaufman D, Boyle R, Hazen KC, et al. Fluconazole prophylaxis against fungal colonization and infection in preterm infants. N Engl J Med 345(23):1660–6, 2001.

100. Uko S, Soghier LM, Vega M, et al. Targeted short-term fluconazole prophylaxis among very low birth weight and extremely low birth weight infants. Pediatrics 117(4):1243–52, 2006.

101. de Louvois J, Halket S, Harvey D. Neonatal meningitis in England and Wales: sequelae at 5 years of age. Eur J Pediatr 164(12):730–4, 2005.

102. Stoll BJ, Hansen NI, Adams-Chapman I, et al. Neurodevelopmental and growth impairment among extremely low-birth-weight infants with neonatal infection. JAMA 292(19):2357–65, 2004.

103. Unhanand M, Mustafa MM, McCracken GH Jr, Nelson JD. Gram-negative enteric bacillary meningitis: a twenty-one-year experience. J Pediatr 122(1):15–21, 1993.

104. Edwards MS, Rench MA, Haffar AA, et al. Long-term sequelae of group B streptococcal meningitis in infants. J Pediatr 106(5):717–22, 1985.

105. Wald ER, Bergman I, Taylor HG, et al. Long-term outcome of group B streptococcal meningitis. Pediatrics 77(2):217–21, 1986.

Chapter 13

Magnetic Resonance Imaging's Role in the Care of the Infant at Risk for Brain Injury

Caroline C. Menache, MD • Petra S. Hüppi, MD

The Term Newborn
The Preterm Infant

Despite marked improvements in antenatal and perinatal care, perinatal brain injury remains one of the most important medical complications in the newborn resulting in chronic handicapping conditions later in life. Remarkable experimental advances in recent years have helped to understand many of the cellular and vascular mechanisms of perinatal brain damage, showing a correlation between the nature of the injury and the maturation of the brain. Early identification of brain injury and appropriate prognostication though remain a major challenge to neonatal care. New diagnostic tools have emerged to detect early brain injury and help predict outcome.

Magnetic resonance (MR) techniques are one of these new diagnostic tools that allow the assessment of the developing brain in detail thanks to their resolving power and their relative noninvasiveness. Their capacity to provide detailed structural as well as metabolic and functional information without the use of ionizing radiation is unique.

Conventional MR imaging (MRI) is therefore now widely used for identifying normal and pathologic brain morphology giving objective information about the structure of the neonatal brain during development. Diffusion-weighted imaging (DWI) (1), magnetic resonance spectroscopy (MRS) (2), and functional MRI (fMRI; blood-oxygenation-dependent (BOLD) imaging) (3) are newer MR techniques that complement conventional MRI and can indicate some of the pathophysiologic mechanisms occurring during brain injury in the newborn and the postinjury plasticity. This chapter will focus on the role of the different MR techniques in the study of perinatal brain injury. The specific patterns of brain injury identified by different imaging techniques will be illustrated by case presentations, followed by the discussion of pathophysiologic and neurodevelopmental outcome associated with the described brain lesion. This approach should allow the reader to make the right choice of imaging method at the right time to decide on intervention, withdrawal of care, and accurate prediction of range of neurofunctional outcome.

THE TERM NEWBORN

Neonatal brain injury in the term infant is most frequently related to hypoperfusion and/or hypoxemia followed by reperfusion as the infant is resuscitated, typically shortly after delivery. This is summarized in the term "asphyxia," progressive hypoxemia, and hypercapnia with significant metabolic acidosis occurring both antenatal, intrapartum, and neonatal (4). Perinatal asphyxia may lead to hypoxic-ischemic encephalopathy (HIE) which is the clinically defined condition of disturbed neurologic function in the term newborn, characterized by insufficient respiration, depression of tone and reflexes, altered level of consciousness, and often seizures (5). The subsequent neurologic deficits of concern are grouped together under the term of cerebral palsy (6, 7), but include different motor deficits, such as spasticity, choreoathetosis, dystonia, and ataxia. Further cognitive deficits and seizures might also be the end result of neonatal HIE. The major varieties of neonatal HIE are listed in Table 13-1.

Selective neuronal necrosis is the most common injury observed in HIE and refers to necrosis of neurons in a characteristic, although often widespread, distribution. The four basic patterns of the topography of the neuronal injury depend on the severity and temporal characteristics of the insult, and on the gestational age. Thus, pontosubicular necrosis occurs more frequently in premature than in term infants and the basal ganglia neurons of the putamen are more likely to be affected in term infants, whereas neurons from the globus pallidus are more frequently affected in premature infants (8).

The reason for which one term infant with ischemia may develop one of the various patterns of selective neuronal necrosis or primarily parasagittal cerebral injury is not entirely clear.

Pre- or postnatal generalized systemic circulatory insufficiency can also generate focal or multifocal ischemic necrosis. However, other etiologies occurring without HIE are also common for this type of focal lesion (see later).

Table 13-1 Major Varieties of Neonatal HIE	
Major neuropathologic varieties of neonatal HIE in the term infant	Characteristics of the usual insult according to the pattern of injury or pathogenesis of the injury
Selective neuronal necrosis: – diffuse – cerebral cortex–deep nuclear – deep nuclear–brainstem – pontosubicular Parasagittal cerebral injury	Characteristics of the insult: – very severe, very prolonged – moderate to severe, prolonged – severe, abrupt – unknown Pathogenesis: Disturbance in cerebral perfusion due to: – parasagittal anatomical factors (arterial border zones and end zones) – impaired cerebrovascular autoregulation (pressure-passive state due to cerebral ischemia)
Focal and multifocal ischemic necrosis	Pathogenesis: Generalized systemic circulatory insufficiency (pre- or postnatal) – intrauterine – neonatal

Modified from Volpe JJ. Neurology of the Newborn. Philadelphia, PA: WB Saunders, 2001.

Table 13-2   Neurologic Syndrome of a Severe HIE

Birth to 12 hours	12–24 hours	24–72 hours	After 72 hours
Deep stupor or coma	Variable change in	Stupor or coma	Persistent but
Periodic breathing or	alertness	Respiratory arrest	diminished stupor
respiratory failure	More seizures	Oculomotor and	Disturbed sucking,
Intact pupillary and	Apneic spells	pupillary	swallowing, gag,
oculomotor	Jitteriness	disturbance	and tongue
response	Weakness (upper		movements
Hypotonia and	limbs in terms; lower		Hypotonia
minimal	limbs in prematures)		> hypertonia
movements/			Weakness (upper
occasionally			limbs in terms;
hypertonia			lower limbs in
Seizures			prematures)

Modified from Volpe JJ. Neurology of the Newborn. Philadelphia, PA: WB Saunders, 2001.

The occurrence of a neonatal neurologic syndrome is one of the important conditions for attributing intrapartum insults as a likely cause for the brain injury. The neurologic symptoms of a severe HIE are described in Table 13-2. Important systemic abnormalities (renal, cardiac, hepatic, etc.) related to ischemia accompany the neurologic manifestations in most cases but show no relation to outcome (9).

Clinicopathologic correlations can be made for the different neuropathologic varieties of neonatal HIE in the term infant and are summarized in Table 13-3.

The following five cases of term perinatal asphyxia illustrate the clinical course, the neuroimaging characteristics, and the subsequent neurodevelopmental outcome and illustrate the role and appropriate timing of MRI in the evaluation of the term newborn after perinatal asphyxia.

CASE 1

History

Term pregnancy with signs of fetal distress, cesarean section, low Apgar score, perinatal acidosis (pH 6.99). On day 1 general hypotonia, tonic deviations of eyes, sucking, smacking "subtle seizures" were noted. Normal neurologic examination on day 10.

Neuroimaging studies

Neonatal head ultrasound performed on day 1 was normal. MRI on day 3 revealed no significant signal abnormalities on T2-weighted images and some signal hyperintensities on T1-weighted images especially in the central cortex (Fig. 13-1A and 13-1B). DWI showed abnormal signal intensities with reduced apparent diffusion coefficient (ADC) bilaterally in the thalamus and internal capsule (Fig. 13-1C). Some discrete areas of reduced ADC were seen in the cortex. A repeat follow-up study on day 10 (see Fig. 13-2) showed the thalami appearing hyperintense on T2-weighted images.

Clinical correlates in the neonatal period

This child developed signs of moderately severe impairment of bilateral hemispheres which characteristically results in diffuse hypotonia. He also presented with neonatal seizures of the "subtle" type which are thought to result from diffuse cortical injury, and could be related to the discrete areas or reduced ADC seen in

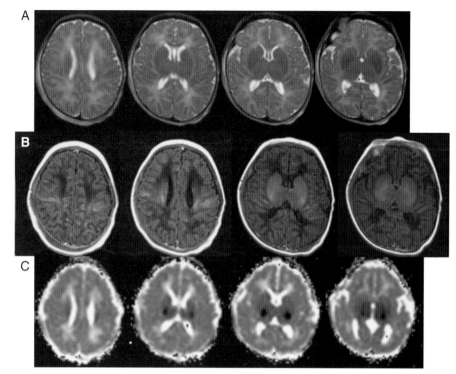

Figure 13-1 Case 1. Infant with perinatal asphyxia and MRI at day 3 of life. (A) T2-weighted images with slight T2-hyperintensity of the thalami; no striking signal abnormalities. (B) T1-weighted images show abnormal high signal intensities in several cortical areas, specifically in the depth of sulci. Thalamic area slightly hypointense. (C) DWI shows striking lesions (dark) with ADC reduction in bilateral thalami and in some discrete central cortical areas.

the cortex. The normalization of the neurologic examination at 10 days of life is usually a good prognostic sign.

Long-term clinical correlates

Ultimately he developed signs of moderate spasticity especially in the upper limbs, but was able to walk unaided at the age of 3 years with a certain degree of truncal hypotonia. His fine motor skills were delayed due to dystonic movements of the arms. The onset of dystonia started around the age of 12 months and became more prominent with time. He had no major cognitive deficits. The mild spasticity is explained by the involvement of the central white matter (seen best on DWI at day 3) and the dystonia is the result of the thalamoputaminal lesions. The relatively

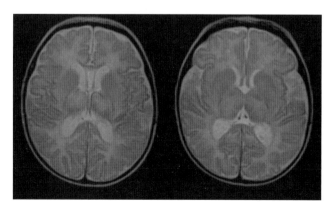

Figure 13-2 Case 1. MRI 10 days after perinatal asphyxia. T2-weighted images show marked hyperintensity in bilateral thalami involving in part the internal capsule and mild ventricular dilatation.

good outcome of this patient was in part predictable from the normalization of his neurologic examination at 10 days of life. The diagnosis still is dystonic cerebral palsy (CP) with a spastic component (see also Table 13-3).

CASE 2

History

Term pregnancy with signs of fetal distress, emergency cesarean section for uterine rupture, meconium aspiration, low Apgar scores ($1^1 3^5 5^{10}$), perinatal acidosis (pH 6.84). There was initial general hypotonia, then hypertonicity, however without seizures.

Neuroimaging studies

Neonatal head ultrasound performed on day 1 was normal. MRI on day 1 revealed no significant signal abnormalities on T2-, T1-weighted images and on DWI. Single voxel ^{1}H-MRS performed on basal ganglia revealed elevated lactate (Lac) resonance at 1.3 ppm with no loss of N-acetyl aspartate (NAA) (see Fig. 13-3). Follow-up MRI at day 10 showed bilateral hyperintense appearing thalami and putamen on T2-weighted images with clear distinction on proton density images and with no cortical signal abnormalities (see Fig. 13-3). Notable on T1-weighted images

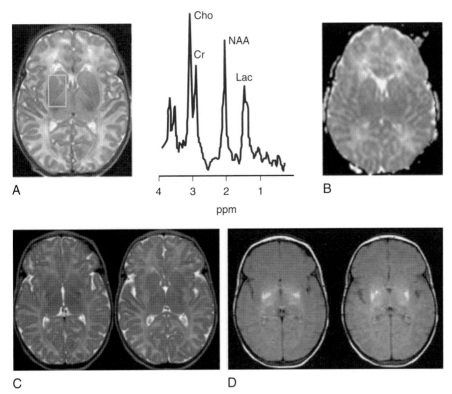

Figure 13-3 Case 2. (A) MR examination obtained at 12 hours after perinatal asphyxia. Axial T2-weighted image shows no signal abnormalities and single voxel ^{1}H-MRS performed over the right basal ganglia shows markedly increased Lac resonance with preserved NAA, Cr, and Cho resonances. (B) DWI with axial ADC map shows no diffusion abnormalities. MRI at 10 days after perinatal asphyxia: (C) axial T2-weighted images show areas of high and low signal intensity in the putamen and thalamus representing clear ischemic-hemorrhagic lesions and (D) axial proton density images with excellent detection of the lesion extension.

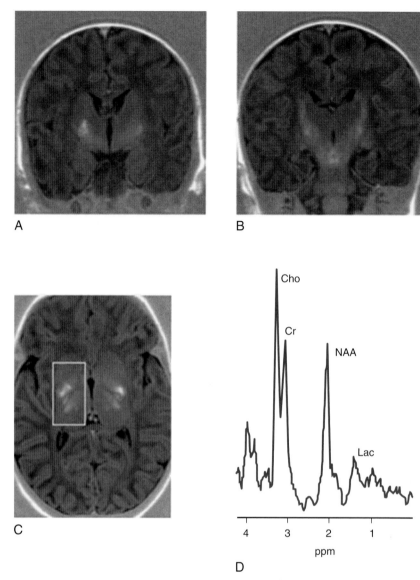

Figure 13-4 Case 2. Coronal and axial inversion recovery sequences with T1-weighted contrast at 10 days after perinatal asphyxia. T1-hyperintensities appear irregular (A, C) (compare to regular distribution of beginning myelination in (B)). (D) ^{1}H-MRS shows normalization of Lac and reduction of NAA compared to ^{1}H-MRS at day 1.

hyperintensities in this region can be confounded by hyperintensities due to myelination (see Fig. 13-4).

Clinical correlates in the neonatal period

After a brief period of hypotonia, corresponding most likely to the bilateral involvement of the reticular activating system in the diencephalon, this child rapidly developed the characteristic hypertonia associated with basal ganglia lesions and involvement of the extrapyramidal system. It is interesting to note that no seizures were observed, most likely in relation to the fact that there were no cortical lesions.

Long-term clinical correlates

This child developed striking truncal hypotonia and severe dystonic posturing of the upper extremities, severely limiting her motor development, although there was no spasticity. She is unable to walk unaided at age 3 years. Her cognitive functions are, however, preserved. The diagnosis is severe CP of the dystonic type (see also Table 13-3).

CASE 3

History

Term pregnancy with intrauterine growth restriction, fetal distress, cesarean section, meconium aspiration perinatal acidosis, persistent pulmonary hypertension, acidosis (pH 7.08).

Neuroimaging studies

Neonatal head ultrasound performed on day 1 was normal. MRI on day 1 revealed no significant signal abnormalities on T2- and T1-weighted images and standard DWIs reveal no striking signal abnormality. ADC values measured in the right basal ganglia (ADC 0.8 μm^2/ms) and central white matter (ADC 0.8 μm^2/ms) reveal markedly reduced ADC values compared to normal term neonates (1.0–1.2/1.4) (see Fig. 13-5) (10). ^{1}H-MRS performed on basal ganglia revealed elevated Lac resonance at 1.3 ppm with no loss of NAA. Follow-up MRI showed marked T2 signal abnormalities in the basal ganglia with involvement of the left internal capsule with extension into the central white matter in a parasagittal distribution (see Fig. 13-6).

Clinical correlates in the neonatal period

This infant did not develop striking neurologic abnormalities in the neonatal period. The only symptom was moderate hypotonia, and some weakness in the upper extremities.

Long-term clinical correlates

Marked right upper extremity palsy developed at the age of 6 months. The child did not reach for objects with the right hand and exhibited a spastic position of the right arm during leg movements. In the ventral position, she was unable to elevate her right arm. These impairments were consistent with the lesions of the left internal capsule. Later, at age 18 months, she showed signs of hyperreflexia in the four limbs, likely a consequence of the bilateral white matter lesions. Notably, spasticity predominated on the right side, as sequelae of the unilateral left internal capsule lesion. Her cognitive performance was mildly delayed. She was able to walk unaided at the age of 2 years. The diagnosis is spastic CP with predominant right-sided involvement (see also Table 13-3).

CASE 4

History

Term pregnancy with uterine rupture at delivery. Perinatal resuscitation with Apgar scores at $0^1 0^5 3^{10}$ and severe perinatal acidosis. On day 1 there was development of a moderate HIE with lethargy and hypotonia. Efforts in arousing the infant resulted in hypertonia and jitteriness. Spontaneous movements were diminished. Convulsions appeared rapidly.

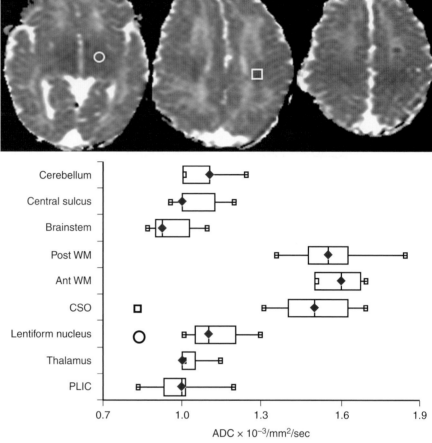

Figure 13-5 Case 3. MRI on day 1 after perinatal asphyxia. Conventional MRI reveals no signal abnormalities (not shown). DWI shows no overt lesions but ADC values measured in the left basal ganglia (ADC 0.8 μm²/ms) (circle) and central white matter (ADC 0.8 μm²/ms) (square) reveal markedly reduced ADC values compared to normal term neonates. The graph shows box plots of ADC distribution in normal full-term newborns in different regions of the brain. (Reproduced with permission from Rutherford M, Counsell S, Allsop J, et al. Diffusion–weighted magnetic resonance imaging in term perinatal brain injury: a comparison with site of lesion and time from birth. Pediatrics 114:1004–14, 2004.)

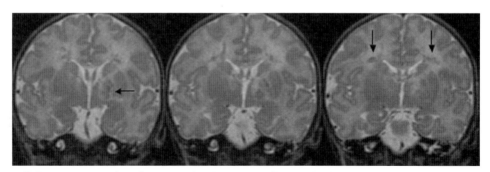

Figure 13-6 Case 3. MRI 7 days after perinatal asphyxia. Coronal T2-weighted images showing T2-hypointensities and T2-hyperintensities in the central white matter with additional left-sided lesions in the internal capsule and lateral thalamus (see arrows).

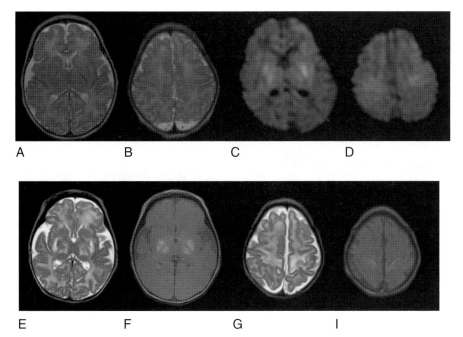

Figure 13-7 Case 4. MRI at day 2 after perinatal asphyxia (A–D). Conventional T2-weighted images at the level of the basal ganglia and the high centrum semiovale show no signal abnormalities (A, B). DWI shows striking hyperintensities within the putamen and thalamus bilaterally (C) and some high signal in the central cortex (D). MRI at 10 days after the insult confirms the distribution of the lesions with hyper- and hypointensities on T2-weighted images (E), typical high signal intensity with good lesion definition in proton density images (F), and the perirolandic cortex shows typical T2 and PD hyperintensity (G–I).

Neuroimaging studies

Neonatal head ultrasound performed on day 1 was normal. MRI on day 2 revealed no significant signal abnormalities on T2- or T1-weighted images. DWIs revealed bilateral reduced ADC in putamen and thalami (see Fig. 13-7). ^{1}H-MRS performed on basal ganglia reveals elevated Lac resonance at 1.3 ppm with no loss of NAA. Follow-up MRI at 17 days showed marked T2 signal abnormalities in the basal ganglia and alteration of the perirolandic cortex bilaterally visible both on proton density images as well as on T2-weighted images (see Fig. 13-7). At 2 months of age additional atrophy and delay in myelination was present (see Fig. 13-8).

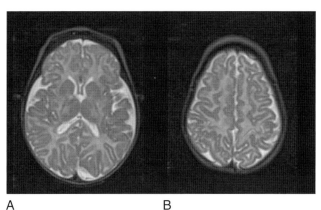

Figure 13-8 Case 4. MRI at 2 months of age reveals the same lesions with marked atrophy and delay in myelination.

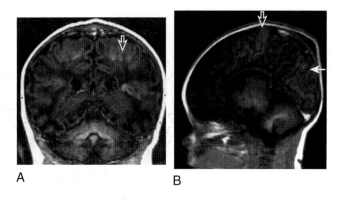

Figure 13-9 Typical parasagittal distribution of T1-hyperintensities within cortical neurons of deep sulcal cortex of another patient with acute perinatal asphyxia.

Clinical correlates in the neonatal period

The infant presented with neonatal seizures and a disturbed level of consciousness which reflected the bilateral cortical lesions.

Long-term clinical correlates

The child developed a severe spastic quadriplegia consistent with the bilateral parasagittal lesions. Additionally, dystonia started around the age of 12–18 months. This extrapyramidal syndrome was the result of the basal ganglia lesions. The child was thus severely disabled and unable to walk unaided. However the cognitive impairment was mild (see also Table 13-3).

CASE 5

History

Term pregnancy with persistent signs of fetal distress, cesarean section, low Apgar score with meconium aspiration and resuscitation.

On day 1 general hypotonia, tonic deviations of eyes, sucking, smacking "subtle seizures" were noted and there was electroencephalographic status epilepticus.

Neuroimaging studies

Neonatal head ultrasound performed on day 1 showed small ventricles and increased parenchymal echogenicity. MRI performed on day 5 showed extensive edema with the cortex roughly isointense with white matter on T2- and T1-weighted images and apparent sparing of the basal ganglia. On DWI there was markedly decreased ADC in cortex, white matter, and basal ganglia (see Figs. 13-10A and 13-10B). Follow-up MRI shows evolution into multicystic encephalopathy with loss of both hemispheric gray and white matter and severe ex vacuo ventriculomegaly (see Figs. 13-10C and 3-10D).

Clinical correlates in the neonatal period

The generalized hypotonia and the seizures reflect the bilateral extensive cortical injuries. The status epilepticus which is not uncommon in the full-term asphyxiated infant is the sign of the severity of the insult.

Long-term clinical correlates

The child developed a severe spastic quadriplegia with mental retardation and microcephaly. Spasticity was a major issue. The seizure disorder remained active

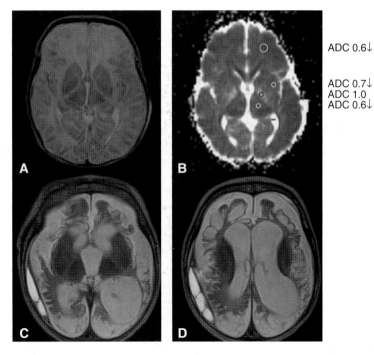

ADC 0.6↓

ADC 0.7↓
ADC 1.0
ADC 0.6↓

Figure 13-10 Case 5. Term newborn with nonreassuring fetal monitoring for several hours, meconium stained fluid, and poor Apgar score requiring delivery room resuscitation. Axial T2-weighted imaging on day 2 shows diffuse T2-hyperintensities with loss of gray–white matter differentiation. DWI with markedly reduced ADC (ADC <1.0 μm²/ms) values throughout the brain (B) indicating ongoing necrosis. Chronic stage T2-weighted images with multicystic encephalopathy and massive ventricular dilatation.

during the first months of life. The EEG remained severely depressed, indicating diffuse cortical necrosis. The diagnosis is severe spastic CP (see also Table 13-3).

Cranial Ultrasonography in the Evaluation of Perinatal Asphyxia or HIE

Neonatal sonography is still the only bedside technique to image the neonatal brain. In term perinatal asphyxia and HIE the most typical findings in the acute phase are represented by poor differentiation of cortical sulci and diffuse increase of parenchymal echogenicity and slit-like ventricles (11). These features can be primarily related to diffuse cerebral edema. Hemorrhagic necrosis in the basal ganglia can lead to hyperechogenic basal ganglia, which have been shown to be predictive of poor outcome (12, 13). But many early ultrasound scans in neonates with HIE lesions are normal or nonspecific, as illustrated in the cases shown. Ultrasound examinations can be considered as a first-step technique; however, an MRI study should follow.

MR Techniques in the Evaluation of Perinatal Asphyxia or HIE

MR has become the technique of choice to evaluate the ischemic brain both in adults and in the newborn (14). Advanced MRI techniques, such as the use of DWI and MRS have further improved the MR capability to investigate the neonatal brain. Generally, to increase the signal-to-noise ratio, a higher field magnet (1.5–3 T) should be used, allowing for high-resolution imaging and increased sensitivity for spectroscopy (15, 16).

Conventional MRI Sequences and Features in HIE

The basic information in conventional MRI is represented by T1- and T2-weighted images. Proton density and FLAIR images help illustrate brain lesions with slightly different contrast than T1- and T2-weighted images. A neonatal MRI protocol should provide good quality T1- and T2-weighted images with a maximum field of view of 16–18 cm and a slice thickness of 3 mm or less. Typically MR sequence parameters for T1-weighted term neonatal images are repetition time (TR) shorter than 600 ms and echo time (TE) shorter than 20 ms, and for T2-weighted images TR of at least 3000 ms and TE of at least 120 ms (14, 17).

SELECTIVE NEURONAL NECROSIS AFTER PERINATAL ASPHYXIA

As shown in the three cases above with a history of acute perinatal asphyxia, selective involvement of areas with advanced maturation and higher energy demands, i.e., the putamen, lateral thalami, and perirolandic cortex, are particularly vulnerable. Characteristic changes representing selective neuronal necrosis in these areas on T1-weighted images are hyperintensities, which become apparent 3–7 days after the insult. These T1-hyperintensities might represent cellular reaction of glial cells and macrophages containing lipid droplets and/or some mineralization of necrotic cells. Some difficulties identifying these lesions arise from the fact that early myelination shows the same image characteristics (18). Thus hyperintensities in the internal capsule due to initial myelination need to be differentiated from lateral thalamic and putamenal lesions. Often the posterior limb appears swollen and has lost its normal T1-hyperintensity/T2-hypointensity, which has a bad prognostic value with spastic hemiplegia often being associated (19). On T2-weighted images the thalami might appear slightly hyperintense in the acute phase (see Case 1) but these subtle signal changes tend to be very difficult to detect. T2-hyperintensities become more apparent in later stage, illustrated also by well-defined lesions on proton density images (see Case 2). Evolution of these lesions is marked by progressive atrophy of the involved area (i.e., putamen, thalami, rolandic cortex) with persistent T2-hyperintensity and possible cavitation (20).

Of note, similar lesions in the bilateral thalami, lenticular nucleus, and globus pallidum can be detected also in premature infants with documented severe anoxic insults, most frequently associated with the typical periventricular white matter injuries (8).

Parasagittal Cerebral Injury. Isolated parasagittal injury refers to a lesion of the cerebral cortex and the subcortical white matter with a defined distribution, i.e., parasagittal, superomedial aspects of the cortical convexities, usually bilateral but often asymmetric in its extension (21). During the acute phase the cortex might show increased T1-weighted signal intensity or little abnormality on conventional MRI (see Fig. 13-9). Chronic changes involve cortical thinning and atrophy.

Multicystic Encephalomalacia. Case 5 shows another form of brain injury associated with HIE. Early on (<2 days), conventional MRI is characterized by a diffuse T1-hypointensity and T2-hyperintensity involving both the cortex and the subcortical white matter but sparing the cerebellum and the more basal structures of the medulla (see Fig. 13-10). Late intrauterine generalized prolonged systemic circulatory insufficiency is probably at the origin of these lesions, which evolve into severe cortical atrophy with cavitation and are invariably associated with a severe neurologic syndrome.

DWI Sequences and Features in HIE

DWI measures the self-diffusion of water. The two primary pieces of information available from DWI studies – water ADC and diffusion anisotropy measures – change dramatically during development, reflecting underlying changes in tissue water content and cytoarchitecture (1). ADC is a quantitative measure (velocity) of overall water diffusion in tissue and anisotropy is a measure of directionality of preferred water diffusion in a given tissue. The developing human brain presents several challenges for the application of DWI. Values for the water diffusion parameters differ markedly between neonatal brain and adult brain and vary with age. As a result, much of the knowledge regarding DWI derived from studies of mature, adult human brain is not directly applicable to the developing brain.

In order to perform DWI, the optimum b value required to make the measurement has to be optimized, as it differs between the newborn and adult brain. In general, a b value corresponding to approximately 1.1/ADC provides the greatest contrast-to-noise ratio for such a measurement (22). In neonatal brain, the high b value is typically of the order of 700–1000 mm^2/s.

DWI parameters also change in response to brain injury. The decrease in water diffusion associated with injury was initially described for animals (23, 24) and adult human stroke (25), and was subsequently confirmed for human infants (10). Cases 1 and 4 clearly show the marked reduction of ADC in the basal ganglia with only slight hyperintensities on T2-weighted images which can be easily missed. DWI in this case detects the lesion more reliably.

There is still debate on the precise mechanism for the decrease in the ADC associated with injury. Changes in ADC following injury are dynamic. ADC values are initially decreased, but subsequently increase so that they are greater than normal and remain so in the chronic phase of injury. During the transition between decreased and increased values there is a brief period during which values are normal, a process referred to as "pseudonormalization." Pseudonormalization takes place roughly 2 days following stroke in a rat model (26) and at approximately 9 days following injury in adult human stroke (27). Preliminary data indicate that the timing of pseudonormalization in human newborns follows more closely that of adult humans than that of rodents, taking place at roughly 7 days following the injury (28). Interpretation of ADC values to detect acute brain injury in the developing brain needs to be adjusted for the regional differences in ADC values according to age (see Fig. 13-5) (10). Case 3 illustrates that without numerical measurement of ADC, acute tissue alteration on diffusion maps can be missed.

Case 2 illustrates that in the human newborn very early (<24 hours) DWI might also miss detection of ischemic injury, which has been reported in several studies (28–30).

From these studies we can summarize the current role of DWI in the evaluation of the term newborn with HIE as follows:

1. DWI obtained less than 24 hours after injury may demonstrate focal abnormalities when measuring ADC values and comparing them to regional age-corresponding values; however, the full extent of lesions might not be detected.
2. DWI with ADC measurement obtained between day 2 and 4 may detect lesions not detected by conventional MRI.
3. DWI at 7–10 days is less sensitive then conventional MRI due to the "pseudonormalization."

Magnetic Resonance Spectroscopy in HIE

Proton magnetic resonance spectroscopy (^{1}H-MRS) has also entered the clinical arena of MR techniques routinely used for the evaluation of the brain and permits the noninvasive study of metabolic alterations in brain tissue.

The physiologist is usually interested in the intracellular concentration of a chemical species in a particular cell type. It must be noted, though, that the in vivo human MR measurement in single voxel MRS is an average (over the sensitive volume) of all tissue types. In the brain, therefore, we generally assess a combination of glial and neuronal cells with different extracellular space depending upon how much white matter, gray matter, or cerebrospinal fluid (CSF) the volume of interest contains.

When oxidative phosphorylation is impaired, energy metabolism follows the alternative route of anaerobic glycolysis and produces lactic acid. Lactate has a chemical shift of 1.3 ppm and presents as a doublet peak in the in vivo ^{1}H-MRS due to coupling effects. Groenendaal et al. first described markedly elevated Lac levels in five infants with severe perinatal asphyxia (31). The five patients died within the neonatal period. ^{1}H-MRS data have been generated that demonstrate regional differences in Lac elevation after hypoxic-ischemic events in newborns. Single volume ^{1}H-MRS in these patients showed greater increase of the Lac/NAA ratio in the basal ganglia than in the occipitoparietal cerebrum (32) This corresponds to the signal abnormalities observed with early DWI after term hypoxia-ischemia. Case 2 illustrates the typical changes in ^{1}H-MRS after term perinatal hypoxia-ischemia.

Early spectroscopy (<18 hours after event) and measurement of high Lac/creatine (Cr) ratio in ^{1}H-MRS correlated well with neurodevelopmental outcome at 1 year (33). This acute phase lactic acidosis is followed by persistently elevated Lac levels not associated with acidosis 1–2 weeks after the event to several weeks after the hypoxic-ischemic event (34–36). However, ^{1}H-MRS performed in the first 24 hours after the insult is sensitive to the presence of hypoxic-ischemic brain injury, and seems to be suitable for the detection of brain injury on the first day when conventional MRI and DWI might not yet detect the injury. Early MRS has recently been shown to predict outcome more accurately than very early DWI alone (37).

As markers of cell integrity other metabolites visible on ^{1}H-MRS can be used for the assessment of HIE. Ratios of NAA/choline (Cho) and NAA/Cr have been used to assess cellular metabolic integrity in neonatal brain injury (2, 38–40). Studies using ^{1}H-MRS at a distance (>1–2 weeks) to the hypoxic-ischemic event showed good correlation between reduced NAA ratios with adverse neurodevelopmental outcome (36, 39–41), whereas in early (acute stage) ^{1}H-MRS NAA ratios are not correlated with outcome.

From these studies we can summarize the current role of ^{1}H-MRS in the evaluation of the term newborn with HIE as follows:

1. MRS can play an important role in the assessment of encephalopathic term infants. Elevated Lac/NAA, Lac/Cr, and Lac/Cho ratios or elevated absolute concentrations of Lac at less than 24 hours reliably indicate cellular injury.
2. MRS might therefore be more useful than DWI techniques in identifying infants who would benefit from early therapeutic interventions.

Focal and Multifocal Ischemic Brain Necrosis without Asphyxia

As mentioned above, focal and multifocal ischemic brain necrosis can also occur without HIE, and the sole presence of these brain lesions also places the neonate in the "high-risk infant" category even if they have not suffered asphyxia. These lesions occur within the distribution of single or multiple major blood vessels. Almost 90% of the infarcts are unilateral, and of these lesions nearly all involve the middle cerebral artery (MCA), 75% of them involving the distribution of the left MCA for a yet unexplained reason.

The neonatal and long-term clinical correlates of HIE are described in Table 13-3. The major etiologies of these infarcts occurring without asphyxia are given in Table 13-4.

Neonatal seizures occur in 80–85% of these patients and are in most cases focal, clonic, contralateral to the lesion. Regarding long-term correlates, hemiparesis

Table 13-3   Neonatal and Long-term Clinical Correlates of the Different Varieties of HIE

Topography of the major injury	Neonatal correlates	Long-term correlates
Selective neuronal necrosis of the *diffuse* type	Stupor and coma (cortical injury) Seizures (cortical injury) often of the subtle type Hypotonia (cortical or anterior horn injury) Oculomotor disturbance (cranial nerve nuclei injury) Disturbed sucking, swallowing (brainstem involvement)	Intellectual retardation (cortical injury) Spastic quadriparesis (cortical injury) Seizure disorder (10–30%) (cortical injury) Impairment of cortical visual function Precocious puberty (10%) (hypothalamus) Impairment of sucking, swallowing, drooling, fixed facial expression (bulbar or pseudobulbar palsy) Hearing deficits (cochlear neurons) Atonic cerebral palsy (rare) (anterior horn cells)
Selective neuronal necrosis of *cortical–deep nuclear* type	Same symptoms except that the tone is usually increased, especially with stimulation	Same symptoms Additionally: delayed onset of dystonia (6–12 months and even as late as 7–14 years of age)
Selective neuronal necrosis of *deep nuclear–brainstem* type	Same symptoms as above + ptosis, facial diparesis, ventilatory disturbances	Prolonged difficulties with feeding Normal cognition in 50%
Parasagittal cerebral injury	Proximal weakness predominant in the upper limbs Seizures (variable) Disturbed level of alertness (variable)	Spastic quadriparesis Intellectual deficits (often "specific")
Focal and multifocal brain necrosis (cortical and subcortical)	Seizures, usually focal Hemiparesis or quadriparesis if bilateral	Spastic hemiparesis or quadriparesis Cognitive deficits Seizure disorder

Modified from Volpe JJ. Neurology of the Newborn. Philadelphia, PA: WB Saunders, 2001.

occurs only in 25% of patients with unilateral lesion. The likelihood of hemiparesis depends on the extent of the lesion or on the involvement, even if not severe, of the contralateral hemisphere or both (42). Thus hemiparesis is almost certain if the distribution of the stem of the MCA is affected, or if there are bilateral lesions. However, if only a cortical branch or lenticulostriate vessels are affected, the likelihood of hemiparesis is around 10%. This relatively good outcome in unilateral lesions is probably related to the ability of the opposite hemisphere to reestablish ipsilateral corticospinal tract innervation (brain plasticity). Seizure disorders occur in approximately 10% of infants. Cognitive function is impaired if lesions are bilateral. In unilateral lesions, only 20–25% of infants develop cognitive problems.

CASE 6

History

The pregnancy was uneventful. During spontaneous labor, the cardiotocogram showed variable decelerations with signs of fetal distress and emergency cesarean section was performed for acute fetal bradycardia. The Apgar score was noted to be $5^1 9^5 9^{10}$ with rapid clinical recovery. The infant was transferred to the neonatal

Table 13-4   Etiologies of Focal and Multifocal Ischemic Lesions

Etiologies of focal and multifocal ischemic brain necrosis occurring without asphyxia

Idiopathic (majority of cases)
Vascular maldevelopment
Vasculopathy
Vasospasm (e.g., with cocaine use)
Vascular distortion (obstetrical trauma to head and neck)
Vascular manipulation-ligation (i.e., for extracorporeal membrane oxygenation)
Embolus:
   – placental thrombosis or tissue fragments (twin pregnancy with death of co-twin)
   – involuting fetal vessels (thrombi)
   – catheterized vessels (thrombi or air)
   – cardiac: myxoma or rhabdomyoma, right to left shunt, patent foramen ovale
Thrombus:
   – meningitis with arteritis or phlebitis
   – trauma
   – disseminated intravascular coagulation
   – polycythemia
   – hypercoagulable state: protein C, protein S, antithrombin III deficiency, antiphospholipid antibodies, factor V Leiden mutation
   – hypernatremia–dehydration

Modified from Volpe JJ. Neurology of the Newborn. Philadelphia, PA: WB Saunders, 2001.

unit for surveillance. On day 3 of life the infant developed apneic attacks and convulsions were noted with head deviation.

Neuroimaging studies

MRI on day 4 reveals significant signal abnormalities on the ADC maps and DWIs during the acute phase. DWI showed a striking reduction of diffusivity and ADC in the left temporoparieto-occipital region with involvement also of the basal ganglia and internal capsule, consistent with an acute infarction (see Fig. 13-11). Thus, the mean value for ADC in the intact right hemisphere was 1.68 ± 0.12 $\mu m^2/ms$, whereas in the corresponding left hemisphere, the ADC was 0.60 ± 0.04 $\mu m^2/ms$, reflecting the dramatic decline in ADC during acute ischemic injury. MR angiography showed permeable vessels on both sides. On day 8 of life, the ADC was 1.69 ± 0.09 $\mu m^2/ms$ in the right hemisphere and 0.93 ± 0.19 $\mu m^2/ms$ in the left hemisphere. The MRI at 6 weeks of age showed tissue dissolution in the left posterior cerebral region with an increased ADC of 2.85 ± 0.15 $\mu m^2/ms$, compared to normal ADC of 1.44 ± 0.16 $\mu m^2/ms$ in the right hemisphere. T2-weighted images at 6 weeks of age showed that the lesion had evolved with tissue dissolution (see Fig. 13-11). At 13 weeks diffusion tensor images (DTI) showed loss of optic radiation fibers and loss of cortical visual response on fMRI (not shown). At 12 and 20 months of age, DTI with fiber tracking illustrates recovery of optic radiation fibers and preserved anterior cerebral activation upon visual stimulation in the lesioned hemisphere (see Fig.13-12).

Clinical correlates in the neonatal period

This is a typical case of focal infarction where the seizure usually presents after 2–3 days of life, without other neurologic signs. In particular, no hypotonia or lethargy

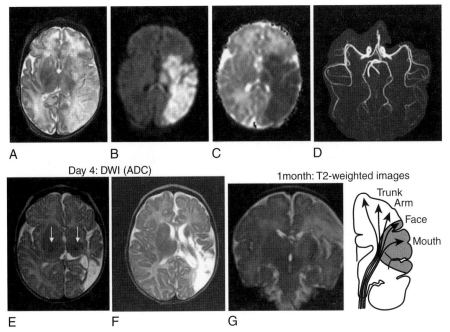

Day 4: DWI (ADC)

1month: T2-weighted images

Trunk
Arm
Face
Mouth

Figure 13-11 Case 6. Acute left middle cerebral artery infarction. (A) Axial T2-weighted image where infarction appears as "missed cortex" with absence of cortical–subcortical differentiation due to acute edema. (B) DWI and (C) ADC map with clear demarcation of ischemic zone. (D) Reperfused middle cerebral artery on the left with MR angiography. (E, F) Axial T2-weighted images in the chronic phase of infarction with cystic transformation of the initial ischemic zone and absence of left-sided myelination in the posterior limb of internal capsule (arrows). (G) Coronal T2-weighted image corresponding to figure representing corticospinal tracts and innervation. Lesion predicts hemiplegia with predominant involvement of arm and face.

was described. In this situation the seizures are the result of a focal cortical lesion and not due to diffuse cortical involvement.

Long-term clinical correlates

This child developed hemiplegia contralateral to the side of the lesion, which was expected due to the extent of the lesion. Alteration of the visual field in the area of the infarct also occurred. Some degree of intellectual impairment developed as well, as was predictable from the size of the lesion (see also Table 13-3).

MR Techniques in the Evaluation of Focal Ischemic Infarction in the Term Newborn

MRI is the technique of choice for evaluating focal neonatal cerebral infarctions, as ultrasonography only shows ill-defined slight hyperechogenecity with difficulty to evaluate peripheral cortical extension.

Conventional MRI shows loss of corticosubcortical differentiation in both T1- and T2-weighted imaging due to the increase of T2 signal intensity in the edematous cortex, thus approaching the signal intensity of the unmyelinated white matter. This sign is also called the "disappeared cortex" sign. The best modality to identify a focal ischemic infarct is DWI, with striking reduction of ADC in the acute phase with normalization by 6–10 days and tissue dissolution thereafter, which results in a porencephalic cyst with T2 characteristics of CSF.

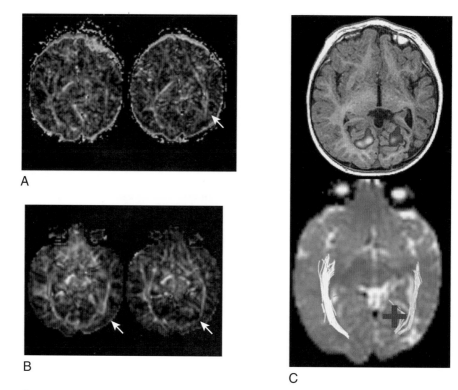

Figure 13-12 Case 6. Diffusion tensor imaging with anisotropy maps at 12 months (A) and 20 months (B). Arrows indicate recovery of optic radiation fibers visualized by DTI. (C) fMRI response to visual stimulation at 20 months of age shows recovery of cortical vision in the area of tract recovery.

As outlined in the clinical description, focal ischemic infarction may have less severe neurologic sequelae probably due to the brain's potential for plasticity (42, 43).

Advanced MR techniques such as *DTI* and *fMRI* have recently been shown to be of use in the study of postinjury plasticity (44). The geometric nature of the diffusion tensor can be used to display the architecture of the brain white matter fiber tracts illustrating them by vector images. fMRI can illustrate functional brain activation by measuring changes in local perfusion based on the BOLD contrast. In a case of perinatal middle cerebral artery stroke (Case 6) at 20 months of age, event-related fMRI showed significant activation in the visual cortex of the injured left hemisphere that was not observed at 3 months of age (45). DTI vector maps suggest recovery of the optic radiation in the vicinity of the lesion. Optic radiations in the injured hemisphere were more prominent in DTI at 20 months of age than in DTI at 12 months of age which indicates that functional cortical recovery is supported by structural modifications that concern major pathways of the visual system.

Traumatic Brain Lesions of the Posterior Fossa

Intracranial hemorrhage as such is another important brain lesion in the neonatal period, particularly affecting the preterm infant but also occurring in the full-term infant in certain situations. In particular, traumatic brain lesions of the posterior fossa in the term newborn associated with massive hemorrhage can cause serious neurologic sequelae. The mechanism responsible for this lesion is occipital osteo-diastasis. This consists of traumatic separation of the cartilaginous joint between the squamous and lateral portions of the occipital bone. In the most severe forms, the dura and the occipital sinus are torn resulting in massive subdural hemorrhage in the posterior fossa and cerebellar laceration. Risk factors are breech delivery, vacuum extraction, primiparity, and fetomaternal disproportion.

Clinical manifestations in the most severe cases are immediate signs of brainstem compression (stupor or coma, oculomotor and pupillary abnormalities, nuchal rigidity with opisthotonos, respiratory abnormalities, bradycardia, and then respiratory arrest) and this syndrome is rapidly lethal. In less severe forms, neurologic signs can be absent in the first hours, then symptoms of increased intracranial pressure develop due to ventricular dilatation (block of the CSF flow in the posterior fossa). The signs of brainstem compression due to the posterior fossa hematoma appear afterwards. In addition, seizures occur in the majority of patients, most likely due to the accompanying subarachnoid blood. Long-term outcome is poor in severe occipital diastasis. If the posterior fossa hemorrhage is less pronounced, the outcome is more variable, depending on the rate of rapidity of diagnosis and intervention. With extension of the hemorrhage into the cerebellum, cerebellar deficits due to destruction of the cerebellar tissue are almost invariably present (intention tremor, dysmetria, truncal ataxia, and hypotonia). Hydrocephalus requiring ventriculoperitoneal shunts occurs in 50% of cases. Cognitive deficits are also variably present.

CASE 7

History

Term pregnancy with vaginal delivery instrumented by vacuum for nonprogression of labor, Apgar scores were $9^1 9^5 10^{10}$ (pH 7.23). On day 1 there was general hypotonia, tonico-clonic seizure, with subsequent tonic seizures.

Neuroimaging studies

Neonatal head ultrasound performed on day 2 showed posterior fossa hemorrhage with enlarged ventricles. MRI on day 2 revealed a large T2-hypointense lesion in the posterior fossa involving the cerebellar vermis with concomitant ventricular dilatation. On the sagittal images the vein of Galen can be identified. MR angiogram shows no arterial or venous malformation. Tonsillar herniation of the cerebellum was present. On follow-up T2-weighted images, marked cerebellar lesions were visualized (see Fig. 13-13).

Clinical correlates in the neonatal period

This child presented with hypotonia which could be due to brainstem compression and seizures due to cortical "irritation" by the subarachnoid blood. The brainstem compression signs which are common in this situation had not yet taken place when the diagnosis was made as a consequence of seizures which resulted in the emergency neuroimaging. Surgical removal of the hematoma was then performed. The child developed a cardiac arrest during surgery due to the massive blood loss and was immediately, successfully, resuscitated.

Long-term clinical correlates

The patient presented with severe truncal hypotonia and truncal ataxia with delayed spontaneous walking. This child also developed mild spasticity in the lower extremities, most likely as sequelae of a mild cortical injury which happened during the short cardiac arrest during surgery. Her cognitive function is normal at the age of 5 years. However, the cerebellar deficits are still very significant (intention tremor, dysmetria, and truncal ataxia).

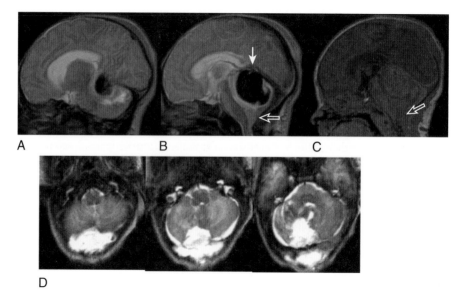

A   B   C

D

Figure 13-13 Case 7. Sagittal T2-weighted images acquired on day 2 reveals a large T2-hypointense lesion in the posterior fossa involving the cerebellum with concomitant ventricular dilatation (A, B). In (B) the vein of Galen can be identified (small arrow). Tonsillar herniation of the cerebellum is present (large arrows) (B). (C, D) Axial T2-weighted images with residual cerebellar lesion.

MR Techniques in the Evaluation of Traumatic Brain Injury in the Term Newborn

As the posterior fossa is the primary site of subdural hemorrhage after traumatic birth, cranial ultrasound through the anterior fontanel has limited capacity in the detection of the extent of posterior fossa lesions. The MRI appearance of blood is dependent on the oxidative state of hemoglobin and its environment. Acute hemorrhage (3 hours to 10 days) therefore shows isointensity to slight hyperintensity on T1-weighted images (gradient-echo sequences preferred) and low signal intensity on T2-weighted images (see Fig. 13-13) with evolution to high signal intensity on T2-weighted images between 10 days and 3 weeks after the hemorrhage (Fig. 13-13). MR angiography can exclude vein of Galen malformations or sinus thrombosis. Sagittal image planes are necessary to look for cerebellar tonsillar herniation in the presence of posterior fossa hemorrhage.

THE PRETERM INFANT

Brain injury in the premature infant is composed of multiple lesions, principally described as germinal matrix intraventricular hemorrhage (IVH), venous hemorrhagic infarction, posthemorrhagic hydrocephalus, and periventricular leukomalacia (PVL). However, many preterm infants show neurodevelopmental delay without having been diagnosed with any of these typical perinatal brain injuries.

The site of origin of IVH is the subependymal germinal matrix, which is a very cellular, gelatinous, highly vascularized region. The exact site of the hemorrhage seems to be the capillary-venule or small venule level (46). In 80% of cases the blood enters then the lateral ventricles and spread occurs through the ventricular system. The presence of blood may create an obliterative arachnoiditis over days to weeks with obstruction of CSF flow. The blood clot can also lead to impaired CSF circulation at the aqueduct of Sylvius and the arachnoid villi. One of the possible consequences of this phenomenon is the development of progressive ventricular dilation and hydrocephalus which may require shunting. Posthemorrhagic hydrocephalus may happen in an acute, subacute, or chronic way. Approximately 15% of infants also develop a characteristic parenchymal lesion, with a triangular shape, in the white matter situated dorsally and laterally to the external angle of the lateral ventricle. This lesion corresponds to a hemorrhagic infarction (47). The current prevailing hypothesis regarding its pathogenesis is that the dilatation of the lateral ventricle by the IVH creates an obstruction of the terminal vein and impaired blood flow in the medullary veins, resulting in hemorrhagic venous infarction which is usually unilateral. Indeed, the terminal vein draining the medullary veins runs essentially within the germinal matrix. The venous congestion creates a periventricular ischemia, leading to the periventricular hemorrhagic infarction (PVHI) which is a very different lesion from the PVL (see Table 13-5). The long-term neurologic prognosis is mostly dictated by the extent of the intraparenchymal lesion. Neurologic sequelae mostly consist of spastic hemiparesis or asymmetrical quadriparesis with cognitive deficits. Posthemorrhagic hydrocephalus is more likely to occur if the IVH is severe and can contribute to the neurologic sequelae in some cases.

PVL has classically been described as a disorder characterized by multifocal areas of necrosis, forming cysts in the deep periventricular cerebral white matter, which are often symmetrical and occur adjacent to the lateral ventricles. The earliest neuropathologic changes are of *coagulation necrosis* of all cellular elements with loss of cytoarchitecture and tissue vacuolation (48). *Axonal swelling* and intense activated *microglial reactivity* and proliferation are observed as early as 3 hours after insult (49, 50). In addition in the periphery of these focal lesions a marked *astrocytic and vascular endothelial hyperplasia* characterizes the brain tissue reaction at the end of the first week. After 1–2 weeks *macrophage activity with characteristic lipid laden macrophages* is predominant over the astrocytic reactivity, with progressive cavitation of the tissue and cyst formation thereafter. During subacute and chronic stages of PVL, swollen axons calcify, accumulate iron, and degenerate particularly at the periphery of the injured zone. The deep focal necrotic lesions of PVL occur in areas that are considered arterial end zones. The state of development of the periventricular vessels is a function of gestational age, and the degree of ischemia required to produce these focal lesions may vary depending upon the state of development of these vessels and thus upon gestational age (51).

These *focal* necrotic lesions correlate well with the development of spastic CP in very low birth weight (VLBW) infants, whereas the increasingly large number of VLBW infants with mild motor impairment and cognitive and behavioral deficits (52) may relate to a more *diffuse* injury to the developing white matter which has only recently been recognized. Diffuse white matter damage is macroscopically

Table 13-5 White Matter Lesions in the Premature Infant

Lesion	Circulation affected	Massive hemorrhage	Unilateral in most cases	Long-term outcome in most cases
PVHI	Venous	Yes	Yes	Spastic hemiparesis or asymmetrical spastic quadriparesis
PVL	Arterial	No	No	Spastic diplegia

Modified from Shah P, Riphagen S, Beyene J, Perlman M. Multiorgan dysfunction in infants with post-asphyxial hypoxic-ischaemic encephalopathy. Arch Dis Child Fetal Neonatal Ed 89:F152–5, 2004.

characterized by a paucity of white matter, thinning of the corpus callosum, and, in later stages, ventriculomegaly and delayed myelination.

The pathogenesis of the more diffuse lesions may relate in part to the development of the penetrating vessels more peripherally. These diffuse lesions also seem to be related to less severe ischemia than the focal ones. In sick prematures the cerebral circulation tends to become pressure passive, i.e., when blood pressure falls, so does the cerebral blood flow. This mechanism adds on to ischemia in the pathogenesis of cerebral white matter injury. Neuropathologic findings of the diffuse type of cerebral injury in the preterm infant further include preferential death of preoligodendrocytes (53, 54), axonal damage (49), and death of the transitory subplate neurons (55) through mechanisms of oxidative injury, glutamate toxicity, and the presence of cytotoxic cytokines produced by infection and inflammation (see Chapter 2). These inflammatory factors are likely to be more important in the pathogenesis of the more diffuse type PVL. *Diffuse neuronal loss*, especially in lower cortical layers, the hippocampus, and in the cerebellar Purkinje cell layer, is described in preterm brain neuropathologic studies (56).

The clinical correlates of PVL are described in Table 13-6.

At least some of the cognitive deficits associated with PVL may be due to subsequent disturbance of cortical neuronal organization, because of injury to subplate neurons, to late migrating astrocytes, or to axons with retrograde disturbances in dendritic development (55, 57, 58).

The role of MRI in the diagnosis and prognosis of these lesions will be illustrated with four cases.

CASE 8

History

This was a premature infant of 27 weeks gestational age, with hyaline membrane disease, pneumothorax, and neonatal sepsis.

Neuroimaging studies

Neonatal head ultrasound performed on day 5 showed bilaterally increased periventricular echodensities. At day 12 there were persistent periventricular echodensities with the appearance of small echolucencies (Fig. 13-14). MRI at term showed

Table 13-6 Clinical Correlates of PVL		
Topography of the injury	**Neonatal correlates**	**Long-term correlates**
Periventricular white matter (descending motor fibers, optic radiations, and association fibers)	Probable lower limb weakness (difficult to objectivate in the sick premature)	Spastic diplegia Visual deficits In the more severe forms: involvement of upper extremities and intellectual impairment Epilepsy in 3% Intellectual and visual deficits can also occur in infants without motor deficits in the more diffuse form of PVL

Modified from Volpe JJ. Neurology of the Newborn. Philadelphia, PA: WB Saunders, 2001.

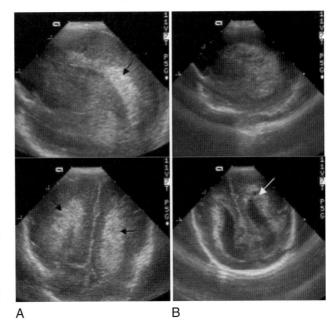

Figure 13-14 Case 8. (A) Head ultrasound examination on day 5 of life with increased slightly irregular periventricular hyperechogenicity (arrows). (B) Head ultrasound at day 10 with persisting periventricular hyperechogenicity and appearance of echolucencies (white arrow). Typical ultrasound images of evolving periventricular leukomalacia.

periventricular cysts surrounded by hyperintense areas on T1-weighted images consistent with gliosis (Fig. 13-15). The lateral ventricles are enlarged and irregularly shaped. There is overall volume reduction of the white matter especially posteriorly.

Clinical correlates in the neonatal period

There was no definite neurologic syndrome in the neonatal period.

Long-term clinical correlates

The child developed spastic diplegia as a sequela of the bilateral PVL. This is a good example of a PVL occurring in the setting of hemodynamic alterations but also inflammation due to the neonatal sepsis. The spastic diplegia was severe, so walking with aid was achieved at age 3 years. There was mild intellectual impairment. The child also presented with a strabismus.

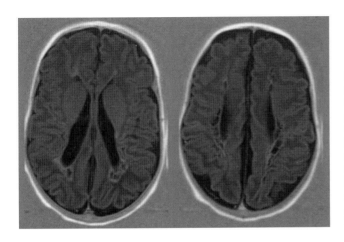

Figure 13-15 Case 8. MRI examination at term age with inversion recovery sequence and T1-weighted contrast illustrating the periventricular cysts surrounded by hyperintense areas on T1-weighted images consistent with gliosis. The lateral ventricles are enlarged and irregularly shaped with squared-off posterior horns. There seems to be overall volume reduction of the white matter especially posteriorly. These findings are typical for late-stage periventricular leukomalacia.

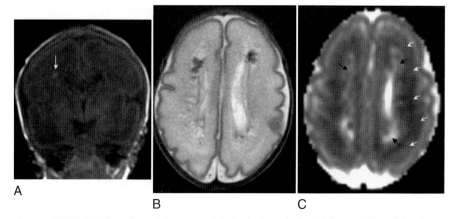

Figure 13-16 MRI in early evolving periventricular leukomalacia. (A) Coronal T1-weighted conventional MRI shows small hyperintense lesion (white arrow) in the periventricular white matter, representing small hemorrhagic component seen as hypointensities on T2-weighted images. (B) Axial T2-weighted MRI shows diffuse hyperintensities of the white matter difficult to interpret in the immature brain. (C) DWI with axial ADC map shows diffuse restriction of water diffusion with ADC values measured <1 μm^2/ms in the periventricular white matter (white arrows) and areas of increased ADC (black arrows) representing areas of beginning liquefaction.

CASE 9

History

This was a preterm infant of 29 weeks gestation, delivered via emergency caesarean section for signs of placental abruption; after resuscitation he presented with acidosis, and respiratory distress syndrome.

Neuroimaging studies

Neonatal head ultrasound performed on day 2 showed bilateral IVH with mild ventricular dilatation and local extension into frontal white matter indicative of periventricular venous infarction. MRI on day 2 confirmed intraventricular hemorrhage with unilateral venous infarction with large T2-hypointense ventricles and T2-hyperintensities adjacent to the ventricle with typical flaring pattern (Fig. 13-17A). The rest of the white matter parenchyma showed no focal T2 abnormalities, but DWI measurements revealed abnormally low ADC (0.8 μm^2/ms) in the periventricular white matter (Fig. 13-17B). Follow-up MRI 3 weeks later showed tissue dissolution in the peripheral white matter with T2 signal similar to CSF, residual IVH illustrated by T2–hypointensities, and hydrocephalus (Fig. 13-17C).

Clinical correlates in the neonatal period

There was no major neurologic syndrome in the neonatal period.

Long-term clinical correlates

This child had a very poor outcome with severe spastic quadriplegia, epilepsy, and visual and cognitive impairment. All these sequelae are due to the severe bilateral cystic leukomalacia and not to the bilateral IVH or the unilateral PVHI. This is a good example of early leukomalacia detectable only by ADC measurements which clearly changes neurologic prognosis early on. The hydrocephalus (possibly ventriculomegaly) in this case is due to tissue loss surrounding the ventricles (ex vacuo hydrocephalus).

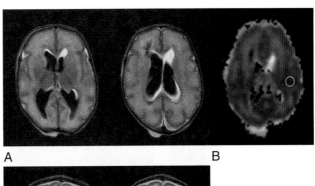

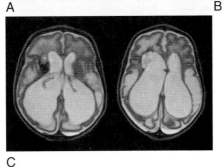

A   B

C

Figure 13-17 Case 9. Axial T2-weighted images (A) with ventricles filled with blood (low intensity) of an acute intraventricular hemorrhage with periventricular hemorrhagic infarction into frontal parenchyma (arrows) with normal appearing adjacent white matter. DWI in (B) shows reduced ADC values (circle; 0.8 μm^2/ms) in the parietal white matter. Evolution after 3 weeks shows multicystic encephalopathy with marked hydrocephalus on axial T2-weighted images.

CASE 10

History

This was a triplet pregnancy with preterm labor at 24–26 weeks gestation and premature rupture of membranes at 30 weeks gestation. Reduced growth of one triplet and alteration of umbilical Doppler measurements led to caesarean section at 33 weeks gestation. Triplet 1 was small for gestational age, and with normal Apgar score.

Neuroimaging studies

Neonatal ultrasonography on day 2 revealed bilateral periventricular hyperechogenecity (Fig. 13-18). Conventional MR imaging at term revealed multiple areas of diffuse T2-hyperintensities (DEHSI) in the white matter and subcortical white matter cysts as well as some T2-hyperintensities/T1-hyperintensities corresponding to gliotic changes in the periventricular white matter (Figs. 13-19 and 13-20).

Clinical correlates in the neonatal period

There was no major neurologic syndrome in the neonatal period.

Long-term clinical correlates

This patient developed increased tone in the four extremities, predominately affecting the lower limbs with hyperreflexia and moderate spasticity of both legs, consistent with the white matter cysts visualized on neuroimaging. He was however able to walk without help at age 2 years. His intellectual performances were markedly delayed, most likely as a sequela of the more diffuse white matter alterations. This case illustrates the fact that white matter injuries of both types (cystic and diffuse) can also occur in utero as a sequela of poor perfusion and/or inflammation.

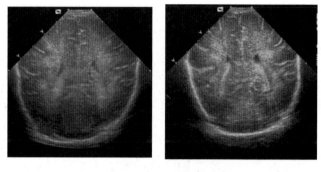

Figure 13-18 Case 10. Cranial ultrasound images acquired in the first week of life. Mild diffuse white matter hyperechogenecity.

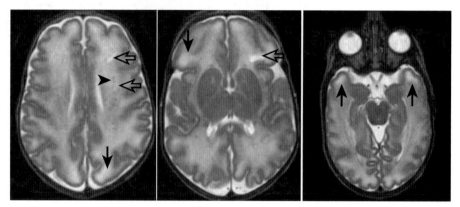

Figure 13-19 Case 10. MRI examination at term. Axial T2-weighted images show diffuse excessive hyperintense white matter (DEHSI) (small arrows) with some small cystic lesions (wide arrow) in periventricular white matter. In the periventricular white matter there are small punctate hypointense lesions (triangle).

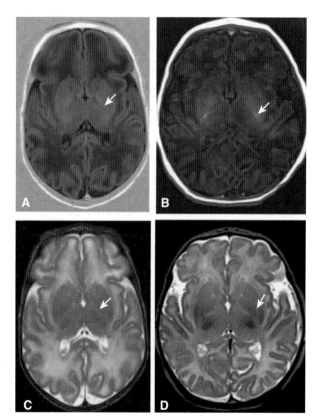

Figure 13-20 Case 10. MRI at term age (A, C). Axial inversion recovery sequence with T1-weighted contrast showing absence of myelination in the posterior limb of the internal capsule (A) compared to full-term infant (B) with typical T1-hyperintensity in the posterior limb of internal capsule. Axial T2-weighted images of Case 8 with absence of T2-hypointensity in the posterior limb of the internal capsule (C) compared to presence of T2-hypointensities in the full-term infant (D). Note also the difference in complexity of cortical folding between the preterm at term (A, C) and full-term newborn (B, D).

CASE 11

History

This was a preterm infant with gestational age at birth of 25 weeks and birth weight of 650 g. Neonatal course was significant for respiratory distress syndrome with subsequent chronic lung disease, patent ductus arteriosus ligation, necrotizing enterocolitis, and nosocomial sepsis.

Neuroimaging studies

Neonatal ultrasonography was normal throughout neonatal period. Conventional MRI at term revealed diffuse T2-hyperintensities and T1-hypointensities in the white matter with poor cortical gyrification and on DWI markedly elevated ADC values (ADC >1.8 μm^2/ms throughout the central white matter).

Clinical correlates in the neonatal period

There was no major neurologic syndrome in the neonatal period.

Long-term clinical correlates

General neurodevelopmental delay was noted at follow-up with increased tone in all four extremities and poor fine motor performance. At 24 months of corrected age there was a marked delay in motor development (assessed at the 16 month level), as well as a marked delay in the cognitive development (assessed at the 15 month level). In addition there was poor attention control. He received special neuro-developmental interventions since birth. This case is a good illustration of diffuse white matter alteration which has not been visualized by cranial ultrasound.

Cranial Ultrasonography in the Preterm Infant

Neonatal sonography is the one major bedside technique available to image the neonatal brain. Leviton and Paneth postulated in 1990 that ultrasonographic white matter echodensities and echolucencies in low birth weight infants predicted later handicap more accurately than any other antecedent (59). Unlike IVH, damage to the white matter can have different appearances and depending on the timing of the injury the imaging characteristics can be nonspecific with generally an increase in echogenicity in the acute phase of the injury (Figs. 13-14 and 13-18). In clinical practice, at least in the older preterm infant, the condition of white matter is judged by its echogenic potential as compared to choroid plexus. Generally the echogenicity found in early PVL is similar in intensity to choroids plexus, with a bilateral but slightly asymmetric appearance, can be sharply delineated, and may have nodular components. This has to be differentiated from normal peritrigonal flaring which is perfectly symmetric and with a radial appearance. Evolution of such hyperechogenecity can be twofold: either complete disappearance or evolution into cysts and/or ventricular dilatation. Cyst formation in analog to neuropathology is a process typical for the second week (10–40 days) after the insult. DeVries et al. (60) postulated an ultrasound-based classification for PVL of four grades, increasing grades being associated with increasing neurodevelopmental handicap. Grade I is the transient (>7 days) periventricular densities without cyst formation. If cysts develop and are few in number, localized primarily in frontal and frontoparietal white matter, this is classified as Grade II. When they are widespread and extend into the parieto-occipital region they are referred to as Grade III; they may grow

Table 13-7	Ultrasound Classification of PVL (60)
Grade I	Transient periventricular echodensities (PVE) (>7 days)
Grade II	PVE evolving into localized frontoparietal cystic lesions
Grade III	PVE evolving into extensive periventricular cystic lesions
Grade IV	Echodensities evolving into extensive periventricular and subcortical cysts

and gradually disappear leaving an irregularly dilated lateral ventricle. If cysts are present all the way into the subcortical area resembling porencephaly, this is referred to as Grade IV (Table 13-7).

Classification needs longitudinal assessment with daily to weekly ultrasound evaluations.

Ultrasound can be viewed as the ideal mode of imaging to detect cystic PVL, but has very limited value for detecting diffuse white matter injury, as shown in studies comparing neonatal sonography with MRI (61–65).

Conventional MRI in the Preterm Infant

Conventional MRI features of chronic white matter injury in the immature brain are characterized not only by cysts similar to ultrasound but also and more importantly by a persistent high signal intensity of the white matter in T2-weighted images representing diffuse white matter injury (66) (see Figs. 13-16, 13-19, and 13-20). This imaging characteristic is later associated with the thinning of the corpus callosum and loss of white matter volume as a result (see later). In several recent studies on preterm infant brains, diffuse excessive high signal intensity (DEHSI) in the cerebral white matter on T2-weighted imaging was reported to be present in up to 40 to 75% of low birthweight preterm infants imaged at term (67) (Fig. 13-19). MRI is further ideally equipped to assess delayed myelination. The absence of myelination in the posterior limb of the internal capsule (missing T1 high signal intensity, T2 low signal intensity) at term age is a good indicator of later neuromotor impairment (Fig. 13-20) (68, 69).

Conventional T1- and T2-weighted imaging can also show other signal abnormalities in the periventricular white matter. In the subacute phase of white matter injury, MRI detects punctate periventricular areas of T1 signal hyperintensities (see Fig. 13-21). The precise neuropathologic correlate of these signal abnormalities is not completely known but may be due to some hemorrhagic components of the lesion but most likely represents the cellular reaction of glial cells and macrophages, which are known to contain lipid droplets (see neuropathology description) which explain perfectly the high signal intensity in T1-weighted MR images (70).

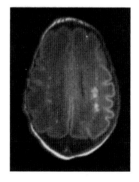

Figure 13-21 White matter abnormalities in the centrum semiovale characterized by chain-like T1-hyperintensities in a preterm infant.

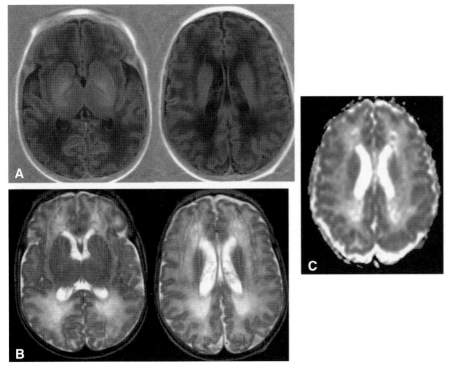

Figure 13-22 Case 11. MRI examination at term of a 25-week gestation preterm infant. Normal cranial ultrasounds throughout perinatal period (A). Axial inversion recovery sequence with T1-weighted contrast shows low signal intensity in the white matter which corresponds in the T2-weighted images to high signal intensity throughout the white matter with moderately dilated ventricles and poor cortical folding (B). ADC values (C) of the central white matter are diffusely elevated with values >1.8 μm²/ms. Also note the poor cortical gyrification with simple gyri that most likely represent secondary rather than tertiary sulci.

Conventional MRI can qualitatively appreciate cortical differentiation and preterm infants with diffuse white matter abnormalities often show poor cortical gyrification at term with simple appearing gyri and sulci compared to complex tertiary sulci seen in the full-term infant (Figs. 13-20 and 13-22). Quantification of these changes can be assessed by three-dimensional quantitative MRI (3D-MRI) techniques described later.

Diffusion MRI in the Preterm Infant

Early assessment of periventricular white matter in preterm infants with DWI can reveal bilateral periventricular diffusion restriction similar to the typical distribution of PVL when ultrasound and conventional MRI show no or nonspecific abnormalities (71) (see Fig. 13-16). A reduced ADC in an otherwise normal preterm brain is considered an early indicator of white matter damage (just as a reduced ADC is seen shortly after the onset of an acute cerebral ischemic lesion in the full-term newborn). The typical histologic changes in the acute phase of PVL outlined above like cellular and axonal swelling and astrocytic hyperplasia are characterized by some of the same mechanisms leading to restriction of water diffusivity. This considerably changes the microstructure of white matter and therefore changes water diffusivity.

The diffuse T2-hyperintensities or DEHSI as indicators of the chronic phase of white matter injury are associated with higher ADC values which confirms the locally higher tissue water content and loss of microstructure impeding water diffusion in those areas (72–74) (see Fig. 13-22). These high ADC values are similar to those seen in the very immature healthy white matter; therefore a potential explanation for the failure of ADC to decline from high levels in the extremely premature infant to lower levels in the term infant in the presence of DEHSI might be related to prior injury with destruction of normal cellular elements (e.g., preoligodendrocytes) (75). Further quantitative measures of diffusion at term among premature infants with perinatal white matter lesions, when compared to preterm infants without white matter injury, showed lower anisotropy values in the area of the previous injury, i.e., central periventricular white matter, but also in the underlying posterior limb of internal capsule (73, 76). The lower anisotropy in the injured cerebral white matter suggests that white matter fiber tracts were destroyed or their subsequent development was impaired. The lower anisotropy in the internal capsule further suggests a disturbance in the development of the descending corticospinal tracts (77). This finding might well be the basis for the reduction in myelination in the posterior limb of the internal capsule observed in conventional MRI which was shown to be highly correlated with development of motor deficits. DWI with DTI has provided new insights into the microstructural white matter development and seems to be an ideal tool to assess alteration of white matter pathways in neurologic disease.

Magnetic Resonance Spectroscopy in the Preterm Infant

The biochemical characteristics of white matter damage in preterm infants have been studied in vivo using MRS (78, 79). Similar to the high diagnostic value of MRS in term asphyxia, MRS in acute phase immature white matter injury can detect indicators of anaerobic glycolysis with increased intracerebral lactate (32). Preliminary results show that white matter damage in the preterm infant studied around term gestational age resulted in high Lac/Cr and high Myo-Inositol/Cr ratios (79). The increased presence of lactate at this chronic stage was not associated with changes in pH, while NAA, as a marker of neuroaxonal integrity, was reduced in the damaged periventricular white matter. Astrocytes further play a variety of complex nutritive and supportive roles in relation to neuronal metabolic homeostasis. For example, astrocytes take up glutamate and convert it to glutamine; this removal of glutamate from the extracellular space protects surrounding cells from excitotoxicity from glutamate. Glutamate uptake into astrocytes further stimulates glycolysis within the astrocyte with production of lactate that can be used by neurons as energy substrate (80). Given that chronic phase white matter injury is characterized by widespread cerebral white matter astrocytosis, this change in metabolite composition might be an expression of altered cellular composition and substrate utilization.

Advanced Quantitative MRI with Image Analysis Tools

Only recently 3D-MRI methods combined with image postprocessing techniques have been developed, which allow volumetric assessment of brain development and an absolute quantitation of myelination in the newborn (81–83). These techniques allow exact definition of brain volume and can therefore accurately monitor brain growth, and measure CSF volume and volume changes in white matter and cortical gray matter. 3D-MRI volumetric techniques were used to evaluate the effect on subsequent brain development of early white matter injury in premature infants. In the premature infants with preceding white matter injury, the volume of myelinated white matter at term was significantly lower than in the premature infants without prior white matter injury and the infants born at term measuring the degree of delay of myelination. Furthermore this study showed a marked decrease in cortical gray matter volume in the preterm infants with prior periventricular white matter injury indicating impaired cerebral cortical development after early white matter injury (84). In a recent population study similar volumetric changes of overall brain development in preterm infants was confirmed with significant reduction of myelinated white matter and cortical gray matter in preterm infants compared to full-term infants, with a reduction also of deep nuclear gray matter (basal ganglia) most pronounced in the lowest gestational ages (82). Assessing moderately preterm infants without signs of white matter injury cortical development was similar to full-term infants (85). Regional assessment of white matter myelination in preterm infants further revealed particular delay in myelination in the central and posterior part of the brain (86). When assessing cerebellar volume at term there was a significant reduction of cerebellar volume of preterm infants when compared to term infants (87). Unilateral cerebral white matter lesions resulted in contralateral reduction of cerebellar volume indicating the trophic interplay due to loss of cerebrocerebellar connectivity (88).

Long-term follow-up studies of preterm infants have confirmed the permanent character of these disruptive/adaptive changes in brain development. Recent evaluations of 8-year-old preterm infants with volumetric brain assessment showed persistence of cortical gray matter reduction in preterm infants accompanied with a reduction in the volume of hippocampus, which correlated with cognitive scores indicating long-term functional consequences (89). Both cortical volume and cortical thickness were shown to be reduced in 15-year-old adolescents born prematurely (90).

In conclusion, the main advantages of MR techniques in the evaluation of the preterm infant are as follows:

1. Abnormal signal intensities in the white matter are more reliably detected by MRI than by ultrasound.
2. More widespread nonhemorrhagic white matter injury in the presence of IVH is more readily diagnosed with MR techniques than with ultrasound in both the acute as well as chronic phase.
3. Diffuse white matter injury without frank cystic development can be detected by MRI by both conventional MRI (DEHSI) as well as DWI with measurement of ADC.
4. Myelination pattern at term defined by inversion recovery, T1- and T2-weighted MR sequences can predict neuromotor outcome.
5. More advanced MRI tools such as DTI, 3D volumetric MRI, and fMRI can define plasticity and predict functional outcome of more complex brain functions.

Acknowledgment

The authors acknowledge support by the Swiss National Foundation (SNF: 3200-056927/102127).

REFERENCES

1. Neil J, Miller J, Mukherjee P, Hüppi PS. Diffusion tensor imaging of normal and injured developing human brain: a technical review. NMR Biomed 15:543–52, 2002.
2. Hüppi PS, Lazeyras F. Proton magnetic resonance spectroscopy ((1)H-MRS) in neonatal brain injury. Pediatr Res 49:317–20, 2001.
3. Seghier ML, Lazeyras F, Hüppi PS. Functional MRI of the newborn. Semin Fetal Neonatal Med 11:479–88, 2006.
4. Volpe JJ. Perinatal brain injury: from pathogenesis to neuroprotection. Ment Retard Dev Disabil Res Rev 7:56–64, 2001.

5. Perlman JM. Summary proceedings from the neurology group on hypoxic-ischemic encephalopathy. Pediatrics 117:S28–33, 2006.
6. Nelson KB, Grether JK. Potentially asphyxiating conditions and spastic cerebral palsy in infants of normal birth weight. Am J Obstet Gynecol 179:507–13, 1998.
7. Perlman JM. Intrapartum asphyxia and cerebral palsy: is there a link? Clin Perinatol 33:335–53, 2006.
8. Barkovich A, Sargent S. Profound asphyxia in the premature infant: imaging findings. AJNR Am J Neuroradiol 16:1837–46, 1995.
9. Shah P, Riphagen S, Beyene J, Perlman M. Multiorgan dysfunction in infants with post-asphyxial hypoxic-ischaemic encephalopathy. Arch Dis Child Fetal Neonatal Ed 89:F152–5, 2004.
10. Rutherford M, Counsell S, Allsop J, et al. Diffusion-weighted magnetic resonance imaging in term perinatal brain injury: a comparison with site of lesion and time from birth. Pediatrics 114:1004–14, 2004.
11. Govaert P, de Vries LS. An Atlas of Neonatal Brain Sonography. Cambridge: Cambridge University Press, 1997, pp. 1–363.
12. Kashman N, Kramer U, Stavorovsky Z, et al. Prognostic significance of hyperechogenic lesions in the basal ganglia and thalamus in neonates. J Child Neurol 16:591–4, 2001.
13. Cabanas F, Pellicer A, Perez-Higueras A, et al. Ultrasonographic findings in thalamus and basal ganglia in term asphyxiated infants. Pediatr Neurol 7:211–15, 1991.
14. Rutherford M. MRI of the Neonatal Brain. Philadelphia, PA: WB Saunders, 2002.
15. Rutherford M, Malamateniou C, Zeka J, Counsell S. MR imaging of the neonatal brain at 3 tesla. Eur J Paediatr Neurol 8:281–9, 2004.
16. Hüppi PS, Lazeyras F. MR spectroscopy. In Tortori-Donati P (ed). Pediatric Neuroradiology Brain. Berlin: Springer, 2005, pp. 1049–72.
17. Triulzi F, Baldoli C, Parazzini C. Neonatal MR imaging. Magn Reson Imaging Clin N Am 9:57–82, viii, 2001.
18. McArdle CB, Richardson CJ, Nicholas DA. Developmental features of the neonatal brain: MR imaging: I. Gray–white matter differentiation and myelination. Radiology 162:223–9, 1987.
19. Rutherford MA, Pennock JM, Counsell SJ, et al. Abnormal magnetic resonance signal in the internal capsule predicts poor neurodevelopmental outcome in infants with hypoxic-ischemic encephalopathy. Pediatrics 102:323–8, 1998.
20. Rutherford M, Ward P, Allsop J, et al. Magnetic resonance imaging in neonatal encephalopathy. Early Hum Dev 81:13–25, 2005.
21. Pasternak JF. Parasagittal infarction in neonatal asphyxia. Ann Neurol 21:202–4, 1987.
22. Conturo TE, McKinstry RC, Aronovitz JA, Neil JJ. Diffusion MRI: precision, accuracy and flow effects. NMR Biomed 8:307–32, 1995.
23. Moseley M, Cohen Y, Kucharczyk J, et al. Diffusion-weighted MR-imaging of anisotropic water diffusion in cat central nervous system. Radiology 176:439–45, 1990.
24. Rumpel H, Ferrini B, Martin E. Lasting cytotoxic edema as an indicator of irreversible brain damage: a case of neonatal stroke. Neurosci Behav 19:1636–8, 1998.
25. Warach S, Chien D, Li W. Fast magnetic resonance diffusion-weighted imaging of acute human stroke. Neurology 42:1717–23, 1992.
26. Li F, Han SS, Tatlisumak T, et al. Reversal of acute apparent diffusion coefficient abnormalities and delayed neuronal death following transient focal cerebral ischemia in rats. Ann Neurol 46:333–42, 1999.
27. Copen WA, Schwamm LH, Gonzalez RG, et al. Ischemic stroke: effects of etiology and patient age on the time course of the core apparent diffusion coefficient. Radiology 221:27–34, 2001.
28. McKinstry RC, Miller JH, Snyder AZ, et al. A prospective, longitudinal diffusion tensor imaging study of brain injury in newborns. Neurology 59:824–33, 2002.
29. Robertson R, Ben-Sira L, Barnes P, et al. MR line-scan diffusion-weighted imaging of term neonates with perinatal brain ischemia. AJNR Am J Neuroradiol 20:1658–70, 1999.
30. Soul JS, Robertson RL, Tzika AA, et al. Time course of changes in diffusion-weighted magnetic resonance imaging in a case of neonatal encephalopathy with defined onset and duration of hypoxic-ischemic insult. Pediatrics 108:1211–14, 2001.
31. Groenendaal F, Veehoven R, van der Grond J, et al. Cerebral lactate and N-acetylaspartate/choline ratios in asphyxiated full-term neonates demonstrated in vivo using proton magnetic resonance spectroscopy. Pediatr Res 35:148–51, 1994.
32. Penrice J, Cady E, Lorek A, et al. Proton magnetic resonance spectroscopy of the brain in normal preterm and term infants, and early changes after perinatal hypoxia-ischemia. Pediatr Res 40:6–14, 1996.
33. Hanrahan J, Cox I, Azzopardi D, et al. Relation between proton magnetic resonance spectroscopy within 18 hours of birth asphyxia and neurodevelopment at 1 year of age. Dev Med Child Neurol 41:76–82, 1999.
34. Hanrahan J, Cox I, Edwards A, et al. Persistent increases in cerebral lactate concentration after birth asphyxia. Pediatr Res 44:304–11, 1998.
35. Robertson NJ, Cowan FM, Cox IJ, Edwards AD. Brain alkaline intracellular pH after neonatal encephalopathy. Ann Neurol 52:732–42, 2002.
36. Robertson N, Cox IJ, Cowan FM, et al. Cerebral intracellular lactic alkalosis persisting months after neonatal encephalopathy measured by magnetic resonance spectroscopy. Pediatr Res 46:287–96, 1999.
37. Zarifi MK, Astrakas LG, Poussaint TY, et al. Prediction of adverse outcome with cerebral lactate level and apparent diffusion coefficient in infants with perinatal asphyxia. Radiology 225:859–70, 2002.

38. Groenendaal F, Roelants-Van Rijn AM, van Der GJ, et al. Glutamate in cerebral tissue of asphyxiated neonates during the first week of life demonstrated in vivo using proton magnetic resonance spectroscopy. Biol Neonate 79:254–7, 2001.

39. Roelants-Van Rijn AM, van Der GJ, de Vries LS, Groenendaal F. Value of (1)H-MRS using different echo times in neonates with cerebral hypoxia-ischemia. Pediatr Res 49:356–62, 2001.

40. Peden C, Rutherford M, Sargentoni J, et al. Proton spectroscopy of the neonatal brain following hypoxic-ischemic injury. Dev Med Child Neurol 34:285–95, 1993.

41. Shu S, Ashwal S, Holshauser B, et al. Prognostic value of 1H-MRS in perinatal CNS insults. Pediatr Neurol 17:309–18, 1997.

42. Boardman JP, Ganesan V, Rutherford MA, et al. Magnetic resonance image correlates of hemiparesis after neonatal and childhood middle cerebral artery stroke. Pediatrics 115:321–6, 2005.

43. de Vries LS, van Der GJ, van Haastert IC, Groenendaal F. Prediction of outcome in new-born infants with arterial ischaemic stroke using diffusion-weighted magnetic resonance imaging. Neuropediatrics 36:12–20, 2005.

44. Seghier ML, Lazeyras F, Zimine S, et al. Combination of event-related fMRI and diffusion tensor imaging in an infant with perinatal stroke. Neuroimage 21:463–72, 2004.

45. Seghier ML, Lazeyras F, Zimine S, et al. Visual recovery after perinatal stroke evidenced by functional and diffusion MRI: case report. BMC Neurol 5:17, 2005.

46. Ghazi-Birry HS, Brown WR, Moody DM, et al. Human germinal matrix: venous origin of hemorrhage and vascular characteristics. AJNR Am J Neuroradiol 18:219–29, 1997.

47. Gould SJ, Howard S, Hope PL, Reynolds EO. Periventricular intraparenchymal cerebral haemorrhage in preterm infants: the role of venous infarction. J Pathol 151:197–202, 1987.

48. Deguchi K, Oguchi K, Takashima S. Characteristic neuropathology of leukomalacia in extremely low birth weight infants. Pediatr Neurol 16:296–300, 1997.

49. Hirayama A, Okoshi Y, Hachiya Y, et al. Early immunohistochemical detection of axonal damage and glial activation in extremely immature brains with periventricular leukomalacia. Clin Neuropathol 20:87–91, 2001.

50. Deguchi K, Oguchi K, Matsuura N, et al. Periventricular leukomalacia: relation to gestational age and axonal injury. Pediatr Neurol 20:370–4, 1999.

51. Takashima S, Tanaka K. Development of cerebrovascular architecture and its relationship to periventricular leukomalacia. Arch Neurol 35:11–16, 1978.

52. Taylor HG, Minich N, Bangert B, et al. Long-term neuropsychological outcomes of very low birth weight: associations with early risks for periventricular brain insults. J Int Neuropsychol Soc 10:987–1004, 2004.

53. Back SA, Han BH, Luo NL, et al. Selective vulnerability of late oligodendrocyte progenitors to hypoxia-ischemia. J Neurosci 22:455–63, 2002.

54. Haynes RL, Folkerth RD, Keefe RJ, et al. Nitrosative and oxidative injury to premyelinating oligodendrocytes in periventricular leukomalacia. J Neuropathol Exp Neurol 62:441–50, 2003.

55. McQuillen PS, Sheldon RA, Shatz CJ, Ferriero DM. Selective vulnerability of subplate neurons after early neonatal hypoxia-ischemia. J Neurosci 23:3308–15, 2003.

56. Marin-Padilla M. Developmental neuropathology and impact of perinatal brain damage: II. White matter lesions of the neocortex. J Neuropathol Exp Neurol 56:219–35, 1997.

57. Volpe J. Subplate neurons-missing link in brain injury of the premature infant? Pediatrics 97: 112–3, 1996.

58. Gressens P, Richelme C, Kadhim HJ, et al. The germinative zone produces the most cortical astrocytes after neuronal migration in the developing mammalian brain. Biol Neonate 61:4–24, 1992.

59. Leviton A, Paneth N. White matter damage in preterm newborns: an epidemiologic perspective. Early Hum Dev 24:1–22, 1990.

60. DeVries L, Eken P, Dubowitz L. The spectrum of leukomalacia using cranial ultrasound. Behav Brain Res 49:1–6, 1992.

61. Maalouf EF, Duggan PJ, Counsell SJ, et al. Comparison of findings on cranial ultrasound and magnetic resonance imaging in preterm infants. Pediatrics 107:719–27, 2001.

62. Childs AM, Cornette L, Ramenghi LA, et al. Magnetic resonance and cranial ultrasound characteristics of periventricular white matter abnormalities in newborn infants. Clin Radiol 56:647–55, 2001.

63. DeVries L, Eken P, Groenendaal F, et al. Correlation between the degree of periventricular leukomalacia diagnosed using cranial ultrasound and MRI later in infancy in children with cerebral palsy. Neuropediatrics 24:263–8, 1993.

64. Rijn AM, Groenendaal F, Beek FJ, et al. Parenchymal brain injury in the preterm infant: comparison of cranial ultrasound, MRI and neurodevelopmental outcome. Neuropediatrics 32:80–9, 2001.

65. Inder TE, Anderson NJ, Spencer C, et al. White matter injury in the premature infant: a comparison between serial cranial sonographic and MR findings at term. AJNR Am J Neuroradiol 24: 805–9, 2003.

66. Hüppi PS. Advances in postnatal neuroimaging: relevance to pathogenesis and treatment of brain injury. Clin Perinatol 29:827–56, 2002.

67. Maalouf EF, Duggan PJ, Rutherford MA, et al. Magnetic resonance imaging of the brain in a cohort of extremely preterm infants. J Pediatr 135:351–7, 1999.

68. de Vries LS, Groenendaal F, van Haastert IC, et al. Asymmetrical myelination of the posterior limb of the internal capsule in infants with periventricular haemorrhagic infarction: an early predictor of hemiplegia. Neuropediatrics 30:314–9, 1999.

69. Aida N, Nishimura G, Hachiya Y, et al. MR imaging of perinatal brain damage: comparison of clinical outcome with initial and follow-up findings. Am J Neuroradiol 19:1909–21, 1998.

70. Schouman-Claeys E, Henry-Feugeas MC, Roset F, et al. Periventricular leukomalacia: correlation between MR imaging and autopsy findings during the first 2 months of life. Radiology 189:59–64, 1993.
71. Inder T, Hüppi P, Zientara G, et al. Early detection of periventricular leukomalacia by diffusion-weighted magnetic resonance imaging techniques. J Pediatr 134:631–4, 1999.
72. Counsell SJ, Allsop JM, Harrison MC, et al. Diffusion-weighted imaging of the brain in preterm infants with focal and diffuse white matter abnormality. Pediatrics 112:1–7, 2003.
73. Hüppi P, Murphy B, Maier S, et al. Microstructural brain development after perinatal cerebral white matter injury assessed by diffusion tensor magnetic resonance imaging. Pediatrics 107:455–60, 2001.
74. Miller SP, Vigneron DB, Henry RG, et al. Serial quantitative diffusion tensor MRI of the premature brain: development in newborns with and without injury. J Magn Reson Imaging 16:621–32, 2002.
75. Counsell SJ, Shen Y, Boardman JP, et al. Axial and radial diffusivity in preterm infants who have diffuse white matter changes on magnetic resonance imaging at term-equivalent age. Pediatrics 117:376–86, 2006.
76. Hüppi PS, Dubois J. Diffusion tensor imaging of brain development. Semin Fetal Neonatal Med 11:489–97, 2006.
77. Mazumdar A, Mukherjee P, Miller JH, et al. Diffusion-weighted imaging of acute corticospinal tract injury preceding Wallerian degeneration in the maturing human brain. AJNR Am J Neuroradiol 24:1057–66, 2003.
78. Groenendaal F, van de Grond J, Eken P, et al. Early cerebral proton MRS and neurodevelopmental outcome in infants with cystic leukomalacia. Dev Med Child Neurol 39:373–9, 1997.
79. Robertson N, Kuint J, Counsell T, et al. Characterization of cerebral white matter damage in the preterm infant using 1H and 31P magnetic resonance spectroscopy. J Cereb Blood Flow Metab 20:1446–56, 2000.
80. Pellerin L, Pellegri G, Martin J, Magistretti P. Expression of monocarboxylate transporter mRNAs in mouse brain: support for a distinct role of lactate as an energy substrate for the neonatal vs. the adult brain. Proc Natl Acad Sci USA 95:3990–5, 1998.
81. Hüppi P, Warfield S, Kikinis R, et al. Quantitative magnetic resonance imaging of brain development in premature and mature newborns. Ann Neurol 43:224–35, 1998.
82. Inder TE, Warfield SK, Wang H, et al. Abnormal cerebral structure is present at term in premature infants. Pediatrics 115:286–94, 2005.
83. Prastawa M, Gilmore JH, Lin W, Gerig G. Automatic segmentation of MR images of the developing newborn brain. Med Image Anal 9:457–66, 2005.
84. Inder T, Hüppi P, Warfield S, et al. Periventricular white matter injury in the premature infant is associated with a reduction in cerebral cortical gray matter volume at term. Ann Neurol 46:755–60, 1999.
85. Zacharia A, Zimine S, Lovblad KO, et al. Early assessment of brain maturation by MR imaging segmentation in neonates and premature infants. AJNR Am J Neuroradiol 27:972–7, 2006.
86. Mewes AU, Hüppi PS, Als H, et al. Regional brain development in serial magnetic resonance imaging of low-risk preterm infants. Pediatrics 118:23–33, 2006.
87. Limperopoulos C, Soul JS, Gauvreau K, et al. Late gestation cerebellar growth is rapid and impeded by premature birth. Pediatrics 115:688–95, 2005.
88. Limperopoulos C, Soul JS, Haidar H, et al. Impaired trophic interactions between the cerebellum and the cerebrum among preterm infants. Pediatrics 116:844–50, 2005.
89. Lodygensky GA, Rademaker K, Zimine S, et al. Structural and functional brain development after hydrocortisone treatment for neonatal chronic lung disease. Pediatrics 116:1–7, 2005.
90. Martinussen M, Fischl B, Larsson HB, et al. Cerebral cortex thickness in 15-year-old adolescents with low birth weight measured by an automated MRI-based method. Brain 128:2588–96, 2005.

Chapter 14

Long-term Follow-up of Very Low Birth Weight Infants

Betty R. Vohr, MD

Modern neonatal intensive care has had major therapeutic advances in the past 10 years which have resulted in a dramatic improvement in survival of extremely low birth weight (ELBW; <1000 g) infants (1–4). This has been most significant among infants at the limits of viability (23–24 weeks) (3–5). These infants have increased neonatal morbidities (6–10), increased complex medical morbidities (respiratory, gastrointestinal, feeding, growth failure), and increased neurodevelopmental morbidities (neurologic, sensory, developmental, and behavioral) after discharge from the neonatal intensive care unit (NICU) (7–13). There are numerous reports of neurodevelopmental abnormalities in ex-ELBW infants in early childhood, but increasing evidence is accumulating of adverse outcomes and special healthcare needs at school age (14–18) and in the young adult (19–21).

The responsibilities for neonatal follow-up programs at tertiary care centers include surveillance of NICU quality indicators, research, and education of fellows and residents (22), and in some programs, clinical management post discharge. Important neurodevelopmental outcomes (quality indicators for a NICU) include cerebral palsy, retardation, vision impairment, and hearing impairment rates. Communication of findings to the primary care provider and facilitation of referrals to necessary support services are important components of the clinical program. One of the challenges of follow-up is to identify the optimal age of assessment to determine the "true outcome" and functional ability of the child. Because of the challenges, costs, and feasibility of long-term tracking, most follow-up studies currently are short term (≤2 years) which may limit the interpretation of the neurodevelopmental outcome data. This chapter will discuss four outcome ages: 18–24 months, 3–6 years, school age, and adolescent/young adult. The discussion will cover two outcome areas: (i) cerebral palsy and other neurologic morbidities and (ii) developmental delays and cognitive impairments. A case report will be provided for each of the four age categories to illustrate some of the challenges encountered in evaluating the neurodevelopmental outcomes of ELBW NICU graduates.

OUTCOME: CEREBRAL PALSY AND OTHER NEUROLOGIC OR SENSORY SEQUELAE

An outcome of major concern for both pediatricians and parents of ELBW infants is cerebral palsy (CP). ELBW infants are at significant risk for brain injury secondary to the effects of hypoxia-ischemia, inflammatory disorders including sepsis, necrotizing enterocolitis, and meningitis, and undernutrition superimposed on a vulnerable immature brain (23–26). Radiographic evidence of brain injury (intraventricular hemorrhage (IVH) (27), periventricular leukomalacia (PVL) (8), and ventriculomegaly (28)) is associated with adverse neurodevelopmental outcomes, including CP. The strongest predictor of CP is PVL (29) Neonatologists use this radiographic information to provide feedback to families on the relative risk of neurodevelopmental sequelae. The sensitivity and specificity of an abnormal cranial ultrasound, however, remain weak, and Laptook et al. (7) reported that the rate of CP among infants <1000 g with a normal cranial ultrasound was 9.4%. The ability to accurately predict outcome is complicated by the fact that other morbidities (7) and interventions (1, 30–33) may be associated positively or negatively with neurodevelopmental sequelae. Two perinatal interventions (antenatal steroids (1) and prophylactic indomethacin (30, 31)) are associated with a decreased risk of IVH. Postnatal steroid administration which may increase the risk of CP (33) is used therapeutically to wean premature infants with chronic lung disease from assisted ventilation. Laptook et al. (7) identified that within a cohort of ELBW infants with a normal head ultrasound, male gender and multiple birth were independently associated with CP. Cerebral palsy, unfortunately, remains a major neurologic sequelae among ELBW survivors, affecting 9–17% of survivors (34–41). Prompt diagnosis of the infant with CP to ensure appropriate intervention services and supports for the child and family is paramount. There are, however, some challenges associated with recognizing the clinical signs, particularly if the disorder is mild, or there are mixed findings.

An early definition of CP was published by Bax (42) in 1964. He described CP as "a disorder of movement and posture due to a defect or lesion of the immature brain." The definition used by the National Institute of Child Health and Human Development (NICHD) Network (13) at 18–22 months corrected age (CA) includes the following three components: (i) abnormalities of tone, reflexes, coordination, and movement; (ii) delay in motor milestones; and (iii) aberrations in primitive reflexes (retention >6 months) or failure of postural reflexes to emerge >6 months. The traditional CP diagnosis is based on findings of abnormal tone and posture and is classified by the number of limbs involved (4 = quadriplegia, 3 = triplegia, 2 legs = diplegia, right or left arm and leg = hemiplegia, and 1 extremity = monoplegia). The classification of CP based on topology has been linked to ultimate motor prognosis (13). Children with hemiplegia and diplegia are able to eventually attain functional mobility, while children with triplegia and quadriplegia often struggle with motor performance. Another classification of CP (40) is based specifically on the tone and reflexes and has the following categories: spastic ($\uparrow$ tone and $\uparrow$ reflexes), choreoathetotic ($\pm \downarrow$ tone and $\uparrow$ reflexes), dystonic ($\pm \uparrow$ tone and stiff movements), ataxic ($\downarrow$ tone and ataxia), and mixed CP. Fortunately for physicians there is a mixed category since many children do not fit nicely into a specific category (43). Severity of CP may be classified as: (i) mild (impairment interferes with but does not prevent age-appropriate function – includes nonfluent walking), moderate (walks with assistive device or does not walk, sits independently or with support), or severe (no ambulation, no sitting, and no supported sitting) (41); (ii) nondisabling versus disabling (39); and (iii) by gross motor performance (43–45). A Gross Motor Functional Measure (GMFCS) (44, 45) has been developed to systematically evaluate functional skills in prone, rolling, sitting, crawling, standing, walking, jumping, and running (43–46). Wood and Rosenbaum (43) have shown that the GMFCS has stability over time in children with CP.

THE 18- TO 24-MONTH-OLD CHILD

The majority of neurodevelopmental follow-up studies in multicenter networks evaluate infants to 18 or 24 months CA. Current understanding is that a definitive diagnosis of CP can be made at these ages in most children; an exception may be very mild CP. We will try to analyze some of the issues that arise when making the diagnosis.

Drillien (47) published a classic study in 1972 of 300 infants <1250 g. She described early neurologic signs which she called "transient dystonia." There were four categories of neurologic signs: (i) irritability, ↑ crying, feeding difficulty; (ii) jittery, easily startled; (iii) ↑ tone, fisting, arching; and (iv) standing on toes. Infants were categorized in the first year of life as mild (1–2 signs <2 months), moderate (>2 signs after 2 months), and severe (>2 signs at 4–8 months). She demonstrated that the percent of infants with "moderate to severe" signs decreased with increasing age, from 46% at 2 months, 18% at 8 months, to 6% at 12 months. Those infants with persisting severe findings were likely to develop CP; those who "lost" the findings were likely to not have CP. The transient presence of abnormal neurologic findings in ELBW infants in the first year of life has been observed by others (48). Neurologic findings in ELBW infants in the first 6 to 12 months may indicate a need for early intervention services but, unless suspect or abnormal findings persist, they lack specificity relative to long-term outcome.

Other phenomena in the first year of life that aid in making the diagnosis include the fading of primitive reflexes and the emergence of postural reflexes in infants developing normally. In addition, the normality or abnormality of muscle tone often has not fully declared itself until 18–24 months of age since myelination continues during this time. For these reasons follow-up studies reported at 12 months of age or earlier do not provide reliable CP data. Even at older ages, making a definitive diagnosis for children with mild CP may be challenging. Paneth et al. (49) demonstrated that pediatrician reliability in discriminating disabling CP from nondisabling CP and no CP was weak, but improved significantly when as assessment of gross motor functional skills was added to the traditional neurologic examination. Therefore, for optimal clinical management and to ensure accurate diagnoses and appropriate interventions are in place, serial comprehensive assessments of both neurologic signs and motor skills by trained observers are indicated for ELBW infants.

In a NICHD Network study of ELBW infants born 1995–1998, CP was identified in 12.3% and other abnormal neurologic findings in 10.3% of ELBW infant survivors at 18 to 22 months CA. "Other" neurologic findings included hypertonia, hypotonia, seizure disorder, monoplegia, dyspraxia, or dystonia without a specific diagnosis of CP. The study demonstrated that ELBW children with CP are at increased risk of having other neurosensory morbidities, and children with quadriplegia are at greatest risk compared to children with other types of CP or no CP. For the 53 children with quadriplegia, 9.8% had seizures, 18.9% had shunts for hydrocephalus, 21.6% had severe visual impairment (i.e., legal blindness or vision worse than 20/200 in one or both eyes), 9.8% had severe hearing impairment (i.e., deafness or hearing loss requiring amplification in both ears), and 97.9% had a Bayley mental developmental index <70.

The assessment used by the NICHD neonatal research network at 18 to 22 months CA consists of an interim medical history, updated social, demographic, and health data, neurologic assessment, assessment with the Gross Motor

Classification System (44), and a developmental assessment with the Bayley Scales of Infant Development (50). The neurologic examination at 18–22 months is based on the assessment of Amiel-Tison (51) and is performed by certified developmentalists who have been trained to reliability.

Assessment of vision for ELBW infants begins in the NICU with standard assessments by an ophthalmologist skilled in evaluating and treating infants with retinopathy of prematurity, and continues post discharge. During follow-up visits, vision status information is obtained from parent history and ophthalmologist reports of postdischarge eye examinations, and a standard pediatric eye examination is performed to evaluate the presence of strabismus, nystagmus, light reflex, tracking ability, and roving or dysconjugate eye movements. Rates of vision impairment (glasses, strabismus, nystagmus) in ELBW infants at NICHD centers admitted to NICUs in 1993–1994 ranged from 9 to 20%, and rates of unilateral blindness ranged from none to 2% and bilateral blindness ranged from none to 5% (9).

As regards assessment of hearing, currently close to 100% of neonates in NICUs in the USA are screened for hearing loss prior to discharge. It is recommended that NICU infants be screened with automated auditory brainstem response (AABR) or AABR in combination with otoacoustic emissions (OAE) so that all types of sensorineural hearing loss including auditory dyssynchrony (52) are not missed. The current recommendation (53) is that infants screened in the NICU have a diagnostic evaluation by an audiologist by 3 months of age and participate in appropriate early intervention services by 6 months of age. Since some NICU infants may be missed because of multiple hospital transfers or illness severity and some infants who pass newborn hearing screening will later demonstrate delayed-onset permanent hearing loss (54), follow-up of all very low birth weight (VLBW) infants by an audiologist skilled in assessing and treating infants and young children is indicated. Infants with in utero infections such as cytomegalovirus, herpes, rubella, syphilis, and toxoplasmosis are at increased risk of delayed-onset permanent hearing loss (55–61). Since it has been demonstrated that infants with a permanent hearing loss who receive intervention services prior to 6 months of age have significantly better language outcomes than infants diagnosed after 6 months (62, 63), hearing status should be confirmed as soon as possible post discharge. Rates of any hearing impairment, including conductive or unilateral, for ELBW infants at NICHD centers for infants born 1993–1994 ranged from none to 28%, and rates of hearing impairment requiring bilateral amplification ranged from none to 9% at 18 to 22 months CA (9).

Traditional early developmental assessments divide skills into mental (precursor of cognitive) and motor (gross motor and fine motor) domains. Although major cognitive deficits can be detected in early infancy, more common subtle cognitive deficits and learning difficulties are difficult to detect. In addition, some infants fail to progress or deteriorate in level of function or recover with increasing age (64).

Between birth and 24–30 months most investigators use corrected age to evaluate development and interpret test scores. Corrected age is the sum of chronologic age in weeks minus the difference between gestational age at birth and 40 weeks gestation. Although the duration of correction may be controversial, this correction is generally accepted until 30 months of age (22, 65, 66).

Most studies in the USA use the Bayley Scales of Infant Development II (BSID-II) (50), which includes a Mental Developmental Index (MDI), a Psychomotor Developmental Index (PDI), and a Behavior Rating Scale (BRS) to assess developmental outcomes of high-risk infants in the first 3 years of life. Within the NICHD Neonatal Network the Bayley tests are administered by certified examiners trained to reliability by gold standard examiners. Bayley scores of 100 ± 15 represent the mean $\pm$ standard deviation of population of normal infants born at term. A score <70 (2 standard deviations below the mean) is used as evidence of significant developmental delay. The Bayley BRS is an assessment of child behavior during the administration of the BSID-II. Percentile scores ≥25% on the Bayley BRS are within normal limits. An infant is classified as having neurodevelopmental impairment (NDI) if any of the following are present: moderate to severe CP, MDI or PDI <70, blind in both eyes, or hearing impairment requiring bilateral amplification. The BSID-II has been limited by having two primary scores, the MDI and PDI. Therefore, it is unable to differentiate gross motor from fine motor delays and cognitive from language delays. In all likelihood, the new BSID-III (67) which has five domains including receptive language, expressive language, fine motor, gross motor, and cognitive will be used in future studies.

Data from the NICHD Neonatal Network on large cohorts indicate that there is significant evidence of subnormal cognitive performance among ELBW infants at 18–22 months CA. In the NICHD multicenter study of neurodevelopmental outcome, the center rate for a Bayley MDI <70 ranged from a low of 17% to a high of 62% for infants <1000 g (9).

CASE 1

Case report at 18 to 24 months (summarized in Table 14-1). A 33-year-old G1P2 with an IVF pregnancy delivered twin A (520 g) and twin B (630 g) at 23 6/7 weeks.

Although twin A had a milder neonatal course than twin B, he developed severe BPD and was discharged on oxygen. At discharge, he had evidence of ventriculomegaly and increased tone. At the first follow-up visit at 28 days CA, he was reported to have good focus, brief tracking, increased tone, jerky movements, and reflux. At 6 months 28 days CA his Bayley MDI score was 81 and his PDI was 65 (significant delay). His tone subsequently gradually improved and by 9 months CA his neurologic exam was considered normal. By 19 months CA he had normal vision and hearing, and a normal neurologic exam, was walking and running, had good fine motor skills, and speech delay. His Bayley MDI, however, was 57 and PDI was 74. He had received early intervention since hospital discharge and was referred at 19 months CA for speech therapy. His head growth is of interest. He was the smaller of the twins with an initial head circumference at the 10th percentile. Head growth recovered and by 9 months 14 days CA his head circumference was at the 50th percentile. Catch-up of head circumference in the first year of life has been shown to be associated with developmental recovery and higher IQ (68, 69). We recall that he had ventriculomegaly and an abnormal neurologic exam at discharge which have been shown to be associated with abnormal neurologic outcome (28). Although twin A does not have CP, he has significant cognitive and motor delay at 19 months CA.

The neonatal course for twin B was more severe with bilateral IVH (grade 4 on the left and grade 2 on the right), seizures, and posthemorrhagic hydrocephalus requiring repeated ventricular taps by neurosurgery. Although his hydrocephalus resolved prior to discharge, he also had severe BPD requiring oxygen at discharge, and ROP with plus disease which was treated with laser therapy. At discharge, twin B was reported to have seizures, tremors, increased tone, and questionable vision. At his first visit to follow-up at 1 month 27 days CA, he is noted to have motor asymmetry, torticollis, only brief tracking, increased tone, jerky movements, and seizures. This combination of multiple abnormal findings is very worrisome. At his 4 month 26 day CA visit his head circumference had dropped to the 15th percentile. By 6 months 28 days CA, tone in all four extremities is severely spastic, his Bayley MDI and PDI are both 49, and he has limited responses to visual or auditory stimuli. A diagnosis is made of spastic quadriplegia. Over the next few months he has limited head growth and by 11 months 18 days CA, his head circumference has fallen below the 3rd percentile. His weight gain is also dropping because of poor feeding and a G-tube is recommended to facilitate feeds. His parents finally agree and he has surgery prior to his 19 month 4 day CA visit.

Table 14-1   Two-year Follow-up of ELBW Twins With and Without IVH

31 years G1P2, IVF, married, 12th grade education	Twin A	Twin B
23 6/7 w gestation Discharge	520g, no IVH, right ventriculomegaly, BPD ↑ extensor tone, O₂, 111days	630 g, IVH 4 Lt, IVH 2 Rt, ↑ posthemorrhagic hydrocephalus, tapped by neurosurgery, resolved, seizures, Phenobarbital, ROP with Plus, Rx laser, tremors, ↑ tone, O₂, feeding problems, Zantac 117 days
Chronologic 4m 14d Corrected 28d	Suspect neurologic exam, good focus, brief tracking, ↑ tone, jerky movements, reflux, on O₂, EI, HC 10th %	Suspect neurologic exam, brief tracking, ↑ tone, jerky movements, seizures, Phenobarbital, feeding problems, Zantac, on O₂, EI, HC 25th %
Chronologic 5m 18d Corrected 1m 27d	Suspect neurologic exam, tracks 180°, ↑ tone, jerky movements, on O₂, EI, HC 10th %	Suspect neurologic exam, torticollis Rt, eyes Rt, brief tracking, ↑ tone, jerky movements, seizures, Phenobarbital, Zantac, on O₂, EI, HC 30th %
Chronologic 7m 7d Corrected 3m 16d	Suspect neurologic exam, tracks 180°, ↑ tone, on O₂, EI, HC 30th %	Suspect neurologic exam, poor tracking, ↑ tone uppers and lowers, jerky movements, feeding problems, seizures, Phenobarbital, on O₂, EI, HC 40th %
Chronologic 8m 17d Corrected 4m 26d	Suspect neurologic exam, tracks 180°, mild ↑ tone, on O₂, EI, HC 30th %	Suspect neurologic exam, random eye movements, ↑ tone uppers and lowers, jerky movements, feeding problems, seizures, Phenobarbital, on O₂, EI, HC 15th %
Chronologic 10m 19d Corrected 6m 28d	Suspect neurologic exam, tracks 180°, varying tone in legs, on O₂, EI, HC 30th % Bayley MDI 81, Bayley PDI 65	Abnormal neurologic exam, roving eye movements, ↑ tone uppers and lowers, jerky movements, seizures, Phenobarbital, on O₂, EI Dx: spastic quadriplegia, MDI 49, PDI 49, HC 20th %
Chronologic 13m 5d Corrected 9m14d	Normal neurologic exam, tracks 180°, O₂ at night only, EI, HC 50th %	Abnormal neurologic exam, poor tracking, ↑ tone, spastic quadriplegia, dyskinetic, movements, seizures, Phenobarbital on O₂, EI, HC 10th %
Chronologic 15m 9d Corrected 11m18d	Normal neurologic exam, tracks 180°, off oxygen, EI, HC 50th %, cruising	Abnormal neurologic exam, poor tracking, ↑ tone, spastic quadriplegia, jerky, dyskinetic movements, daily seizures/ Phenobarbital and Topomax, seizures, O₂ on standby, EI, Pediasure, wt and HC <3rd %
Chronologic 16m 16d Corrected 13m 5d	Not seen	Abnormal neurologic exam, poor tracking, ↑ tone, spastic quadriplegia, dyskinetic movements, seizures, Phenobarbital and Topomax, no O₂, EI, Pediasure, wt and HC <3rd %
Chronologic 22m 25d Corrected 19m 4d	Normal neurologic exam, tracks 180°, walking, good pincer, good fine motor skills, not running, "Mama, Dada, baby," EI, HC 55th %, wt 3rd %, Bayley MDI 57, Bayley PDI 74, speech therapy recommended	Abnormal neurologic exam, poor tracking, smiles and laughs, nystagmus, esotropia, seizures/ Phenobarbital and Zanagram, ↑ tone, spastic quadriplegia, dyskinetic movements, seizure disorder, EI, PT, OT, G-tube feeds begun, Pediasure, wt and HC <3rd %

At that visit he is noted to have significantly increased tone in all four extremities with poor movement control. His diagnosis is severe spastic quadriplegia with dystonic movements, seizure disorder, and retardation.

The twins were chosen for the 18–24 month presentation for three reasons. The first was to illustrate some of the "early" neurologic findings seen in ELBW infants. Second, we have twins in which one has grade 4 IVH and the other has ventriculomegaly but no IVH so we can contrast their neurodevelopmental progress over time. Third, the twins had 9 to 10 assessments completed by 19 months CA so that their changing neurologic and developmental status with increasing age is available.

Important Lessons for Diagnosis and Intervention

1. Monitoring head growth is an important component of the neurologic exam.
2. Persistence of "multiple" abnormal neurologic signs in the first 12–18 months is ominous.
3. Emergence of "other" findings (vision impairments, seizures, feeding issues) is associated with poor outcome.
4. Serial assessments are needed to ensure that appropriate interventions are in place.
5. Loss of abnormal neurologic findings in the first 12 months is associated with better neurologic outcome.

THE 3- TO 6-YEAR-OLD CHILD

A conventional neurologic assessment (51) can be administered in conjunction with gross motor classification system at 3 to 6 years of age. By 3½ years of age "intelligence" and preacademic skills can be assessed and CA is no longer used. By age 6 (first grade) a variety of tests can be used to evaluate cognition, attention, and achievement (22). Assessment may include the Beery Test of Vision Motor Integration (70), an intelligence test such as the WISC IV (71) or Stanford Binet (72), and a receptive vocabulary test such as the Peabody Picture Vocabulary Test (73). The assessment of behavior may include the Child Behavior Checklist (74) or the Conners' Rating Scales (75) which are both parent interviews. A further assessment of functional domains can be obtained with the WeeFIM (76), Vineland (77), or PEDI (78). There are fewer outcome studies of ELBW infants evaluated at 3–6 years of age than at 18–24 months. Ment et al. (79) reported on a cohort of 337 preterm infants seen at 4½ years of age as part of the follow-up of the Indomethacin Trial. Children who had received indomethacin had better outcomes than children who received saline: IQ <70 12% versus 17%, respectively (79). Peterson et al. (69) reported on 128 VLBW children who underwent a comprehensive neuropsychologic academic and behavioral assessment at 6.8 years of life. They reported that subnormal head circumference was significantly associated with lower IQ and poorer perceptual motor skills, academic achievement, and adaptive behavior. In addition, the VLBW cohort had significantly more cognitive and academic difficulties than term controls.

CASE 2

Case report at 6 years (Table 14-2). This age of evaluation was chosen because it is the critical age of school entry, and success or failure in school for ex-ELBW infants may be dependent upon the provision of appropriate support services as part of an individualized education plan (IEP). Baby B was born to a 37-year-old G4P4 married mother with a graduate degree and private health insurance. Delivery was at 24 3/7 week. Birth weight was 655 g and complications included cardiomyopathy, bilateral pneumothoraces, seizures, bilateral grade 4 IVH, multiple ventricular

Table 14-2   Five-year Follow-up of ELBW Infant: An Example of Recovery Over Time

36 years G4P4, married, graduate degrees, private insurance	
24 3/7 w gestation	655 g, BPD, cardiomyopathy, bilateral pneumothoraces, seizures, bilateral grade 4 IVH, multiple ventricular taps, ROP stable
Discharge	Normal tone, positive suck, positive grasp, hydrocephalus considered stable, 120 days
2 months postdischarge	Shunt placed for progressive hydrocephalus
Chronologic 6m 18d Corrected 3m 0d	Suspect neurologic exam, tracks 180°, early intervention (EI), ↑ tone, slight head lag, prone 90°, HC 85th %, shunt functioning on right, reflux, on Zantac
Chronologic 10m 21d Corrected 7m 4d	Suspect neurologic exam, tracks 180°, shunt, ↑ tone lowers, slight head lag, likes to push back, some arching, prone 90°, good grasp and release, cooing, EI, PT, OT HC 75th %, Bayley MDI 83, Bayley PDI <62
Chronologic 21m 23d Corrected 18m 5d	Abnormal neurologic exam, tracks 180°, ↑ tone lowers, mild uppers, limited supination of forearms, knee jerks 3+, ± babinskiis, tight ankles, sits, pulls to stand, diagnosis: spastic diplegia, eating well, has asthma, 8 episodes of otitis media, EI, PT, OT HC 95th %, Bayley MDI 95, Bayley PDI <50
Chronologic 36m 29d Corrected 33m 11d	History of two seizures since last visit, not placed on medication. Abnormal neurologic exam, consistent with mild spastic diplegia, has AFOs, getting Botox injections × 2, wears glasses for far-sightedness, charming boy now walking, tracks 180°, has IEP and is getting OT and PT HC 98th %, Bayley MDI 82, Bayley PDI <70, Peabody receptive vocabulary 24 %, Beery VMI 4th %
Chronologic 5y 3m	Seizure disorder now treated with Tegretol, getting Botox q 8m, tone in uppers appears normal, mild ↑ tone in lowers, ↓ balance but can walk independently, glasses, AFOs, IEP, and integrated kindergarten WPPSI IQ 98, Peabody receptive vocabulary 63 %, Beery VMI 16th %, CBCL and Connors WNL, HC 98th %

taps to relieve pressure, and ROP which stabilized. The discharge exam reported at 120 days was consistent with normal tone, good suck, and positive grasp, and the hydrocephalus was considered stable. Post discharge, progressive hydrocephalus developed, however, and a shunt was placed on the right 2 months after discharge.

At 3 months CA, the baby presented with reflux which was treated with Zantac. He was tracking to 180°, had slight head lag, increased tone, and when prone elevated to 90°. The shunt was functioning well and head circumference was at the 85th percentile. At 7 months CA, he still had increased tone in the lower extremities, slight head lag, some arching, but good grasp and release of the hands, and was cooing. Head circumference was at 75th percentile. His Bayley MDI was 83 and PDI was 62. At 18 months CA his neurologic exam was consistent with mild spastic diplegia. He had increased tone, greater in the lower extremities, tight heel cords, and limited supination of the forearms. He good sitting balance and could pull to stand but was not yet cruising. Head circumference was at 95th percentile, and the shunt was functioning well. Bayley MDI was 95 and PDI <50 (significant delay). In this child's situation, we were confident with the diagnosis of classic spastic diplegia at 18 months CA. At 33 months, he presented with some additional findings. He had had two seizures since his last visit and the neurologist's decision had been not to treat with anticonvulsants. He also had been diagnosed with far-sightedness and was wearing glasses. He was now walking, wore bilateral ankle foot orthoses (AFOs), had received two Botox injections, had an IEP, and was getting occupational therapy (OT) and physical therapy (PT). His head circumference was at the 98th percentile and the shunt was functioning fine. His test scores were as follows: Bayley MDI, 82; PDI, 70; Peabody Picture Vocabulary Test (73), 24th percentile; and Beery Vision Motor Index (VMI) (70), 4th percentile. The findings at 33 months demonstrate that additional neurosensory findings can present or be diagnosed at older ages than 18 months and recovery of Bayley motor scores can occur between 18 and 33 months CA. This motor recovery is probably in part a response to the Botox injections, use of AFOs, and ongoing PT and OT. His Peabody vocabulary score, however, is low. Language delays are frequent among ELBW infants and may still be evident at 33–36 months CA, despite early intervention. The low Beery VMI could reflect impaired fine motor function, but in a child with hydrocephalus this may represent a vision perception motor integration problem. At 5 years 3 months CA he presented as a social and charming boy who walked independently with AFOs but had some minor problems with balance. His seizure disorder was now being treated with Tegretal, he was getting Botox injections every 8 months, he wore corrective lenses, and continued to have findings consistent with a mild diplegia. He had an IEP and had been placed in an integrated kindergarten with children with and without disabilities. All of his test scores had improved since his last visit. His WPPSI IQ was 98, Peabody receptive vocabulary was at the 63%, Beery VMI was at the 16%, and his mother's responses to the Child Behavior Checklist and the Connors suggested no behavior problems. This is a wonderful example of excellent recovery of a child with bilateral grade 4 IVH. Why he is doing so well and our twin with unilateral grade 4 is not doing well is not completely clear. Both boys reside in stable home environments and have received multiple support services. This reminds us of the relatively poor predictive validity of neonatal cranial ultrasound.

Important Lesions for Diagnosis and Intervention

1. The outcome of infants with grade 4 IVH is not always ominous.
2. Persistent posthemorrhagic hydrocephalus may require shunting post discharge.
3. Recovery of Bayley cognitive and motor scores may continue during the first 5 years.
4. Follow-up outcomes at 5 to 6 years may provide us with a more stable "quality indicator" reflective of NICU care than 18- to 24-month outcomes.
5. Seizure disorders and sensory deficits may present late.
6. There can be a disconnect between motor impairments and cognitive impairments.
7. Diagnostic magnetic resonance imaging (MRI) prior to discharge may provide better neurologic prognostic information than cranial head ultrasound.
8. Provision of comprehensive support, therapeutic, and educational services is associated with recovery.

THE SCHOOL AGE CHILD

By age 8 (third grade), intelligence, neuropsychologic function, school performance, behavior problems, memory skills, sensorimotor function, language, functional skills, and learning disabilities can be identified (22). A conventional neurologic assessment is administered (51).

A number of studies have reported that approximately 50% of VLBW children require educational resources at school age. Vohr et al. (12) performed assessments at 8 years of age on ex-VLBW (600–1250 g) infants who participated in the longitudinal follow-up of the Indomethacin Trial (12). Within this cohort, rates of educational resource needs for children without IVH were 48%. However, rates ranged from 62 to

79% for children with IVH. The children with IVH also had significantly greater requirements for the number of individual resources needed, a self-contained class-room, and speech/language therapy. Within this cohort of VLBW children evaluated at 3, 4½, 6, and 8 years of age, significant improvement in cognitive and language test scores was observed between 3 and 8 years (80). Improvements in test scores were associated with higher maternal education, two-parent household, and early inter-vention services if the mother had less than a 12th grade education. Hack et al. (81) also reported that rates of impairment defined as MDI or KABC <70 dropped from 39% at 20 months CA to 16% at 8 years for ELBW infants.

CASE 3

Case report at school age. Table 14-3 shows the neurodevelopmental findings over 12 years of a boy born at 27 weeks who had normal cranial ultrasounds during his hospitalization. At 3 months CA he was noted to have increased tone, tremors, and jerky movements. Findings continued to be abnormal and by 12 months CA a diagnosis of spastic diplegia is made. Note that between 6 and 12 months CA his developmental scores have dropped and his Bayley MDI and PDI are both <49 and remain <49 at 18 months CA. Subsequently we observe steady improvement on his cognitive skills, so that by 12 years his verbal IQ is 123, performance IQ is 106, and full scale IQ is 116. He has exceptional vocabulary skills. His diagnosis remains spastic diplegia requiring multiple therapeutic and educational support services. He is, however, reported to have difficulty socializing with peers. A number of studies suggest that children who have been of VLBW are more likely to have emotional and behavior problems at school age than full-term children (82, 83).

Important Lessons for Diagnosis and Intervention

This child's history illustrates a number of important points:

1. Infants with a normal neonatal cranial ultrasound can develop CP and have evidence of early and persistent motor delay.
2. Cognitive skills may improve with increasing age for children in a favorable home environment who receive comprehensive intervention, and education support services. We observe steady improvement in scores for this boy between 18 months and 12 years of age.
3. Despite a high IQ and excellent verbal skills at 12 years of age, a number of resources within the school system continue to be needed including OT and PT.
4. At school age, ELBW children have an increased incidence of behavior problems.

THE ADOLESCENT AND YOUNG ADULT

Adolescent outcome studies indicate that former ELBW infants are at increased risk of neurologic abnormalities, sensory impairments, lower IQs, motor impairments, and poor academic performance (84–88).

Adolescents also have increased rates of health problems especially asthma (2, 89–91), and they have also been shown to have a higher incidence of behavioral problems and psychopathology (20). Saigal et al. (92) have investigated preferences of adolescents compared to professionals and parents relative to their health outcomes. They found that despite the higher rates of morbidities, both adolescents and their parents rated health-related quality of life higher than healthcare professionals.

Outcomes studies of VLBW infants as young adults are rare. These studies are extremely difficult to accomplish because of long-term tracking and the associated

Table 14-3	Eight-year Follow-up of Infant With Normal Cranial Ultrasound	
30 years G2 P3, married, partial college, private insurance	Medical and neurologic exam findings	Test scores
27w gestation	1040 g, RDS, PDA, bowel perforation, normal cranial ultrasound	
Discharge	Hosp. 111 days, neurologic findings not reported	
3m CA	Suspect neurologic exam, tracks 180°, early intervention (EI), ↑ tone, tremors, jerky movements	
6m CA	Suspect neurologic exam, tracks 180°, ↑ tone lowers, HC 60th %	Bayley MDI 63, Bayley PDI 73
12m CA	Abnormal neurologic exam, tracks 180°, ↑ tone lowers, mild uppers, limited supination of forearms, knee jerks 3+, ±babinskiis, tight ankles, sits, pulls to stand, diagnosis: spastic diplegia, EI, PT, OT, HC 95th %	Bayley MDI 49, Bayley PDI <49
18m	History of two seizures since last visit not placed on medication. Abnormal neurologic exam, consistent with mild spastic diplegia has AFOs	Bayley MDI 49, Bayley PDI <49
3y CA	q 8m, tone in uppers appears normal, mild ↑ tone in lowers, ↓ balance but can walks with walker, ataxic, poor balance, poor fine motor skills, AFOs, IEP, Special Ed placement, HC 60th %, PT, OT	Peabody 2y 10m, Beery VMI – unable to do Stanford Binet 83
4½ years	Abnormal, CP, AFOs, walker, IEP, Special Ed placement, PT, OT	Peabody 4y 2m
6y 2m	Abnormal, CP, AFOs, walker IEP, Special Ed placement, PT, OT	Performance IQ 87 Beery 5y 10m Verbal IQ 92 Full Scale IQ 89
8 years	Abnormal, CP, AFOs, IEP, walker, Special Ed resources, PT, OT	Performance IQ 115 Verbal IQ 119 Full scale IQ 119
12 years	Abnormal, CP, AFOs, IEP, walker, Special Ed services Difficulties socializing, PT, OT	Verbal IQ 123 Performance IQ 106 Full scale IQ 116 Peabody vocabulary 33y 8m

costs. Hack et al. (21) has reported outcomes of VLBW infants at 20 years of age compared to term controls. VLBW adults were less likely to have graduated from high school or to be enrolled in a secondary school, and they had lower IQs, more sensory impairments, and were shorter in stature. The findings of Saigal et al. (93) in a population of ELBW infants followed to young adulthood (22–25 years) in Canada were more favorable. They found no significant differences compared to controls in education or employment status. This better outcome may be related to a higher socioeconomic status of the Canadian population.

CASE 4

Case report of young adult. The final case report presented in Table 14-4 is of a VLBW (1300 g) infant with a relatively benign course in the NICU including a normal cranial ultrasound. Her parents are married, college educated, and had private insurance. She consistently does well during follow-up assessments on neurologic, developmental, and cognitive testing from 6 weeks to 6 years 11 months of

Table 14-4   Adult Outcome of VLBW Infant

29 years G1P1, married, college, private insurance	Medical and neurologic exam findings	Test scores
31w gestation	1300 g, female, RDS, hyperbilirubinemia, apnea, feeding problems, normal cranial ultrasound	
Discharge	Hosp. 45 days, neurological findings normal	
6w CA	Normal neurologic exam, tracks 180°, minimal head lag, overall normal, HC <3rd %	
3m CA	Normal neurologic exam, tracks 180°, HC 25th %	
9m 21d CA	Normal neurologic exam, HC 45th %	Bayley MDI 11.7 m Bayley PDI 9.4 m
21.5m CA	Normal neurologic exam, HC 45th %	Bayley MDI 22.5 Bayley PDI 22.5
3y CA	Normal neurologic exam, HC 50th %	Stanford Binet IQ 132
6y 11m	Normal neurologic exam, HC 50th %	Stanford Binet IQ 111 Riley Motor Skills Normal
29 years	Presents in the WIH NICU as a senior medical student. Calls to say she was in a follow-up study as an infant	
30 years	Resident in pediatrics	Excellent outcome

age. At age 29 she does a medical school rotation in the NICU in which she was a VLBW patient, and a year later she is a pediatric resident.

Important Lessons for Diagnosis and Intervention

1. The combination of optimal antenatal and neonatal care, a benign course in the NICU, an optimal home environment, and appropriate interventions can result in very good long-term outcomes for VLBW infants.

GAPS IN KNOWLEDGE

1. Refinement of a systematic, easy-to-administer neurologic assessment in the first year of life to achieve better predictive validity is needed.
2. Identification of the specific environmental factors associated with recovery. We know that higher maternal education is an important predictor.
3. Identification of genetic factors associated with recovery.
4. Further investigation of postnatal interventions (massage, human milk, probiotics, thyroxine) associated with good outcomes and recovery.
5. Further development and ease of obtaining MRI prior to NICU discharge.
6. Adolescent and adult outcome studies of infants at the limits of viability are indicated.
7. Investigation of the relationships between neonatal morbidities and adult disease.

CONCLUSIONS

ELBW infants without evidence of significant neonatal brain injury can recover from the stresses of preterm birth and prolonged NICU care when exposed to a nurturing home environment and comprehensive early intervention services. In contrast, ELBW infants in poor home environments with limited access to services do not do well. Meticulous longitudinal serial neurologic assessments, developmental assessments, and functional assessments are needed to evaluate ongoing neurodevelopmental status to ensure appropriate intervention and educational services are in place, to evaluate changing neurodevelopmental status with increasing age, and to better predict long-term outcome. Assessment at school age provides more reliable outcome data than preschool assessment.

REFERENCES

1. National Institutes of Health (NIH). Consensus Development Conference: effects of corticosteroids for fetal maturation on perinatal outcomes. Am J Obstet 173:246–8, 1995.
2. Fanaroff AA, Hack M, Walsh MC. The NICHD neonatal research network: changes in practice and outcomes during the first 15 years. Semin Perinatol 27:281–7, 2003.
3. El-Metwally D, Vohr B, Tucker R. Survival and neonatal morbidity at the limits of viability in the mid 1990s: 22 to 25 weeks. J Pediatr 137:616–22, 2000.
4. Hintz SR, Poole WK, Wright LL, et al. Changes in mortality and morbidities among infants born at less than 25 weeks during the post-surfactant era. Arch Dis Child Fetal Neonatal Ed 90:F128–33, 2005.
5. Hintz SR, Kendrick DE, Vohr BR, et al. Changes in neurodevelopmental outcomes at 18 to 22 months' corrected age among infants of less than 25 weeks' gestational age born in 1993–1999. Pediatrics 115:1645–51, 2005.
6. Blakely ML, Lally KP, McDonald S, et al. Postoperative outcomes of extremely low birthweight infants with necrotizing enterocolitis or isolated intestinal perforation: a prospective cohort study by the NICHD Neonatal Research Network. Ann Surg 241:984–9; discussion 989–94, 2005.
7. Laptook AR, O'Shea TM, Shankaran S, et al. Adverse neurodevelopmental outcomes among extremely low birth weight infants with a normal head ultrasound: prevalence and antecedents. Pediatrics 115:673–80, 2005.
8. Shankaran S, Johnson Y, Langer JC, et al. Outcome of extremely-low-birth-weight infants at highest risk: gestational age < or = 24 weeks, birth weight < or = 750 g, and 1-minute Apgar < or = 3. Am J Obstet Gynecol 191:1084–91, 2004.
9. Vohr BR, Wright LL, Dusick AM, et al. Center differences and outcomes of extremely low birth weight infants. Pediatrics 113:781–9, 2004.
10. Walsh MC, Morris BH, Wrage LA, et al. Extremely low birthweight neonates with protracted ventilation: mortality and 18-month neurodevelopmental outcomes. J Pediatr 146:798–804, 2005.
11. Schmidt B, Asztalos EV, Roberts RS, et al. Impact of bronchopulmonary dysplasia, brain injury, and severe retinopathy on the outcome of extremely low-birth-weight infants at 18 months: results from the trial of indomethacin prophylaxis in preterms. JAMA 289:1124–9, 2003.
12. Vohr BR, Allan WC, Westerveld M, et al. School-age outcomes of very low birth weight infants in the indomethacin intraventricular hemorrhage prevention trial. Pediatrics 111:e340–6, 2003.
13. Vohr BR, Msall ME, Wilson D, et al. Spectrum of gross motor function in extremely low birth weight children with cerebral palsy at 18 months of age. Pediatrics 116:123–9, 2005.
14. Taylor HG, Klein N, Minich NM, et al. Middle-school-age outcomes in children with very low birthweight. Child Dev 71:1495–511, 2000.
15. Litt J, Taylor HG, Klein N, et al. Learning disabilities in children with very low birthweight: prevalence, neuropsychological correlates, and educational interventions. J Learn Disabil 38: 130–41, 2005.
16. Sherlock RL, Anderson PJ, Doyle LW. Neurodevelopmental sequelae of intraventricular haemorrhage at 8 years of age in a regional cohort of ELBW/very preterm infants. Early Hum Dev 81: 909–16, 2005.
17. Doyle LW and Anderson PJ. Improved neurosensory outcome at 8 years of age of extremely low birthweight children born in Victoria over three distinct eras. Arch Dis Child Fetal Neonatal Ed 90:F484–8, 2005.
18. Marlow N, Wolke D, Bracewell MA, et al. Neurologic and developmental disability at six years of age after extremely preterm birth. N Engl J Med 352:9–19, 2005.
19. Hack M and Klein N. Young adult attainments of preterm infants. JAMA 295:695–6, 2006.
20. Hack M, Youngstrom EA, Cartar L, et al. Behavioral outcomes and evidence of psychopathology among very low birth weight infants at age 20 years. Pediatrics 114:932–40, 2004.
21. Hack M, Flannery DJ, Schluchter M, et al. Outcomes in young adulthood for very-low-birth-weight infants. N Engl J Med 346:149–57, 2002.
22. Vohr BR, Wright LL, Hack M, et al. Follow-up care of high-risk infants. Pediatrics Suppl 114, 2004.
23. Vohr BR, Wright LL, Dusick AM, et al. Effects of site differences at 12 participating NICHD centers on 18 month outcomes of extremely low birth weight (ELBW) <1000 gram infants. The NICHD Neonatal Research Network Follow-up Study. Pediatrics 113(4):781–9, 2004.
24. Perlman JM. Summary proceedings from the neurology group on hypoxic-ischemic encephalopathy. Pediatrics 117:S28–33, 2006.
25. Shalak L and Perlman JM. Hemorrhagic-ischemic cerebral injury in the preterm infant: current concepts. Clin Perinatol 29:745–63, 2002.

26. Chamnanvanakij S, Margraf LR, Burns D, et al. Apoptosis and white matter injury in preterm infants. Pediatr Dev Pathol 5:184–9, 2002.

27. Papile LA, Burstein J, Burstein R, et al. Incidence and evolution of subependymal and intraventricular hemorrhage: a study of infants with birth weights less than 1,500 gm. J Pediatr 92:529–34, 1978.

28. Ment LR, Vohr B, Allan W, et al. The etiology and outcome of cerebral ventriculomegaly at term in very low birth weight preterm infants. Pediatrics 104:243–8, 1999.

29. Ancel PY, Livinec F, Larroque B, et al. Cerebral palsy among very preterm children in relation to gestational age and neonatal ultrasound abnormalities: the EPIPAGE cohort study. Pediatrics 117:828–35, 2006.

30. Ment LR, Oh W, Ehrenkranz RA, et al. Low-dose indomethacin and prevention of intraventricular hemorrhage: a multicenter randomized trial. Pediatrics 93:543–50, 1994.

31. Schmidt B, Davis P, Moddemann D, et al. Long-term effects of indomethacin prophylaxis in extremely-low-birth-weight infants. N Engl J Med 344:1966–72, 2001.

32. Yeh TF, Lin YJ, Lin HC, et al. Outcomes at school age after postnatal dexamethasone therapy for lung disease of prematurity. N Engl J Med 350:1349–51, 2004.

33. Yeh TF, Lin YJ, Lin HC, et al. Outcomes at school age after postnatal dexamethasone therapy for lung disease of prematurity. N Engl J Med 350:1304–13, 2004.

34. Hagberg B, Hagberg G. The changing panorama of cerebral palsy: bilateral spastic forms in particular. Acta Paediatr Suppl 416:48–52, 1996.

35. Powell B, Hagberg G, Olow I. The changing panorama of cerebral palsy in Sweden: VI. Prevalence and origin during the birth year period 1983–1986. Acta Paediatr 82:387–93, 1993.

36. Stanley F, Watson L. The cerebral palsies in western Australia: trends, 1968 to1981. Am J Obstet Gynecol 158:89–93, 1988.

37. Piecuch RE, Leonard CH, Cooper BA, et al. Outcome of infants born at 24–26 weeks' gestation: II. Neurodevelopmental outcome. Obstet Gynecol 90:809–14, 1997.

38. Surman G, Newdick H, Johnson A. Cerebral palsy rates among low-birthweight infants fell in the 1990s. Dev Med Child Neurol 45:456–62, 2003.

39. Pinto-Martin JA, Riolo S, Cnaan A, et al. Cranial ultrasound prediction of disabling and nondisabling cerebral palsy at age two in a low birth weight population. Pediatrics 95:249–54, 1995.

40. Prevalence and characteristics of children with cerebral palsy in Europe. Dev Med Child Neurol 44:633–40, 2002.

41. Vohr BR, Wright LL, Dusick AM, et al. Neurodevelopmental and functional outcomes of extremely low birth weight infants in the National Institute of Child Health and Human Development Neonatal Research Network, 1993–1994. Pediatrics 105:1216–26, 2000.

42. Bax MC. Terminology and classification of cerebral palsy. Dev Med Child Neurol 11:295–7, 1964.

43. Wood E, Rosenbaum P. The gross motor function classification system for cerebral palsy: a study of reliability and stability over time. Dev Med Child Neurol 42:292–6, 2000.

44. Palisano R, Rosenbaum P, Walter S, et al. Development and reliability of a system to classify gross motor function in children with cerebral palsy. Dev Med Child Neurol 39:214–23, 1997.

45. Russell DJ, Avery LM, Rosenbaum P, et al. Improved scaling of the Gross Motor Function Measure for children with cerebral palsy: evidence of reliability and validity. Physical Therapy 80:873–85, 2000.

46. Nordmark E, Jarnlo GB, Hagglund G. Comparison of the Gross Motor Function Measure and Paediatric Evaluation of Disability Inventory in assessing motor function in children undergoing selective dorsal rhizotomy. Dev Med Child Neurol 42:245–52, 2000.

47. Drillien CM. Abnormal neurologic signs in the first year of life in low-birthweight infants: possible prognostic significance. Dev Med Child Neurol 14:575–84, 1972.

48. Vohr BR, Garcia-Coll C, Mayfield S, et al. Neurologic and developmental status related to the evolution of visual-motor abnormalities from birth to 2 years of age in preterm infants with intraventricular hemorrhage. J Pediatr 115:296–302, 1989.

49. Paneth N, Qiu H, Rosenbaum P, et al. Reliability of classification of cerebral palsy in low-birth-weight children in four countries. Dev Med Child Neurol 45:628–33, 2003.

50. Bayley N. Bayley Scales of Infant Development-II. San Antonio, TX: Psychological Corporation, 1993.

51. Amiel-Tison C. Neuromotor status. In Taeusch HW, Yogman MW (eds). Follow-up Management of the High-Risk Infant. Boston, MA: Little, Brown & Company, 1987, 115–26.

52. Berlin CI, Hood L, Morlet T, et al. Auditory neuropathy/dys-synchrony: diagnosis and management. Ment Retard Dev Disabil Res Rev 9:225–31, 2003.

53. Joint Committee on Infant Hearing. Year 2000 position statement: principles and guidelines for early hearing detection and intervention programs. Am J Audiol 9:9–29.

54. Johnson JL, White KR, Widen JE, et al. A multisite study to examine the efficacy of the otoacoustic emission/automated auditory brainstem response newborn hearing screening protocol: introduction and overview of the study. Am J Audiol 14:S178–85, 2005.

55. Fowler KB, Dahle AJ, Boppana SB, et al. Newborn hearing screening: will children with hearing loss caused by congenital cytomegalovirus infection be missed? J Pediatr 135:60–4, 1999.

56. Fowler K, Stagno S, Pass R, et al. The outcome of congenital cytomegalovirus infection in relation to maternal antibody status. N Engl J Med 326:663–7, 1992.

57. Madden C, Wiley S, Schleiss M, et al. Audiometric, clinical and educational outcomes in a pediatric symptomatic congenital cytomegalovirus (CMV) population with sensorineural hearing loss. Int J Pediatr Otorhinolaryngol 68:1191–1198, 2005.

58. Rivera L, Boppana S, Fowler KB, et al. Predictors of hearing loss in children with symptomatic congenital cytomegalovirus infection. Pediatrics 110:762–7, 2002.

59. Nance WE, Lim BG, Dodson KM. Importance of congenital cytomegalovirus infections as a cause for pre-lingual hearing loss. J Clin Virol 35:221–5, 2006.

60. Morton CC, Nance WE. Newborn hearing screening: a silent revolution. N Engl J Med 354: 2151–64, 2006.

61. Pass RF, Fowler KB, Boppana SB, et al. Congenital cytomegalovirus infection following first trimester maternal infection: symptoms at birth and outcome. J Clin Virol 35:216–20, 2006.

62. Yoshinaga-Itano C. From screening to early identification and intervention: discovering predictors to successful outcomes for children with significant hearing loss. J Deaf Stud Deaf Educ 8:11–30, 2003.

63. Moeller MP. Early intervention and language development in children who are deaf and hard of hearing. Pediatrics 106:1–9, 2000.

64. Ment LR, Vohr B, Allan W, et al. Change in cognitive function over time in very low-birth-weight infants. JAMA 289:705–11, 2003.

65. Blasco PA. Preterm birth: to correct or not to correct. Dev Med Child Neurol 31:816–21, 1989.

66. Lems W, Hopkins B, Samson JF. Mental and motor development in preterm infants: the issue of corrected age. Early Hum Dev 34:113–23, 1993.

67. Bayley N. Bayley Scales of Infant Development-III. San Antonio, TX: Psychological Corporation, 2006.

68. Hack M, Breslau N. Very low birth weight infants: effects of brain growth during infancy on intelligence quotient at 3 years of age. Pediatrics 77:196–202, 1986.

69. Peterson J, Taylor HG, Minich N, et al. Subnormal head circumference in very low birth weight children: neonatal correlates and school-age consequences. Early Hum Dev 82:325–34, 2006.

70. Beery K. Developmental Test of Visual Motor Integration, 4th edition. Parsippany, NJ: Modern Curriculum Press, 1997.

71. Wechsler D. The Wechsler Intelligence Scale for Children, 4th edition. San Antonio, TX: The Psychological Corporation, 2003.

72. Roid G. The Stanford-Binet Intelligence Scales, 5th edition. Ithasca, IL: Riverside Publishing, 2003.

73. Dunn LMDL. Peabody Picture Vocabulary Test III. Circle Pines, MN: American Guidance Service, 1997.

74. Achenbach TM. Child Behavior Checklist 2–3. Burlington, VT: University of Vermont, Department of Psychiatry, 1992.

75. Connors Parent Rating Scales Revised. San Antonio, TX: Psychological Corporation, 1996.

76. Ottenbacher KJ, Msall ME, Lyon N, et al. The WeeFIM instrument: its utility in detecting change in children with developmental disabilities. Arch Phys Med Rehabil 81:1317–26, 2000.

77. Sparrow SBD, Cicchetti D. Vineland Adaptive Behavior Scales Interview Edition: Survey Form Manual. A revision of the Vineland Social Maturity Scale by E.A. Doll. Circle Pines, MN: American Guidance Service, 1984.

78. Pediatric Evaluation of Disability Inventory (PEDI). Nashville, TN: Ellsworth and Vandermeer Press, 1997.

79. Ment LR, Vohr B, Allan W, et al. Outcome of children in the indomethacin intraventricular hemorrhage prevention trial. Pediatrics 105:485–91, 2000.

80. (CELF-R) Clinical Evaluation of Language Fundamentals III. San Antonio, TX: Psychological Corporation, 2003.

81. Hack M, Taylor HG, Drotar D, et al. Poor predictive validity of the Bayley Scales of Infant Development for cognitive function of extremely low birth weight children at school age. Pediatrics 116:333–41, 2005.

82. Reijneveld SA, de Kleine MJ, van Baar AL, et al. Behavioural and emotional problems in very preterm and very low birth weight infants at age 5 years. Arch Dis Child Fetal Neonatal Ed 91:F423–8, 2006.

83. Short EJ, Klein NK, Lewis BA, et al. Cognitive and academic consequences of bronchopulmonary dysplasia and very low birth weight: 8-year-old outcomes. Pediatrics 112:e359, 2003.

84. Saigal S, Hoult LA, Streiner DL, et al. School difficulties at adolescence in a regional cohort of children who were extremely low birth weight. Pediatrics 105:325–31, 2000.

85. Doyle LW, Ford GW, Rickards AL, et al. Antenatal corticosteroids and outcome at 14 years of age in children with birth weight less than 1501 grams. Pediatrics 106:E2, 2000.

86. Rushe TM, Rifkin L, Stewart AL, et al. Neuropsychological outcome at adolescence of very preterm birth and its relation to brain structure. Dev Med Child Neurol 43:226–33, 2001.

87. Saigal S, den Ouden L, Wolke D, et al. School-age outcomes in children who were extremely low birth weight from four international population-based cohorts. Pediatrics 112:943–50, 2003.

88. Hack M, Taylor HG, Klein N, et al. School-age outcomes in children with birth weights under 750 g. N Engl J Med 331:753–9, 1994.

89. Korhonen P, Laitinen J, Hyodynmaa E, et al. Respiratory outcome in school-aged, very-low-birth-weight children in the surfactant era. Acta Paediatr 93:316–21, 2004.

90. Anand D, Stevenson CJ, West CR, et al. Lung function and respiratory health in adolescents of very low birth weight. Arch Dis Child 88:135–8, 2003.

91. Johnson A, Bowler U, Yudkin P, et al. Health and school performance of teenagers born before 29 weeks gestation. Arch Dis Child Fetal Neonatal Ed 88:F190–8, 2003.

92. Saigal S, Stoskopf BL, Feeny D, et al. Differences in preferences for neonatal outcomes among health care professionals, parents, and adolescents. JAMA 281:1991–1997, 1999.

93. Saigal S, Stoskopf B, Streiner D, et al. Transition of extremely low-birth-weight infants from adolescence to young adulthood: comparison with normal birth-weight controls. JAMA 295:667–75, 2006.

Index

Page numbers for figures have suffix **f,** those for tables have suffix **t**